Handbook of Nuclear Medicine and Molecular Imaging for Physicists

Handbook of Nuclear Medicine and Molecular Imaging for Physicists

Modelling, Dosimetry, and Radiation Protection, Volume II

Edited by
Michael Ljungberg

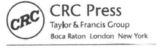

CRC Press
Taylor & Francis Group
Boca Raton London New York

CRC Press is an imprint of the
Taylor & Francis Group, an informa business

First edition published 2022
by CRC Press
6000 Broken Sound Parkway NW, Suite 300, Boca Raton, FL 33487-2742

and by CRC Press
2 Park Square, Milton Park, Abingdon, Oxon, OX14 4RN

Library of Congress Cataloging-in-Publication Data
A catalog record has been requested for this book

ISBN: 978-1-138-59329-9 (hbk)
ISBN: 978-1-032-05954-9 (pbk)
ISBN: 978-0-429-48954-9 (ebk)

DOI: 10.1201/9780429489549

Typeset in Times
by Newgen Publishing UK

Access the Support Material: www.routledge.com/9781138593299

Contents

Preface

During the spring of 2017, I was writing a review of a proposal for a book to potentially be published by CRC Press. Upon closing the discussion with CRC Press regarding the result of this review, I was asked to be an editor for a handbook of nuclear medicine, with focus on physicists of this field. After spending the summer thinking about a relevant table of contents and related potential authors, I formally accepted the offer. I soon realized that the field of nuclear medicine was too extensive to be covered in a single book. After consolidating with the publisher, it was decided that instead of one book it would be best to develop three volumes with the titles, (I) Instrumentation and Imaging Procedures, (II) Modelling, Dosimetry, and Radiation Protection, and (III) Radiopharmaceuticals and Clinical Applications.

My vision was to create state-of-the-art handbooks, encompassing all major aspects relating to the field of Nuclear Medicine. The chapters should describe the theories in detail but also, when applicable, have a practical approach, focusing on procedures and equipment that are either in use today, or could be expected to be of importance in the future. I realized that the topic of each chapter would be broad enough, in principle, to lay the foundation for individual books of their own. As such, the chapters needed only cover the most relevant aspects of each topic. Therefore, this book series will, hopefully, serve as references for different aspects relating to both the academic and the clinical practice of a medical physicist.

I originally struggled with the definition of the word 'handbook'. I did not want the chapters to serve as point-by-point guidelines, but rather to function as independent chapters to be read more or less independently of one another. Consequently, there is some overlap in the content between chapters but, from a pedagogical point of view, I do not see this as a drawback, as repetition of key aspects may aid in the learning.

This second volume of three focuses on mathematical modelling, dosimetry, and radiation protection. Mathematical modelling is an important part of nuclear medicine. Therefore, several chapters of this book have been dedicated towards describing this topic. In these chapters, an emphasis has been put on describing mathematical modelling of radiation transport of photons and electrons, as well as on transportation of radiopharmaceuticals between different organs and compartments. It also includes computer models of patient dosimetry. Two chapters of this book are also devoted towards introducing the concept of biostatistics and radiobiology. These chapters are followed by chapters detailing dosimetry procedures commonly used in the context of diagnostic imaging, as well as patient-specific dosimetry for radiotherapy treatments. For safety reasons, many of the methods used in nuclear medicine and molecular imaging are strictly regulated. Therefore, this book also highlights the basic principles for radiation protection. It also describes the process of how guidelines and regulations aimed at minimizing radiation exposure are determined and implemented by international organizations. Finally, this book describes how different dosimetry methods may be utilized depending on the intended target, including whole-body or organ-specific imaging, as well as small-scale dosimetry down to cellular dosimetry.

These three volumes are the result of the efforts of outstanding authors who, despite the exceptional circumstances related to the COVID-19 pandemic, have managed to keep to the deadline of the project – although, I must admit, there were times when I questioned the feasibility of doing this. As COVID-19 hit, many of us were faced with unexpected tasks to solve: Distance teaching, restrictions and changes in administration, and sometimes also rapid modifications to local procedures at departments and hospitals. Naturally, the combined effect of these interruptions impacted the time available to dedicate to writing. However, despite these many challenges, we all did our utmost to complete the chapters according to the deadline.

I would like to thank all authors for their contributions, which made this book possible. You have all done a phenomenal job, especially considering the extraordinary circumstances we are currently faced with, but also considering the fact that you all have other obligations of high priority. I would especially like to thank Professor Philip Elsinga, who initially helped me define the content of the radiopharmaceutical section being prepared for Volume III. This subtopic of nuclear medicine is the one I have the least knowledge of, and I am therefore very grateful for the kind support I received during the initial planning of Volume III.

I would like to thank CRC Press officials for entrusting me with the position as editor of this series of books. I would also like to thank Kirsten Barr, Rebecca Davies, and Francesca McGowan, who have been the points of contact for me during these years.

It is also important to acknowledge two authors who are sadly no longer with us: Anna Celler, University of British Columbia, Vancouver, Canada, and Lennart Johansson, Umeå University, Sweden. Both were dear friends and great scientists. Throughout the years, their work has made a huge impact in their respective fields of research.

Finally, I would like to dedicate this work to my wife, Karin, as well as to my beloved daughter Johanna, who lives in Brisbane, where she is pursuing her PhD at the University of Queensland. Karin – I am so grateful for your patience, especially during the intense period around Christmastime right before the submission of the manuscript for this volume. I love you both very much.

Michael Ljungberg, PhD
Professor Medical Radiation Physics, Lund
Lund University, Lund, Sweden

Access to colour images and support material: http://www.routledge.com/9781138593299

Editor

Michael Ljungberg is a Professor at Medical Radiation Physics, Lund, Lund University, Sweden. He started his research in the Monte Carlo field in 1983 through a project involving a simulation of whole-body counters but later changed the focus to more general applications in nuclear medicine imaging and SPECT. Parallel to his development of the Monte Carlo code, SIMIND, he began working in 1985 with quantitative SPECT and problems related to attenuation and scatter. After earning his PhD in 1990, he received a research assistant position that allowed him to continue developing SIMIND for quantitative SPECT applications and to establish successful collaborations with international research groups. At this time, the SIMIND program became used world-wide. Dr. Ljungberg became an associate professor in 1994 and, in 2005, after working clinically as a nuclear medicine medical physicist, received a full professorship in the Science Faculty at Lund University. He became the Head of the Department of Medical Radiation Physics at Lund in 2013 and a full professor in the Medical Faculty in 2015.

Aside from the development of SIMIND – including new camera systems such as CZT detectors – his research includes an extensive project in oncological nuclear medicine. In this project, he and colleagues developed dosimetry methods based on quantitative SPECT, Monte Carlo absorbed-dose calculations, and methods for accurate 3D dose planning for internal radionuclide therapy. Lately, his work has focused on implementing Monte Carlo–based image reconstruction in SIMIND. He is also involved in the undergraduate education of medical physicists and bio-medical engineers and supervises MSc and PhD students. In 2012, Professor Ljungberg became a member of the European Association of Nuclear Medicines task group on Dosimetry and served that association for six years. He has published over a hundred original papers, 18 conference proceedings, 18 books and book chapters, and 14 peer-reviewed papers.

Contributors

Martin Andersson
Medical Radiation Physics, Malmö, Lund University,
  Sweden and
Department of Medical Radiation Sciences, Institute
  of Clinical Sciences, Sahlgrenska Cancer Center,
  University of Gothenburg, Sweden

Manuel Bardiès
Institut de Recherche en Cancérologie de Montpellier,
  Université de Montpellier, France

Remco Bastiaannet
Department of Radiology and Radiological Science,
  Johns Hopkins University, School of Medicine,
  Baltimore, USA

Naomi Clayton
Centre de Recherches en Cancérologie de Toulouse,
  Université Toulouse, France

Marta Cremonesi
Istituto Europeo di Oncologia, IRCCS, Milano, Italy

Hugo W.A.M. de Jong
Department of Radiology and Nuclear Medicine,
  University Medical Center, Utrecht, The Netherlands

José M. Fernández-Varea
Facultat de Física (FQA & ICC), Universitat de
  Barcelona, Spain

Jonathan Gear
Joint Department of Physics, The Royal Marsden
  NHSFT, Sutton, United Kingdom

Gerhard Glatting
Klinik für Nuklearmedizin, Universität Ulm, Ulm, Germany

Johan Gustafsson
Medical Radiation Physics Lund, Lund University,
  Lund, Sweden

Heribert Hänscheid
Klinik fuer Nuklearmedizin, Universitaetsklinikum
  Wuerzburg, Wuerzburg, Germany

Cecilia Hindorf
Department of Medical Radiation Physics and
  Nuclear Medicine, Karolinska University Hospital,
  Stockholm, Sweden

Roger W. Howell
Departments of Radiology and Radiation Oncology,
  New Jersey Medical School, Rutgers University,
  Newark, NJ, USA

Lennart Johansson†
Department of Radiation Sciences, Radiation Physics,
  Umeå University, Sweden

Lena Jönsson
Medical Radiation Physics Lund, Lund University,
  Lund, Sweden

Gunjan Kayal
Centre de Recherches en Cancérologie de Toulouse,
  Université Toulouse, France

Michel Koole
Nuclear Medicine and Molecular Imaging, Department
  of Imaging and Pathology, KU Leuven, Leuven,
  Belgium

Michael Lassmann
Klinik fuer Nuklearmedizin, Universitaetsklinikum
  Wuerzburg, Wuerzburg, Germany

Mark Lubberink
Nuclear Medicine and PET, Department of
  Surgical Sciences, Uppsala University,
  Uppsala, Sweden

Sören Mattsson
Medical Radiation Physics Malmö, Lund
  University, Sweden

Markus Nilsson
Clinical Sciences Lund, Radiology, Lund University,
  Lund, Sweden

Stig Palm
Department of Medical Radiation Sciences, Institute
  of Clinical Sciences, Sahlgrenska Academy,
  University of Gothenburg, Sweden

Gian Luca Poli
Dosimetry and Medical Radiation Physics
  Section, International Atomic Energy Agency,
  Vienna, Austria

Michael G. Stabin
RADAR, Inc., Nashville, USA

Lidia Strigari
Department of Medical Physics IRCCS
  Azienda Ospedaliero-Universitaria di Bologna,
  Bologna, Italy

Alex Vergara Gil
Centre de Recherches en Cancérologie de Toulouse,
  Université Toulouse, France

1 Introduction to Biostatistics

Johan Gustafsson and Markus Nilsson

CONTENTS

1.1 INTRODUCTION

At the heart of research lies the ability to draw conclusions from data. In this chapter we will introduce basic concepts concerning acquisition and characterization of data and the foundations of hypothesis testing. We will cover basic parametric and non-parametric statistical tests, survival analysis, and multivariate testing. Hypothesis testing can be a powerful tool to separate facts from fiction, but wrongly used it may as well result in fictitious conclusions. To address this, the end of the chapter will cover concepts such as statistical power, the multiple-comparisons problem, and the limitations of hypothesis testing.

1.2 DATA ACQUISITION

When planning for an experiment and the subsequent data analysis, it is important to consider the scale of the measurement [1–5] and the relationship between a population and a sample from that population. These aspects will determine what analysis methods can be applied to the data.

1.2.1 SCALES OF MEASUREMENT

Four measurement scales are commonly defined, based on what comparative operations can be applied to the data and are referred to as nominal, ordinal, interval, and ratio scales [5]. For the nominal scale, data points can be compared only in terms of equality. Examples include the colour of items or the names of people. For this kind of data, a statement such as two items having the same value (e.g., two people having the same name) is meaningful, while a statement about one item being greater than or smaller than another is not. For the ordinal scale, data points can be meaningfully ordered. An example is the rating of an experience from A to E, with A meaning "very bad" and E meaning "very good". For an interval scale, it is in addition possible to calculate meaningful differences between data points. A typical example is temperature (measured in degrees centigrade or Fahrenheit). For a ratio scale, it is also possible to compute meaningful ratios, with typical examples being mass and length. The different scales of measurement are summarized in Table 1.1.

1.2.2 POPULATION AND SAMPLE

We often want to draw conclusions about a population, but we are only able to acquire information about a sample. For example, we may wish to know whether patients given one treatment survive longer than those given another treatment, but we can only study a limited number of patients. To draw any generalizable conclusions, the sample must be representative of the population. That is, we should not have any preference for including or excluding certain individuals from the sample. This can be achieved by making the sampling procedure random. A non-random sampling may result in the sample being biased and thereby lead to incorrect conclusions. For example, giving only the healthiest patients a new treatment would not provide conclusions that would generalize to the whole population.

A parameter calculated from the sample, such as its average, is unlikely to be equal to the same parameter for the whole population. Furthermore, if the sampling was to be repeated, the value calculated for the new sample would generally be different than for the previous sample. The parameter for the sample can thereby only serve as an estimate of the corresponding parameter for the population and will be subject to random variations due to the random sampling. Parameters computed from smaller samples tend to exhibit larger variation than those computed from larger samples.

1.2.3 STOCHASTIC VARIABLES

Random phenomena can be described by stochastic variables. A distinction is made between a stochastic variable and its observed value. The first is affected by the random nature of the phenomena under consideration, while the latter is the value after the outcome has been observed and is, hence, not subject to random variation. There are two main classes of

TABLE 1.1
Summary of Scales of Measurement

Scale of measurement	Description	Examples
Nominal	Items can be classified into categories	Colour, occupation
Ordinal	Items can be ordered	Material hardness
Interval	Differences can be computed	Temperature (in °C), date
Ratio	Ratios can be computed	Mass, length

stochastic variables. Discrete stochastic variables can only take a discrete number of values, while continuous stochastic variables can take a continuum of values.

A stochastic variable is characterized by its distribution. In the case of a discrete stochastic variable ξ, the distribution can be described by either the probability mass function (PMF) $p(x_k) = P(\xi = x_k)$, where $P(\cdot)$ denotes probability so that $P(\xi = x_k)$ denotes the probability for the stochastic variable to obtain the value x_k, or the cumulative distribution function (CDF) $F(x_k) = P(\xi \leq x_k) = \sum_{j=1}^{k} p(x_k)$. For continuous stochastic variables, associating single values with probabilities would not be meaningful, but the CDF can be defined as $F(x) = P(\xi \leq x) = \int_{-\infty}^{x} f(t)\,dt$ where $f(x)$ is the probability density function (PDF). The probability to observe a value in the interval $[a,b]$ is thereby $P(a \leq \xi \leq b) = F(b) - F(a) = \int_{a}^{b} f(t)\,dt$.

A handful of distributions can be used to describe a wide range of phenomena, at least approximately. Examples of such distributions are presented in Figure 1.1. The binomial distribution and Poisson distribution are examples of discrete distributions. The normal (Gaussian) distribution and log-normal distribution are examples of continuous distributions.

1.2.4 INDEPENDENT AND IDENTICALLY DISTRIBUTED STOCHASTIC VARIABLES

The sampling process can be modelled as observing the values of a set of independent and identically distributed (IID) stochastic variables. Independence means in this context that the observed value for one stochastic variable does not affect the distributions for the other variables. For example, for a roll of two dices the observed outcome of the first roll does not give any information about the value that will be observed for the second one. In contrast, when drawing two cards from a deck of cards the value of the two cards are not independent (for example, they cannot both have the same value). Many common statistical methods are based on the assumption of IID variables.

1.2.5 EXPECTED VALUE AND VARIANCE

Two parameters that can be used to characterize distributions are the expected value and the variance. The expected value is defined (for the case of continuous stochastic variables) as

$$E[\xi] = \mu = \int_{-\infty}^{\infty} x f(x)\,dx. \tag{1.1}$$

and can be seen as the centre-of-mass of the distribution, also referred to as the first moment of the distribution. An alternative to the expected value for describing the global position of the distribution is the median, defined as the value x for which the CDF is equal to 0.5.

The variance is defined as

$$V[\xi] = \sigma^2 = \int_{-\infty}^{\infty} (x - \mu)^2 f(x)\,dx \tag{1.2}$$

and characterizes the width of the distribution. It is also referred to as the second central moment. In reporting, it is common to use the standard deviation, $\sigma = \sqrt{\sigma^2}$, rather than the variance itself.

For linear combinations of stochastic variables ξ_1 and ξ_2, the expected values propagate linearly according to $E[a\xi_1 + b\xi_2] = aE[\xi_1] + bE[\xi_2]$, where a and b are two scalars. The corresponding relationship for the variance is $V[a\xi_1 + b\xi_2] = a^2 V[\xi_1] + b^2 V[\xi_2]$, if the variables are independent. In particular, if the stochastic variables ξ_1 and ξ_2 are independent and follow normal distributions with expectation values μ_1 and μ_2 and standard deviations σ_1 and σ_2, respectively, the stochastic variable $\eta = a\xi_1 + b\xi_2$ will also follow a normal distribution with expectation value $\mu = a\mu_1 + b\mu_2$ and standard deviation $\sigma = \sqrt{a^2\sigma_1^2 + b^2\sigma_2^2}$. The normal distribution is of special importance since a large

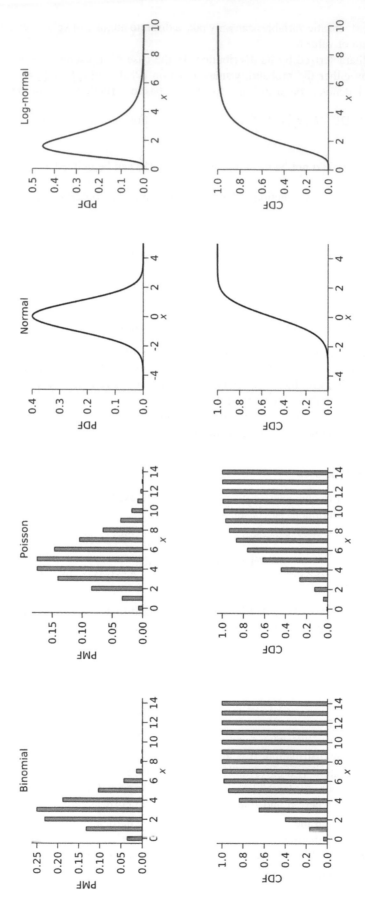

FIGURE 1.1 Examples of PMFs or PDFs and CDFs for some commonly used families of distributions. The upper row shows the PMFs or PDFs and the lower row shows the corresponding CDFs.

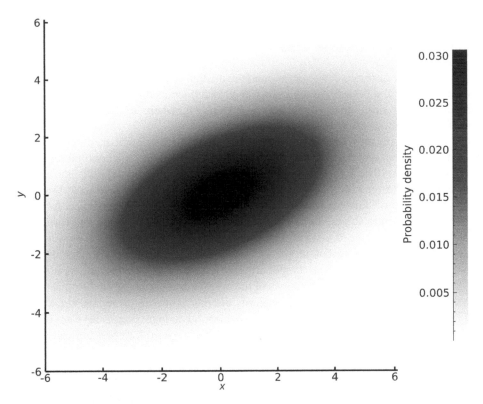

FIGURE 1.2 A bivariate normal distribution. The two stochastic variables governed by this joint probability distribution are not independent and have a non-zero covariance.

number of naturally occurring distributions tend to be well-approximated by a Gaussian. A special case of this principle is the central-limit theorem, stating that the distribution of a sum of IID stochastic variables converges towards a normal distribution.

The concept of probability distributions can also be generalized to the multivariate case. An example of a bivariate normal distribution is shown in Figure 1.2. The joint variation between pairs of stochastic variables can be characterized by the covariance between the variables, which is defined as $\mathrm{cov}[\xi,\eta] = E\big[\big(\xi - E[\xi]\big)\big(\eta - E[\eta]\big)\big]$. A positive covariance indicates that a high observed value for one variable leads to a higher probability to observe a high value also for the second variable, while a negative covariance indicates that a high observed value for the first variable leads to a higher probability to observe a low value (in the sense closer to minus infinity) for the second variable.

1.3 CHARACTERIZATION AND VISUALIZATION OF DATA

Once a sample has been collected, we often characterize it by scalar numbers that represent the average of the whole sample and the variation within it. In short, we are interested in summary statistics. The average is a measure of the central tendency and can be represented by the mean, median, or mode of the sample. The sample mean, here denoted $\bar{x}$, is simply defined as the arithmetic average $\bar{x} = (1/n)\sum_{i=1}^{n} x_i$, and serves as an estimation of the expected value of the underlying distribution. The median, here denoted M, is the middle value in an ordered set of observations, which separates the higher half of the sample from the lower half. The median is closely related to the concept of percentiles: the nth percentile is the value below which n percent of the observations fall, and thus the median is the 50th percentile. Similarly, the first, second and third quartiles show the 25th, 50th and 75th percentiles, respectively. Finally, the mode is the set of observations that appear most often in a sample.

The variation within the sample can similarly be represented by different scalars, such as the sample standard deviation, the median absolute deviation (MAD), the interquartile range (IQR), the range, and the variation ratio.

The sample standard deviation (s) is defined as the square root of the sample variance (s^2), in turn defined as

$$s^2 = \left[1/(n-1)\right]\sum_{i=1}^{n}(x_i - \bar{x})^2,$$ which is also an estimate of the variance of the distribution. The median absolute devi-

ation is defined as the median of absolute deviations around the median ($|x_i - \bar{x}|$). The interquartile range is defined as the difference between the 75th and 25th percentiles. The range is defined as the difference between the maximum and minimum value. Finally, the variation ratio is defined as $v_r = 1 - n_m/n$, where n_m is number of observations equal to the mode, and n is the total number of observations.

To select between the different representations of the average and the variation mentioned above, it is helpful to consider the scale of measurement and the distribution of data. For observations on a nominal scale (without order), the average and variation can be described by the mode and variation ratio. On an ordinal scale, the median can be applied to characterize the average, and range to characterize the variation. It may be tempting to apply the MAD or IQR to such data, but both rely on comparing differences between observations, and are thus inappropriate for ordinal data. Finally, for observations on interval and ratio scales, all of the measures mentioned for averages and variations apply, although to judge whether they are suitable we need to consider the distribution of the data.

For samples drawn from a normal distribution, the average and variation are most commonly characterized by the mean and the sample standard deviation. When samples are drawn from other distributions, as is often the case in practice, it may be relevant to consider other representations of the average and variation. In the presence of outliers, that is, observations which differ substantially from the large majority of other observations representations such as the median for the average and the MAD or the IQR for the variation have clear advantages, since these are insensitive to the magnitude of the outliers. The mode and variation ratio are, however, rarely useful for characterization of data acquired on the interval and ratio scales.

Confidence intervals are also useful for characterizing a sample. In contrast to the scalar representations of averages and variations above, which are so-called point estimates, we may be interested in knowing the interval within which a population parameter can be expected to lie. For example, we may be interested in the mean of a population. It is common to construct a confidence interval for the mean as $\left(\bar{x} - t\cdot s/\sqrt{n}; \bar{x} + t\cdot s/\sqrt{n}\right)$, where n is the sample size and t is determined by the confidence level. For a 95% confidence interval $t \approx 2$ under the assumption of a normal distribution. Sometimes the confidence interval is interpreted as the probability of finding the population parameter in the interval. However, that interpretation is wrong since the population parameter is not subject to random changes and will either be covered by the interval or not. Rather, the confidence interval is such that on average across many samples the confidence interval will cover the population parameter with a specified probability (e.g. 95%).

Visualization is another powerful technique for detecting anomalies and understanding the central tendency and variability in a sample. Figure 1.3 shows an overview of different visualization methods for univariate data. Histograms provide estimates of the probability density functions of continuous variables. It is produced by dividing the range of values in a sample into a series of intervals and counting and charting the number or frequency of samples in each interval. Box plots show groups of data via their quartiles. So-called whiskers can be added to provide box-and-whisker plots, although the meaning of the whiskers is not standardized, and outliers can be showed as isolated data points. Violin plots show groups is data similar to the box-and-whiskers plot, but show a curve similar to a smoothed, rotated, and mirrored histogram instead of the box. Finally, the bee swarm plot shows the full distribution of data points closely packed but sufficiently separated to allow each individual data point to be seen. While the position along the y-axis is determined by the data, the displacement along the x-axis is only a function of the local density of data points.

Other visualization techniques are available for multivariate data, with examples shown in Figure 1.3. Data on an interval or ratio scale from multiple groups can be visualized by stacking box-and-whisker plots, violin plots, or bee swarm plots. Data comprised of pairs of continuous variables can be visualized by scatter plots, and data comprised of triplets, quadruplets or more of continuous variables can be visualized by pair-wise scatter plots along with histograms. Visualizing even more complex data can be done but requires additional and custom procedures. However, this is often worthwhile because patterns in the data often emerge with the right visual representation.

1.4 INFERENCE: HYPOTHESIS TESTING

In hypothesis testing we want to draw conclusions about populations based on samples. For example, we may want to test if two populations have different means, by comparing the averages of samples drawn from the two populations. However, since the sample averages are subject to random variations, a difference between them may not necessarily indicate that there is any difference between the population means.

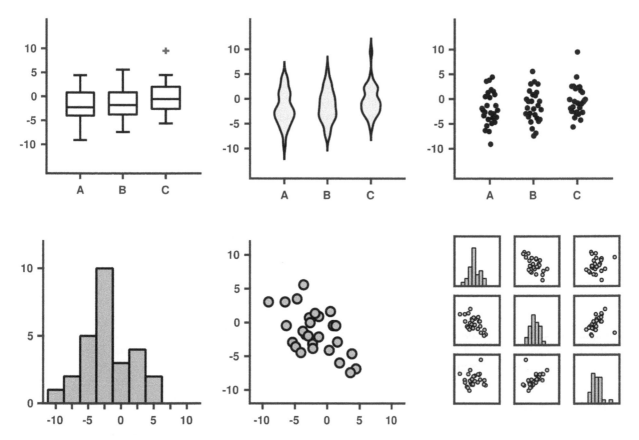

FIGURE 1.3 Examples of data visualizations. The top row shows example visualizations using a box-and-whisker plot, violin plot, and bee-swarm plot, respectively. All plots use the same data from three groups denoted A, B, and C. The cross in the box-and-whisker plot shows an outlier. The bottom row shows a histogram, a scatter plot, and a combination of histograms and scatterplots for visualization of multivariate data. The data from group A was used for the histogram, groups A and B for the scatter plot, and groups A, B, and, C for the multivariate plot. Colour image available at www.routledge.com/9781138593299.

There are three principal steps in hypothesis testing. The first step is to define the hypothesis (H_1) as a statement that can be tested. This means that the negated statement, referred to as the null hypothesis (H_0), can be falsified. A traditional example of a falsifiable statement is "black swans do not exist", which can be falsified by finding a single black swan. In contrast, the statement "black swans exist" is not falsifiable because claims of its invalidity ("no black swan exists") can be met with a trivial objection ("keep looking then"). An example of a more relevant hypothesis is that "patient survival differs between the old and new treatments", coupled with its falsifiable null hypothesis, "patient survival does not differ between the old and new treatments". The point is to construct the hypothesis so that if it is false then the null hypothesis must be true ($\neg H_1 \rightarrow H_0$). If we can prove the null hypothesis to be false, it follows logically that the hypothesis is true ($\neg H_0 \rightarrow H_1$).

The second step is to select a test statistic that can be computed from our samples, and to determine the distribution of this test statistic under the assumption that the null hypothesis is true. For example, we may select as our test statistic the difference in average survival times between two groups of patients undergoing different treatments. The next step would be to determine the distribution of this statistic if the survival did not differ between the groups, as stipulated by the null hypothesis. This null distribution could, in principle, be found by repeating a large number of experiments where the null hypothesis was true – for example, by giving identical treatments to the two groups. This would of course be cumbersome and expensive. To accelerate the process, we make assumptions about how the data were generated, which allows the use of theoretically well-defined distributions of the test statistic. For example, by assuming the survival times to follow normal distributions, we can compute the so-called t-statistic. Under the null hypothesis, this statistic follows Student's t-distribution. The distribution of the test statistic details the range of values that it could reasonably attain without proving the null hypothesis to be false. Formally, this means that if the null hypothesis is true, and the assumptions ('A') used to generate the null distribution are both true, the value of the test statistic lies within some interval with some probability $\left(H_0 \text{ and } A \rightarrow B, \text{ where } B : t \in \left(t_{min}, t_{max} \right) \right)$. If the observed value of the test statistic falls outside this interval, we assume the null hypothesis to be false, because: $\neg B \rightarrow \neg H_0$ (provided that the assumptions hold true). Note that we do not learn anything about the validity of the null hypothesis if the test statistic falls within the allowed interval (knowing B is true allows no inference about H_0).

The third step is to formalize a test of statistical significance. For this purpose, we consider the distribution of the test statistic and define the so-called p-value as the probability of obtaining a value of the test statistic that is equal to that computed from the sample, or a more extreme value, if the null hypothesis and the other assumptions of the test are both true. Formally, we can state this as $p = \int_t^\infty f(t') dt'$, where f is the PDF of the test statistic. If the p-value is lower than the significance threshold, denoted α, the result is said to be statistically significant, and the null hypothesis can be rejected. Accordingly, the original hypothesis is accepted as true. An equivalent procedure is to check whether the test statistic is below or above a critical value corresponding to the significance level. The significance level is normally set to 0.05 or lower, but care is warranted in order to avoid the so-called multiple comparisons problem, which will be discussed later in this chapter.

Several statistical tests appropriate for different kinds of situations are available. A broad division can be made between parametric and nonparametric tests. Parametric tests make use of explicit assumptions on the distribution of the underlying population (typically assuming a normal distribution), whereas nonparametric tests do not rely on such assumptions. The choice between a parametric test and its non-parametric counterpart depends on a number of factors, for example, the scale for measurement for data, assumptions that can safely be made about data, and the sample size. Typically, using a parametric test result in a slightly better ability to reject a false null hypothesis. The probability to reject a false hypothesis is referred to as power.

1.5   TESTS FOR DIFFERENCE IN MEANS

A common objective is to test if the averages of two separate samples reflect a difference between the two populations the samples were drawn from. In this situation, we can use either Student's t-test for testing differences in means [6] or the Mann-Whitney U-test for testing differences in medians [7, 8].

1.5.1   ONE-SAMPLE T-TEST

As a first example, we sample a population to investigate if it has a mean different from a value μ_0. Assuming the population follows a normal distribution, we can define the test statistic

$$t = \frac{\bar{x} - \mu_0}{s / \sqrt{n}}, \qquad (1.3)$$

where n is the sample size, to test the null hypothesis that the population mean is μ_0. The variable t follows the so-called t-distribution with $n-1$ degrees-of-freedom. Under the null hypothesis, the numerator is the observed value of a normal distribution with mean 0 and standard deviation $\sigma / \sqrt{n}$, where σ is the standard deviation of the population. If the denominator were $\sigma / \sqrt{n}$, the test statistics would follow a standard normal distribution, that is, a normal distribution with mean 0 and standard deviation 1. The test would then be referred to as the Z test. Since the denominator is based on the sample standard deviation rather than the population standard deviation, the t-statistics is obtained instead. A t-distribution with a high number of degrees-of-freedom is essentially equal to the standard normal distribution.

1.5.2   ONE-SIDED AND TWO-SIDED TESTS

If a one-sided test is performed, that is, only a large enough positive value of t (caused by the mean of the sample being larger than μ_0) is considered significant. Note that this criterion could just as well be formulated for negative values of t (i.e. the sample mean being smaller than μ_0). The important aspect is that only a deviation in one direction is considered incompatible with the null hypothesis. Alternatively, a two-sided test is performed, that is, a large enough value of t regardless of the direction is considered significant. The difference between one- and two-sided tests is illustrated in Figure 1.4. Note that the critical value of t, $t_{critical}$, that would make the observed difference considered significant

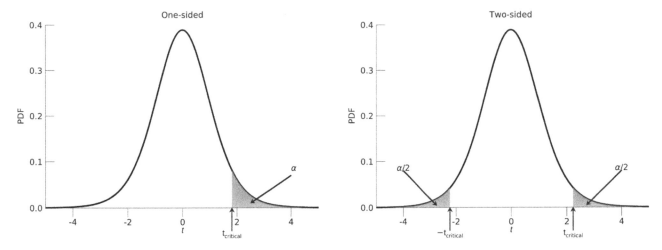

FIGURE 1.4 The difference between one- and two-sided tests. The greyed area is in both cases equal to α but is distributed differently between positive and negative t which leads to different values for the critical values of t beyond which the null hypothesis is rejected.

becomes larger for a two-sided test than for its one-sided counterpart and, hence, significance is achieved for a lower observed difference for a one-sided test than for a two-sided test. Generally, two-sided tests are preferred unless there are good reasons that only a deviation in a pre-determined direction can be considered noteworthy [9].

1.5.3 Two-sample t-test

A similar approach for the one-sample t-test can be used to compare the means of two independent samples. The test is then referred to as a two-sample t-test. The underlying assumptions are that both populations follow normal distributions with equal variances. Under the null hypothesis, that is, that the mean of population 1 is equal to the mean of population 2, the expression

$$t = \frac{\overline{x}_1 - \overline{x}_2}{s_{\text{pooled}} \sqrt{\dfrac{1}{n_1} + \dfrac{1}{n_2}}}, \tag{1.4}$$

where n_1 and n_2 are the sizes of samples 1 and 2, $\overline{x}_1$ and $\overline{x}_2$ are the means of sample 1 and 2, respectively, follows a t-distribution with $n_1 + n_2 - 2$ degrees-of-freedom. s_{pooled} in Equation 1.4 is obtained from

$$s_{\text{pooled}}^2 = \frac{(n_1 - 1)s_1^2 + (n_2 - 1)s_2^2}{n_1 + n_2 - 2} \tag{1.5}$$

and is referred to as a pooled estimation of variance, where s_1 and s_2 are the sample standard deviation for samples 1 and 2, respectively. Here, both samples are used to estimate the standard deviation of the populations in line with the assumption that both populations have the same variance.

1.5.4 Paired t-test

A different situation than the one outlined for a two-sample t-test is if two sets of measurements have been performed on the same sample. A typical example could be that we are interested in the effectiveness of a blood pressure medicine, which is investigated by measuring blood pressures of a group of patients before and after medication. The two sets of measurements cannot be considered independent (since the same patient is measured twice) and, hence, a two-sample t-test would be inappropriate to test for a difference in means. Instead, the paired t-test is used according to

$$t = \frac{\overline{\Delta x}}{s_D / \sqrt{n}}, \tag{1.6}$$

where n is the sample size, $\overline{\Delta x}$ is the average change between the two measurements for the sample, and s_D is the sample standard deviation of that difference, which follows a t-distribution with $n-1$ degrees-of-freedom. The rationale behind constructing a paired study rather than obtaining two independent samples is that variation caused by difference between individuals tends to cancel in a paired construction, thereby decreasing the number of individuals required for a given power.

1.5.5 ROBUSTNESS

The assumptions of underlying normality and, for the two-sample t-test, equal variances for the two populations, might appear to limit the applicability. However, the t-test has been demonstrated to be robust against deviations from normality, provided that the sample sizes are large enough [10–12]. This behaviour can in part be understood by the observation that the formulae are based on the sums of observed values rather than the values individually and application of the central-limit theorem. The details depend on the extent of deviation from normality, but often a sample size between 5 and 15 is considered enough for normality not to be critical, especially for two-sided tests. Also, the two-sample t-test tends to be robust towards deviations from equal variances, in particular if the two sample sizes are equal [10]. If deemed necessary to account for explicitly, there is also a variant of the two-sample t-test where the assumption of equal variances is relaxed, sometimes referred to as Welch's t-test [13].

1.5.6 NON-PARAMETRIC TESTS FOR DIFFERENCES IN MEDIANS

A non-parametric test for the difference between medians for independent samples is the Mann-Whitney U-test [7, 8], or, for paired data, the Wilcoxon signed-rank test [8]. Both these tests are based on the ranking of data rather than on the data values directly and, since they are non-parametric, do not require the underlying population to be normal. If the populations follow normal distributions, the power of a two-sample t-test is higher than the power of the Mann-Whitney U-test for the same significance levels and sample sizes, but the difference is rather modest. If the underlying populations follow non-normal distributions, the U-test may result in a higher power than the t-test [14, 15].

1.6 CORRELATION

Until now we have considered univariate data, but it is common to acquire multivariate data and investigate the relationship (or lack thereof) between variables. For two variables, the covariance has previously been discussed. A negative covariance means that an observed lower value for variable 1 lowered the expected value for variable 2, and vice versa for a positive covariance. It can be shown that for two stochastic variables ξ and η $|\mathrm{cov}(\xi, \eta)| \leq \sigma_\xi \sigma_\eta$, where σ_ξ and σ_η are the standard deviations for ξ and η, respectively. Hence, a measure that is easier to interpret than the covariance is the correlation

$$\mathrm{corr}(\xi, \eta) = \frac{\mathrm{cov}(\xi, \eta)}{\sigma_\xi \sigma_\eta}, \tag{1.7}$$

which will have the property $-1 \leq \mathrm{corr}(\xi, \eta) \leq 1$, with a value of 1 indicating perfect positive correlation between the two variables, a value of -1 indicating a perfect negative correlation between the two variables, and a value of zero indicating that the two variables are uncorrelated.

1.6.1 PEARSON'S CORRELATION COEFFICIENT

For a sample, the Pearson correlation coefficient [16] is calculated as

$$r = \frac{\sum_{i=1}^{n}(x_i - \bar{x})(y_i - \bar{y})}{(n-1)s_x s_y}, \tag{1.8}$$

where s_x is the sample standard deviation for the x-values and s_y is the sample standard deviation for the y-values. The correlation coefficient can be understood in terms of a linear fit between x and y, the sign of r indicating the sign of the slope of the fitted line and the absolute value of r indicating the degree of agreement between a linear regression to the data and the data points.

While the strength of a relationship between two variables is judged from the magnitude of the correlation coefficient, there is also the question of whether an observed correlation is significant, that is, reflects an underlying correlation between the two stochastic variables. This question can also be phrased as if the correlation is statistically different from 0. Even a low correlation coefficient can be statistically different from 0 provided that the sample size is large enough, indicating that the there is a real linear relationship between the two variables, but that there is a considerable scattering of data around that linear relationship. Conversely, it is possible for a relatively large correlation coefficient to occur by chance if only a small sample is considered. One way of performing a test for the significance of Pearson correlation is by using the fact that it can be shown that, for normal data with n data points, the expression

$$t = \frac{r\sqrt{n-2}}{\sqrt{1-r^2}} \tag{1.9}$$

follows a t-distribution with $n-2$ degrees-of-freedom under the null hypothesis that the correlation is 0.

1.6.2 SPEARMAN'S CORRELATION COEFFICIENT

A non-parametric alternative to Pearson's correlation coefficient is Spearman's correlation coefficient [17], which can be defined as Pearson's correlation coefficient applied to the ranking of data. As a result, while Pearson's correlation coefficient measures the strength of a linear relationship between two variables, Spearman's correlation coefficient rather measures the strength of a monotonic relationship between the variables.

1.6.3 CORRELATION AND DEPENDENCE

If two variables are correlated, it implies that they are dependent. However, the converse is not true, since two dependent variables may be uncorrelated. A simple example could be the two stochastic variables ξ and $\eta = \xi^2$ illustrated in Figure 1.5 for a sample of size 100. The two variables are obviously dependent, but their correlation is 0 in both the Pearson and Spearman meanings. This also serves as an example of the importance of visualizing data rather than just relying on summary parameters.

1.6.4 BLAND–ALTMAN PLOTS

When comparing measurement methods, it is not appropriate use a correlation analysis. The reason is that two measurements of the same quantity would be expected to correlate, otherwise at least one of the measurement methods would be extraordinarily poor [18]. A more relevant visualization of the difference between the two methods is achieved by plotting the difference in measurement values as a function of the average of the two. This kind of comparison is referred to as a Bland-Altman plot. The average difference is an indication of systematic difference between the results of the two methods, and the standard deviation of the differences is a measure of random differences between them.

1.7 MULTIVARIATE REGRESSION AND THE F-TEST

So far, we have only considered simple correlations, where the variation in one variable is explained by the variation in another variable. In practice, we often encounter situations where we want to explain the variation in one variable by a set of other variables, or so-called multivariate regression. This can be expressed as

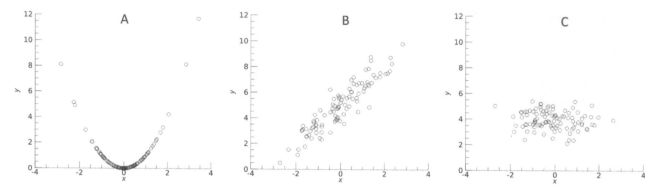

FIGURE 1.5 Examples of dependent, correlated, and independent variables. Subfigure A shows a plot of two variables that are dependent but uncorrelated. Subfigure B is a plot of two variables that are correlated and thereby also dependent, while subfigure C is a plot of two independent variables.

$$Y = \beta_0 + \beta_1 X_1 + \beta_2 X_2 + \cdots \beta_m X_m + \epsilon \qquad (1.10)$$

where Y is the observed value, also known as dependent variable, β_k are referred to as regression coefficients, X_k are the independent variables, also known as, for example, regressors, explanatory variables, and covariates, and ϵ is a stochastic variable representing sampling noise. The values of both the dependent variable and the independent variables are determined during the experiment of the data-collection phase, while the values of the regression coefficients are unknown and determined from the data. If the noise is normally distributed and IID, the regression coefficients can be determined by expressing the equations in a matrix form and performing a so-called pseudo-inverse [19]. Note that the analysis can be applied if the dependent variable is determined on an interval or a ratio scale but not on an ordinal or a nominal scale. The same applies for the independent variables, except that these can be on the nominal scale if only two categories are present. This is the case in a so-called one-way ANOVA analysis.

Multivariate regression can be used for many different purposes. For example, we may want to know if the dependent variable is related to an independent variable. An example of this could be an attempt to explain variation in weight by three covariates: height, age, and sex. A test could be performed to investigate if these three covariates can significantly explain the variation in the dependent variable. To understand how to perform such a test, we need to learn about four concepts: coefficient of determination (r^2), residuals, the F-test, and degrees-of-freedom.

The coefficient of determination is also known as explained variance, and is defined as

$$r^2 = 1 - \frac{SS_{res}}{SS_{tot}}, \qquad (1.11)$$

where SS_{res} and SS_{tot} are the sum-of-squares of the residuals and the total data, respectively. The term residual refers to the difference between the observed values of the dependent variables (Y_i), and the variables predicted by the regression ($\hat{Y}_i$). Thus, $SS_{res} = \sum_{i=1}^n \left(Y_i - \hat{Y}_i\right)^2$. Conversely, $SS_{tot} = \sum_{i=1}^n \left(Y_i - \bar{Y}\right)^2$, which means SS_{tot} quantifies the total variation of the dependent variable around its mean. The r^2 can assume values between zero and unity. Values close to zero mean the regression explains little to none of the variation in the dependent variation, whereas values closer to unity means that nearly all of the variation was explained by the independent variables.

The F-test is designed to compare two pairs of variances, obtained from fitting two different but nested models, and is in its general form defined as

$$F = \frac{(SS_1 - SS_2)/(p_2 - p_1)}{SS_2/(n - p_1)} \qquad (1.12)$$

where SS_1 and SS_2 are the residual sum of squares from the two model fits, p_1 and p_2 are the number of parameters in each of the two models, and n is the number of samples. The models should be arranged so that $p_2 > p_1$ and thus

$SS_1 > SS_2$, for nested models. Just as for the other tests the critical value in the F-test depends on the significance level but also on the degrees-of-freedom of the estimates in the numerator and denominator, which here are $p_2 - p_1$ and $n - p_1$, respectively.

The one-way ANOVA test can be seen as a generalization of the t-test but allows for simultaneous tests across multiple groups. The null hypothesis is that all groups share the same mean, which can be tested using the F-test. The first model assumes the dependent variable to be normally distributed around the common mean and thus $p_1 = 1$, whereas the second model assumes that each group has its own mean, and thus $p_2 = m$, where m is the number of groups. If F is large, it means that the residuals are substantially smaller for the model assuming different means across the groups.

1.8 SURVIVAL DATA

The survival curve $S(t)$ of a stochastic variable is related to the CDF, $F(t)$, of a stochastic variable according to

$$S(t) = 1 - F(t). \tag{1.13}$$

The survival function is a natural way to describe variables that are related to the time at which an event occurs – for example, the time of death for patients.

1.8.1 KAPLAN–MEIER CURVES

Survival functions can be estimated from samples using a technique developed by Kaplan and Meier [20]. The empirical survival function is calculated according to

$$\hat{S}(t) = \prod_{\{i:t_i < t\}} \left(1 - \frac{d_i}{n_i}\right), \tag{1.14}$$

where t_i is the time at which an event (i.e. a death) occurs, d_i is the number of events at time t_i and n_i is the number of individuals at risk of dying at time t_i.

There are two reasons why an individual originally part of the sample may not be part of the individuals at risk at a time t_i. Either the individual has been the cause of a previous event, or information about the status of the individual cannot be accessed beyond a time $t_c < t$. The latter phenomenon is referred to as censoring, that is, the investigator only has partial knowledge about the value of the time when the transition between the two states would occur. Reasons for data to be censored could, for example, be that the individual no longer wishes to participate in the study or that data is compiled before all individuals have died.

Examples of Kaplan-Meier curves for two fictive groups are shown in Figure 1.6 a and b. Censored data, which do not give rise to any event in the generation of the curves, still contribute to the estimation of the survival function by being part of the individuals at risk up until the time they leave the study.

1.8.2 THE LOGRANK TEST

The difference between Kaplan-Meier curves can be tested for significance using the logrank test [21]. The null hypothesis is that the underlying survival curves are equal, and the expected number of events at any given time interval should thereby be in proportion to the number of subjects at risk in the two groups. Under the null hypothesis, the sum of differences between the predicted and observed events approximately follows a χ^2 distribution with one degree-of-freedom for the comparison of two curves, or, in general, the number of groups minus one. A worked example of a logrank test is given by Bland and Altman [22].

The logrank test performs a comparison of the entire survival curves and not just the average survival time. This is important, in particular when the survival time is ill defined due to censored data. The power of the test to detect differences between curves may under some circumstances be low – for example, in the event of two curves intersecting

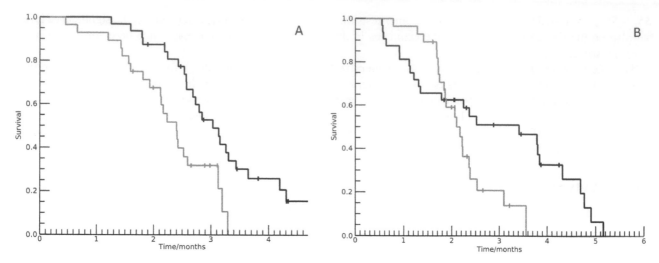

FIGURE 1.6 Fictitious examples of Kaplan-Meier curves. Censored data are marked with vertical lines. In figure B, the two survival curves cross, which may complicate the analysis.

each other [23]. For example, the situation in Figure 1.6a gives a statistically significant difference between the two curves (at the 5% level), while that is not the case for the situation in Figure 1.6b.

1.9 STATISTICAL POWER, TYPE I AND II ERRORS, AND THE MULTIPLE COMPARISONS PROBLEM

Two types of errors can be made in hypothesis testing: type I and type II errors, which generate false positive and false negative findings. A false positive finding occurs when the null hypothesis is rejected despite being true. This means an effect is being reported as present, when it is in fact absent. A false negative finding takes place when the null hypothesis is false but is not rejected. This means an effect is reported as being absent, when it is in fact present. The rate of false positive findings is controlled by the significance threshold. A threshold of $\alpha = 0.05$ means (ideally) that a true null hypothesis will be rejected in 5% of all tests. The false positive rate (β) can be reduced by the use of a stricter (that is, lower) significance threshold, but this would simultaneously inflate the rate of false negative findings because a stricter test means that the effect needs to be larger to be accepted as significant, all other things equal. The false negative rate is thus tightly related to the statistical power ($\pi = 1 - \beta$), which is measured in per cent and defined as the true positive rate. Thus, the power describes the probability of finding an effect as being present (significant) when it is in fact present.

The statistical power increases with the effect size and the sample size. It can be computed for all statistical tests but is here explained for the t-test for equal sample sizes. For this situation t can be defined as

$$t = d / \sqrt{n / 2}, \tag{1.15}$$

where n is the sample size and d is the effect size, referred to as Cohen's d, which is a standardized effect size defined as the ratio between the effect size (difference in population means) and the standard deviation

$$d = \frac{\mu_1 - \mu_2}{\sigma} \tag{1.16}$$

Effect sizes of $d = 0.3$, 0.5, and 0.8 have been referred to as small, medium, and large. The point here is to realize that t is a stochastic variable. Performing an experiment in which samples are collected and computing the value of t from the samples can be seen as drawing a sample from the t-distribution. Each repetition of the whole experiment, if performed on independent samples, would generate a new value of t. The probability by which t will be higher or lower than a critical threshold t_0 and thus indicate a significant difference is referred to as the statistical power. The critical threshold

TABLE 1.2
Group Sizes Required for Different Levels of Statistical Power

Power	Cohen's d				Correlation coefficient (r)			
	0.3	0.5	0.8	1.2	0.3	0.5	0.7	0.9
0.25	38	14	6	4	20	8	5	3
0.50	86	32	13	7	42	15	7	4
0.80	175	64	26	12	85	28	12	6
0.95	290	105	42	19	139	46	19	8

Note: The left group of values shows group sizes per condition for a two-tailed t-test for different effect sizes quantified by Cohen's d. The right group of values shows group sizes for correlation tests for different correlation coefficients.

is defined primarily by the significance level but, to some extent, also by the sample size. The expected value of t, and thus the statistical power, is controlled by a combination of the effect size and the sample size, as seen in Equation 1.15. Small effect sizes thus warrant larger sample sizes than do large effect sizes, if the power is to be kept constant. Table 1.2 shows the required group sizes to achieve different levels of statistical power for variable effect sizes.

The statistical power is also indirectly related to the number of tests performed to assess a certain hypothesis. For example, assume we wanted to test the somewhat silly hypothesis that there is a difference in height between those with surnames starting with the letters 'N' and 'G', and that this was tested by assessing the height of 24 randomly selected persons in each category. Now, assume this test was repeated for randomly selected persons in 100 different countries. In total, 100 tests would be performed and, with a significance threshold of 0.05, we would expect on average 5 tests to show there were significant differences in height. Of course, these would be false positive findings. The problem here is that when we perform m independent tests of the same hypothesis, the effective false positive rate (α_{eff}) grows to

$$\alpha_{eff} = 1 - (1 - \alpha)^m. \tag{1.17}$$

To reduce the effective false positive rate, we can reduce the significance threshold. One way to do this is by so-called Bonferroni correction, where the adjusted threshold α' is set to $\alpha' = \alpha / m$. Alternatively, the so-called Šidák correction can be made by setting α_{eff} to its desired value and then computing α' by solving Equation 1.17.

1.10 SENSITIVITY AND SPECIFICITY

A concept closely related to hypothesis testing is diagnostic testing, where the test can yield a binary answer: positive or negative, often interpreted as diseased or healthy, respectively. For such a test, it is of interest to know its sensitivity and specificity, where the sensitivity is the true positive rate (what fraction of those with the disease that will get a positive test answer) and the specificity is the true negative rate (what fraction of those without the disease will get a negative test answer). In addition to these numbers, it is relevant to know the positive predictive value (PPV) and negative predictive value (NPV). The PPV quantifies the fraction of all with a positive test who in fact have the disease, while the NPV quantifies the fraction of all with a negative test who in fact are healthy. If the disease prevalence in the group that the test is applied to is very low, the PPV tends to be low even for high values of the sensitivity and specificity.

1.11 LIMITATIONS OF HYPOTHESIS TESTING

Hypothesis testing is a powerful tool to help us avoid interpreting random sampling noise as true effects. However, there are multiple ways hypothesis testing can be inadvertently misused. We already mentioned the multiple comparisons problem. A related problem is so-called p-hacking, where data is reanalyzed with different types of tests or pre-processing steps until the p-value falls below a desired level: the significance threshold. This obviously goes against the idea behind hypothesis testing and can happen without malicious intent, for example, when multiple scientists analyze the same data set but with different methods. Regardless, the consequence is that false positive findings will be reported. Another problem is the failure of distinguishing statistical significance from practical significance. With large enough sample sizes, even negligibly small effects may become statistically significant. To prevent this problem, it must be realized that hypothesis testing is just the first step that lets us know whether data indicate the presence of a true effect or just noise. Once this has been established, the data analysis needs to focus on whether the effect has any practical relevance.

Another limitation concerns the topic of generalization. All too often the sample is believed to represent a population much larger and more general than in reality is the case. For example, a study reporting statistically significant effects of a new versus an old treatment on the survival of cancer patients in a certain hospital may be interpreted as applicable to all hospitals around the world. However, until the results of such a study are reproduced in different situations, we cannot know, because the population sampled were not from all around the world, but from the specific hospital. Another limitation is related to the PPV of a hypothesis test. For a diagnostic test, we learned that the PPV is determined by the sensitivity and prevalence, which for hypothesis tests correspond to the power and the a priori probability that the hypothesis is true [24]. This probability is high when reproducing previous findings and, thus, a well-powered study ($\pi = 0.8$) with a conventional significance threshold ($\alpha = 0.05$) that tests a hypothesis with an a priori probability of being true of, let us say, 0.5, the PPV is 0.94. The result of such a study would be trustworthy. For exploratory studies with limited power, however, the situation is different. Assuming a study is performed with low statistical power ($\pi = 0.2$) and an a priori probability of being true of just 1%, we get a value for the PPV of 4%. This means that the vast majority of such studies report significant results that are false despite using technically correct statistical methods.

REFERENCES

[1] J. Gaito, "Measurement scales and statistics: Resurgence of an old misconception," *Psychol. Bull.,* vol. 87, pp. 564–67, 1980.

[2] J. Michell, "Measurement scales and statistics: A clash of paradigms," *Psychol. Bull.,* vol. 100, pp. 398–407, 1986.

[3] J. T. Townsend and F. G. Ashby, "Measurement scales and statistics: The misconception misconceived," *Psychol. Bull.,* pp. 394–401, 1984.

[4] D. J. Hand, "Statistics and the theory of measurement," *J. R. Statist. Soc. A,* vol. 159, Part 3, pp. 445–92, 1996.

[5] S. S. Stevens, "On the theory of scales of measurement," *Science,* vol. 103, pp. 677–80, 1946.

[6] Student, "The probable error of a mean," *Biometrika,* vol. 6, pp. 1–25, 1908.

[7] H. B. Mann and D. R. Whitney, "On a test of whether one of two random variables is stochastically larger than the other," *Ann. Math. Stat.,* vol. 18, pp. 50–60, 1947.

[8] F. Wilcoxon, "Individual comparisons by ranking methods," *Biometrics Bull.,* vol. 1, pp. 80–83, 1945.

[9] J. M. Bland and D. G. Altman, "One and two sided tests of significance," *Brit. Med. J.,* vol. 309, p. 248, 1994.

[10] C. A. Boneau, "The effects of violations of assumptions underlying the *t* test," *Psychological Bulletin,* vol. 57, pp. 49–64, 1960.

[11] E. S. Pearson and N. W. Please, "Relation between the shape of the population distribution and the robustness of four simple test statistics," *Biometrika,* vol. 62, pp. 223–41, 1975.

[12] S. S. Sawilowsky and R. C. Blair, "A more realistic look at the robustness and type II error properties of the t test to departures from population normality," *Psychol. Bull.,* vol. 111, pp. 352–60, 1992.

[13] B. L. Welch, "The generalization of 'Student's' problem when several different population variances are involved," *Biometrika,* vol. 34, pp. 28–35, 1947.

[14] R. C. Blair and J. J. Higgins, "A comparison of the power of Wilcoxon's rank-sum statistic to that of Student's t statistic under various nonnormal distributions," *J. Educ. Stat.,* vol. 5, pp. 309–35, 1980.

[15] J. D. Gibbons and S. Chakraborti, "Comparisons of the Mann-Whitney, Students' t and alternate t tests for means of normal distributions," *J. Exp. Educ.,* vol. 59, pp. 258–67, 1991.

[16] K. Pearson, "VII. Mathematical contributions to the theory of evolution. –III. Regression, heredity, and panmixia," *Philos. T. R. Soc. Lond.,* vol. 187, pp. 253–318, 1896.

[17] C. Spearman, "The proof and measurement of association between two things," *Am. J. Psychol.,* vol. 15, pp. 72–101, 1904.

[18] D. G. Altman and J. M. Bland, "Measurement in medicine: The analysis of method comparison studies," *Statistician,* vol. 32, pp. 307–17, 1983, doi: 10.2307/2987937.

[19] A. Ben-Israel and T. N. E. Greville, *Generalized inverses: Theory and applications,* 2nd ed. New York: Springer, 2003.

[20] E. L. Kaplan and P. Meier, "Nonparametric estimation from incomplete observations," *J. Am. Stat. Assoc.,* vol. 53, pp. 457–81, 1958.

[21] R. Peto and J. Peto, "Asymptotically efficient rank invariant test procedures," *J. R. Statist. Soc. Ser. A-G,* vol. 135, pp. 185–207, 1972.

[22] J. M. Bland and D. G. Altman, "The logrank test," *Brit. Med. J.,* vol. 328, p. 1073, 2004.

[23] D. M. Stablein, W. H. Carter Jr, and J. W. Noval, "Analysis of survival data with nonproportional hazard functions," *Control. Clin. Trials,* vol. 2, pp. 149–59, 1981.

[24] J. P. Ioannidis, "Why most published research findings are false," *PLoS Med.,* vol. 2, p. e124, 2005, doi: 10.1371/journal. pmed.0020124.

2 Radiobiology

Lidia Strigari and Marta Cremonesi

CONTENTS

2.1 INTRODUCTION

Targeted radionuclide therapy (RNT) consists of biologically selective irradiation of malignant cells by means of radio-nuclide labelled tumour-seeking molecules. This therapeutic strategy is undergoing rapid changes due to the availability of new receptor-directed ligands, metabolic precursors, monoclonal antibodies (i.e. radio-immunotherapy) or the development of innovative devices.

A variety of radionuclides, emitting nuclear particles with a range of path lengths from nanometres to millimetres, and novel clinical strategies, are currently used, for which not only the red marrow but also several normal tissues become organs at risk. The basic aspects of radiobiology developed for External Beam Radiotherapy (EBRT) and recently adapted for either brachytherapy or RNT will be illustrated.

2.1.1 THE 'Rs' OF RADIOBIOLOGY

The main features of cell survival models apply both to tumours and to normal tissues and are described using the 'four Rs' of radiobiology [1], initially developed with EBRT and brachytherapy in mind, but applicable to RNT. The 'four Rs' can be summed up as follows [2]:

DOI: 10.1201/9780429489549-2

- **Repair**: DNA is more frequently damaged by 'normal' agents (e.g. temperature, chemicals) than by radiation (factor 1000!) and powerful repair mechanisms counteract these damages. In the case of radiation, the efficiency of these repair pathways is related to Linear Energy Transfer (LET), dose-rate, cell phase, and so forth. The half time for repair (T_{rep}) is in the order of minutes to hours.
- **Repopulation**: In tumours and some normal tissues cell numbers grow during the irradiation, and this effect is partially counteracted by cell killing. Reduction in size enhances oxygenation and tumour growth. Repopulation in normal tissues is also an important mechanism to counteract acute side effects.
- **Reoxygenation**: Oxygen is an important factor to stabilize the effect of radiation. The ratio between the quantitative measure of a given effect in the absence or in presence of oxygen is defined as Oxygen Enhancement Ratio (OER). Indeed, in the centre of the tumours there may be a lack of blood vessels, causing hypoxia and decreasing the cell radiosensitivity. Thus, in order to sterilize hypoxic cells, the tumour needs to be re-oxygenated. This typically happens a few days after the beginning of irradiation. In fact, the removal of more radiosensitive cells from the bulk tumour enables more hypoxic cells to reach the blood vessels, stimulating oxygenation.
- **Redistribution**: Cells have different radio-sensitivity at different phases of the cell cycle. Highest radiation sensitivity is in the early S and late G2/M phase of the cell cycle. Radiation delivered at high doses introduces a block of cells in the G2 phase leading to the synchronization of cells. This produces more radiosensitive cells in tumours and normal tissues and increases the radiation damage, playing an important role in EBRT when the time between fractions is limited to a few hours.

2.2 LINEAR QUADRATIC MODEL

To describe or predict the dose response/damage effect, the Linear Quadratic Model (LQM) has to be extended from EBRT to include different treatment regimens also involving source decay and incorporating the repair of sub-lethal radiation damage [3–7].

The LQ equation for the surviving fraction (sf) of cells after an absorbed dose, D, delivered instantaneously (which is the usual, albeit simplified, description of all RT modalities) is

$$sf(D) = e^{\left(-\alpha D - \beta D^2\right)} \tag{2.1}$$

where α and β are tissue-specific constants, representing the damage induced by DNA irreparable, that is, double strand-breaks (DSB), or reparable, that is, single strand-breaks (SSB) events which, in a semi-logarithmic plot, are linearly and quadratically dependent on absorbed dose D, respectively. Irreparable events simply depend on the absorbed dose D, and they have a probability proportional to D by a term named α. On the contrary, two independent ionizing events (each one reparable) are needed at the same point of the DNA filament and closer in time to generate cellular deaths. This occurrence is proportional to the product of probabilities, that is, to the D^2, by a factor named "β". A pictorial representation of the cell survival curve for the linear and quadratic component is shown in Figure 2.1.

Parameter α corresponds to the initial slope of the sf curve (i.e. the larger values of α correspond to the steeper initial slope) while β determines the degree of downward curvature of the curve (the larger value of β corresponds to the more "bent" curve).

Enzymatic repair mechanisms of reparable events need time to correct a single strand DNA break. Repair time is in competition with additional possible single strand breaks at the same point of the DNA filament. So cellular death from reparable damage depends on the concentration over time of the ionizing events, that is, the dose rate.

When a dose D is delivered over a time "T" (protracted irradiation) the repair mechanism can compete more effectively against radiation damage, therefore the quadratic component must be corrected for repair of sub-lethal damage. A dimensionless function g(T), with a value between 0 and 1, is introduced, describing the decrease in lethality with an increase in the overall treatment time:

$$sf(D) = e^{\left(-\alpha D - \beta D^2\right)} \tag{2.2}$$

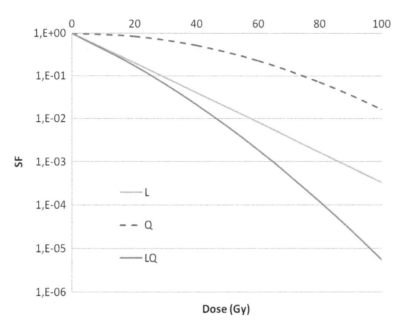

FIGURE 2.1   A pictorial representation of the cell survival curve for the linear (L), quadratic (Q) and the linear-quadratic (LQ) component.

When the duration, T, of the protracted dose delivery becomes significantly long compared to the repair half-time $T \gg T_{rep}$, then g(T) can be approximated by the expression of a dose delivered a constant dose rate:

$$g\left(T \gg T_{rep}\right) \approx \frac{\lambda_e}{\lambda_e + \mu} = \frac{T_{rep}}{T_{rep} + T_{eff}} \tag{2.3}$$

where μ is the rate of repair of sub-lethal damage $\mu = \log(2) / T_{rep}$, T_{rep} representing the repair half-time constant) and λ_e is the effective decay rate of the radioisotope in a tissue ($\lambda_e = \log(2) / T_{eff}$, T_{eff} being the effective half-time of the radioisotope in a tissue) [4, 8]. A continuous low dose rate "spares" the normal tissues much more than the tumour, conferring the same benefits as fractionation.

2.2.1   REPOPULATION

During any irradiation, the cell proliferation rate is in competition with the radio-induced killing rate. In RNT, the repopulation is important since the effective decay lowers the dose rate monotonically. Below a dose-rate threshold, the balance changes in favour of re-grow of the irradiated tissues, and any dose delivered below such a threshold is wasted. Considering this, the biological repopulation factor (BRF)

$$BRF = K \cdot T_{eff} \tag{2.4}$$

where K is the biological dose required to offset each day's worth of tumour repopulation and T is the effective time of treatment expressed in h. Thus, the Biological Effective Dose (BED) can be calculated as follows:

$$BED = D \cdot RE = K \cdot T \tag{2.5}$$

Equation 2.6 allows tacking into consideration that usually fast-repopulating tumours require higher doses to be controlled. The dose heterogeneity decreases efficacy so the targeted radiotherapy would need to be combined with EBRT or chemotherapy [9, 10].

An improvement to the dose-response model at the organ level requires an extensive evaluation of the effects of non-uniform dose distribution in a given tumour or organ [11, 12].

2.3 EQDX FORMALISM

An alternative to the BED for modelling dose-rate effects in radiation therapy is the equi-effective dose [13]. The ICRU defined the equi-effective dose, EQDX, as *the total absorbed dose delivered by the reference treatment plan (fraction size X) that leads to the same biological effect as a test treatment plan that is conducted with absorbed dose per fraction d and total absorbed dose D [13].*

The relation, adapted from the Withers formula [14], is defined as

$$EQDX_{\alpha/\beta} = D \cdot \frac{d + \alpha/\beta}{X + \alpha/\beta} \qquad (2.6)$$

As defined thus far, the quantities BED and EUD account for differences in the temporal and spatial pattern of dose delivery, respectively. Neither quantity accounts for the enhanced biological effects of high linear energy transfer (LET) emissions such as α-particles or Auger electrons.

The quantity, relative biological effectiveness (RBE), has been used to account for the increased biological effect of high LET emissions. The RBE is defined as

$$RBE(X) = \left. \frac{D_{ref}}{D_{test}} \right|_X \qquad (2.7)$$

More recently the formalism has been improved to derive the RBE2(α/β) which is independent of absorbed dose for α-particle emitters, and it provides a more logical framework for data reporting and conversion to equi-effective dose than the conventional dose-dependent definition of RBE [15].

2.3.1 EQUIVALENT UNIFORM DOSE

Based on EBRT the non-uniformity in dose distribution has a crucial role on dose effect response. In particular, O'Donoghue [16] introduced the concept of tumour curability by considering the dose in-homogeneities. The effect of non-uniform dose distribution at the voxel level can be taken into consideration, adopting the Equivalent Uniform Dose EUD [17], defined through the sf and the cell radio-sensitivity as

$$EUD = -\frac{1}{\alpha} \ln \left(sf \left[D_i, V_i \right] \right) \qquad (2.8)$$

where $sf\left[D_i, V_i \right]$ is calculated for each tumour element V_i where dose deposition D_i is considered uniform. Based on Equation 2.9 the EUD is defined as the spatial distribution of absorbed doses which, if delivered uniformly to the tumour, would yield a surviving fraction equal to that obtained from the actual distribution.

Following the derivations by Niemierko, O'Donoghue, and Hobbs [16, 18, 19], the equation for EUD can be written as

$$EUD = \left(\sum_i D_i^{1/n} V_i \right)^n \qquad (2.9)$$

where n is a parameter depending on the type of tissue architecture (for parallel organ n=1 and EUD=mean dose). The following equation provides the EUD for a single tumour with a given distribution of $N\, BED_i$ values [20]:

$$EUD = -\frac{1}{\alpha} ln \left(\frac{\sum_{i=1}^{N} e^{-\alpha BED_i}}{N} \right) \qquad (2.10)$$

2.3.2 RADIOBIOLOGICAL PARAMETERS AND THEIR UNCERTAINTIES

The influence of radiobiological parameter uncertainty on the linear quadratic model prediction has been investigated by many authors [21, 22]. However, Chiesa and colleagues [21] have shown that the error on absorbed dose has a far higher impact than the uncertainty on radiobiological parameters. The variation of surviving fraction against dose at various α/β ratios and at various T_{rep} values have been investigated [23], suggesting that uncertainties in some radiobiological parameters produce acceptable variations of biological effective dose, which represents a robust and efficient approach to the estimate effect of different treatments.

2.4 TUMOUR CONTROL PROBABILITY (TCP)

In a region, receiving a BED, the TCP is given by

$$TCP(BED) = e^{-N^* \cdot e^{-\alpha BED}} \tag{2.11}$$

where N^* is the initial number of clonogenic cells able to proliferate and give rise to a tumour. Usually N^* is proportional to the tumour volume V, ρ being the number of clonogenic cells per cubic centimetre: $N^* = \rho \cdot V$. The value of ρ depends strongly on the type of tumour and on the patient [24]. Tumour cells may be in a bulk primary tumour, in draining lymph nodes and/or in small microscopic spread. Palpable tumours are usually characterized by 10^9 cells/cm^3. A large mass could therefore contain as many as 10^{12} cells and its eradication require higher doses, while microscopic tumours or micrometastasis containing about 10^6 cells require lower doses. As might be expected TCP decreases when the number of initial cells increase. Equation 2.8 is based on the Poisson statistic which assumes that all clonogenic cells are independent: killing a cell does not effect other cells.

Tumour treatment is complex. Indeed, besides absorbed dose (the radionuclide and its microscopic localization and residence time), biological response to radiation depends mainly on LET, dose rate, OER, cell cycle and target population/size and tumour characteristics (intrinsic radiosensitivity plus the "four Rs"), as well as on the presence of other agents given concurrently (e.g. chemotherapy).

Furthermore, tumours with high proliferative activity and a high rate of cell loss diminish in size quickly, while more indolent tumours may take months and remain detectable for weeks or for months (hepato-cellular carcinomas, i.e. HCC) after radiotherapy and, yet, ultimately disappear and never recur [2]. This behaviour can be explained by the fact that the radio-induced cellular damage remains latent until the cells try to replicate with mitosis, when the latent DNA damage prevents its replication, and cell death occurs. So, tumour shrinkage (or organ failure, see later) happens after a latency time that is linked to the proliferation rate in that tissue.

In addition, hypoxic cells are the main obstacle to tumour curability. However, the LQM predicts that dose fractionation influences the control rate only in a minority of tumours, when the overall treatment time is sufficient for re-oxygenation of hypoxic tumour cells.

2.4.1 NORMAL TISSUE CONTROL PROBABILITY (NTCP)

During therapy some doses are inevitably delivered to normal tissues, which might suffer damage according to their tissue architecture (roughly classified into serial and parallel) and a given complication cannot occur unless the fractional volume damaged exceeds the threshold value. In a serial organ the damage to any single small component results in an organ complication, while in a parallel organ the damage occurs when a given dose is delivered to a volume larger than the organ reserve. In other words, in serial organs even a small volume irradiated beyond the threshold can lead to whole organ failure (e.g. spinal cord, oesophagus or gastro-intestinal tract). Parallel organs are assumed to be constituted by Functional Sub-Units (FSUs), working independently; thus, organ failure arises from the inactivation of a certain fraction of FSU (organ reserve), irrespective of location. If the organ reserve is preserved from irradiation, the target portion could receive any dose without risk of organ failure. Similarly, in parallel organs the effect depends on the volume of normal tissue irradiated (the greater the volume the smaller the dose should be, that is, the higher the doses the higher the chance that a whole organ fails). Typical examples of parallel behaviour are found in the liver, kidney sub-organ regions, and lungs.

For most tissue types, sub-lethal radiation damage, β component of LQM, is repaired after about one hour. So normal tissues are greatly advantaged by fractionation (e.g. multi-fractionated treatments), as well as by low dose-rate irradiation. Given the above, mathematical models, such as NTCP, can be used to predict the incidence of complications for both serial and parallel organs.

Tolerance values should be obtained from NTCP analysis, which requires several cases of toxicity, distributed for different absorbed doses. Note, however, that the predictive power of NTCP always has a statistical implication, even in the best case, that is, two patients treated with the same absorbed dose may have a different outcome, according to their individual radio-sensitivity.

Many NTCP models have been proposed, however the most frequently used approach is the Lyman model, which predicts the observed effect after a uniform irradiation of the organ given at 2 Gy per fraction. $NTD_{2,eff}$ given at 2 Gy/fraction can be calculated from BED using the following equation:

$$NTD_{2,eff} = \frac{BED}{1 + \frac{2}{\alpha/\beta}} \tag{2.12}$$

Thus, given an effective uniform irradiation of the organ to total dose $NTD_{2,eff}$ the NTCP can be calculated by

$$NTCP = 0.5 + 0.5 \cdot erf\left(\frac{s}{\sqrt{2}}\right) \tag{2.13}$$

where $erf()$ is the error function and s is defined as:

$$s = \frac{NTD_{2,eff} - TD_{50}(1)}{m \cdot TD_{50}(1)} \tag{2.14}$$

and m is the slope of NTCP versus dose, while $TD_{50}(1)$ is the tolerance dose to the whole organ leading to a 50 per cent complication probability. These normal tissue tolerance data are defined for uniformly irradiated volumes of normal tissues and organs only for conventional EBRT fractionation schedules (of 2 Gy/fraction, 5 fractions/week) [25].

The NTCP model can be improved taking into account heterogeneous dose distribution using Dose Volume Histograms (DVHs) and appropriate reduction methods [25].

2.5 CLINICAL APPLICATIONS AND PROPOSED DOSE-EFFECT RELATIONSHIPS

The applicability of dose-response data from EBRT to RNT agents is still under investigation [26]. In the following paragraphs the toxicity of critical organs, as well as the radiobiological considerations are reported. Some toxicities are observed in organs "new", as a result of the development of new therapies, while the red marrow remains the tissue more typically/frequently involved in toxicity [27]. The development of dose-response models demands considerable data collection; nevertheless, these models are complex and often poorly understood.

In addition, normal tissues show a radiation-response latency proportional to their proliferation rate and depending on dose rate. When large volumes of the bone marrow are exposed, damage may be signalled by a fall in platelets and the white cell count within a few days. Slowly proliferating tissue such as kidney, lung, and so forth show signs of damage only months or years after exposure [2].

2.5.1 LIVER TOXICITY

After the introduction of radioembolization, a treatment in which radioactive spheres are trapped into vessel, various dose-effect models have been investigated mainly including the liver failure. In the package insert for resin spheres, a mean dose of 80Gy is recommended for non-tumour tissue requires, reduced to 70Gy for cirrhotic patients.

All models used to fit experimental NTCP in EBRT were based on the assumption of the liver as a parallel organ. According to [28], the fraction of liver when inactivated, would result in organ failure is $F_{50} = 40$ per cent. In the inactivated fraction (25%) no complication would occur, not even for extremely high absorbed dose. This so-called volume effect, that is, the advantage of partial liver volume irradiation, has been remarked on by Dawson [29], with different tolerances with respect to the reference paper by Emami and colleagues [30] for underlying liver disease [31]. Strigari and colleagues [32], retrospectively analysed 73 HCC patients treated with resin spheres and developed a modified Lyman-Burman-Kutcher model for obtaining the parameters of liver NTCP curve. A similar dose-effect curve has been obtained based on HCC patients treated with glass spheres [33]. A mechanistic model has been developed by Warland and colleagues [34].

To summarize, the evidence emerging from non-tumour tissue irradiation with microspheres is that [35, 36]

- volume effect is confirmed. The more selective is the administration, the higher the tolerable dose;
- a new kind of toxicity seems to appear after irradiation;
- a timing argument has to be introduced to try to differentiate radio-induced liver decompensation from the natural history of the disease;
- basal liver status (basal bilirubin level) and non-tumour parenchyma absorbed dose are the two main risk factors for toxicity;
- the toxicity threshold is lower for resin spheres (40–50 Gy) than for glass spheres.

2.5.2 LUNG IRRADIATION

According to EBRT [30] the TD5/5 and TD50/5 are 17.5 Gy and 24.5 Gy, respectively, for whole lung irradiation. The lung is often a metastatic site for differentiated thyroid cancer. Radio-induced pneumonitis was observed in the pioneering activity escalation study by Benua and colleagues [37] in 1962. They stated that, in order to avoid radio-induced pneumonitis, the total body activity in cases of diffuse micro-metastatic involvement should be kept below 3 GBq (80mCi) at 48 h. In 2006, Song and colleagues [38] argued against this historical rule, since this activity limit is actually a dose-rate limit rather than an absorbed-dose limit. Song took an absorbed-dose limit of 27.25 Gy to whole lung from an observed case of pneumonitis after myeloablative radio-immunotherapy of B-cell lymphoma [39], including both healthy and metastatic parenchyma.

Leung and colleagues [40] demonstrated that radiation pneumonitis in 6.3 per cent of 80 patients was correlated to the lung shunt fraction. The same group, after the observation of 5 cases of radiation pneumonitis, established the threshold for radiation pneumonitis from resin spheres at 30 Gy for a single administration, and 50 Gy cumulative for multiple administrations, non-attenuation corrected (NAC) value. Salem and colleagues [41] with glass spheres delivered more than NAC 30Gy to the lungs in 58/403 patients, and 53 were followed up with imaging. Only 10/53 exhibited grade 1 lung toxicity. Again, lower biological effects were observed with glass spheres at the same absorbed dose. All these authors neglected the difference in photon attenuation between liver and lung, and the number of photons escaping from lung, as well as the absorbed dose, was largely overestimated. The real lung dose and its limit was actually about 60 per cent of the reported value.

2.5.3 KIDNEYS

The kidneys are dose limiting organs for several radiation therapies, such as Peptide Receptor Radionuclide Therapy (PRRT) – addressed to neuro-endocrine tumours (NET), and EBRT as well – for the treatment of upper abdominal cancers or for total body irradiation (TBI). The incidence of radiation-induced impairment to the kidneys is difficult to report and/or identify, as effects occur most often with progressive dysfunction over years after therapy.

The experience of EBRT with dose-effect investigations over several decades covers also the issue of radiation-induced damage to the kidneys and predictive models have been modified and reinforced over time. Among the New Quantitative Analyses of Normal Tissue Effects in the Clinic (QUANTEC) guidelines recently published for the safe treatment of cancer with RT, the paper by Dawson and colleagues [42] provided in particular a review of the data concerning the kidney injury after EBRT. This includes the association with a variety of parameters such age, previous chemotherapy, dose-volume data, mono-bilateral irradiation, by TBI and transplantation, patient- and treatment-related factors. The evolution of predictive models, the matter of toxicity scoring, and areas for future study such as the effect of mitigating factors and radioprotectors, are presented showing the advances, the improved knowledge, and the drawbacks as well.

The Lyman model for the NTCP applied in case of EBRT at a conventional fractionation and bilateral whole kidney irradiation, was able to describe the data provided by different authors [30, 43]. Tolerance doses of 23 Gy and 28 Gy were associated to a 5 per cent ($TD_{5/5}$) and 50 per cent $T(D_{50/5})$ of probability to cause late side effects within 5 years.

A less-steep dose response curve was found, with a $TD_{5/5}$ of 9.8 Gy, when considering a TBI procedure delivering 12 Gy in 6 fractions twice daily.

In case of partial kidney irradiation, greater doses have been shown to be safely deliverable, although quantitative data would be required to support more refined models; there is evidence of dose-volume effects, although only in a few studies have patients been followed for more than ten years. Different absorbed-dose limits were expected to apply to RNT (and in particular to PRRT) as compared to EBRT, due to intrinsic different dose rates and microscopical distribution delivered by the two radiation modalities. The first clinical experiences in PRRT with standardised dosimetry methods failed in giving good correlations between kidney-absorbed dose and toxicity. The improvement of dose estimates with the individual kidney volume assessed by CT allowed to derive good a dose-effect relationship for kidney nephropathy in patients treated with ^{90}Y-peptides.The trend of the curve was similar to the NTCP curve derived for EBRT, but with higher-dose threshold and values for certain effects [44], as expected. The LQM [45, 46] enhanced the correlation and marked several steps similar to those observed in EBRT.

The use of the LQM allowed to account for the differences in ^{90}Y-PRRT administration schemes and to compare the renal toxicity induced by radionuclide therapy with that of EBRT. Absorbed doses were converted into BED with representative radiobiological parameters for kidneys ($T_{1/2eff}$ ~42 h and ~53 h for ^{90}Y- and ^{177}Lu-peptides; $T_{1/2\,rep}$= 2.8 h; α/β= 2.5 Gy) [47]. The endpoint considered was a creatinine clearance loss >20 per cent per year, found to be an indicator of end-stage renal disease. Joining the results from different protocol schemes and applying the Lyman model to BED versus renal toxicity, a BED threshold of 33 Gy for kidney radiation damage and a BED_{50} of 44 Gy were found for PRRT, nicely fitting also the data from EBRT.

The clinical evidence that multiple-cycle schemes decrease the nephrotoxicity rate in case of ^{90}Y-PRRT is adequately interpreted by the BED concept [47, 48]. For a same cumulative dose, the higher the number of cycles, the lower the cumulative BED, and the higher the BED sparing. Similarly for increasing number of cycles, increasing cumulative absorbed doses are associated to the same BED value, thus to the same radiation induced effect to the kidneys. Multiple cycles allow increasing the dose to the kidneys keeping fixed the BED values, suggesting also the possibility to heighten the administered activity without varying the induced effect. This subject proposes an explanation to the high incidence of severe renal damage reported by Imhof and colleagues [49] when 2 cycles of ^{90}Y-peptides were given with activities as high as 6.4 GBq per cycle in a standard male.

Figure 2.2 compares the sf curves for renal cells after ^{90}Y-PRRT at the same cumulative activity of 12.6 GBq given in 2 or in 6 cycles. SF of renal cells are obtained by means of the LQM with a representative kidney dose (2.26 Gy/GBq, median value from the literature) and reference parameters. In this case, after 2 cycles of PRRT, the renal sf value undergoes 20 per cent, which is supposed to lead to renal failure, while the same cumulative activity given in 6 cycles leads remaining well over this 20 per cent threshold value (MIRD 20 [45]). The high incidence of kidney toxicity grade 4 and 5 observed in patients undergoing such a protocol is not surprising, though. The study indicated initial kidney uptake

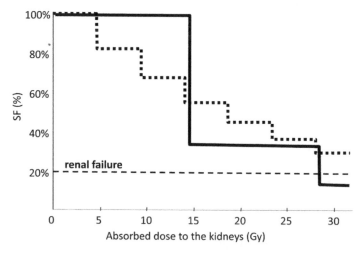

FIGURE 2.2 SF of the renal cells as a function of mean absorbed dose to the kidneys. Comparison is made for a same cumulative activity of 12.6 GBq of ^{90}Y-peptides administered in 2 cycles (continuous line) and 6 cycles (dotted line) and a representative kidney dose factor of 2.26 Gy/GBq. sf was calculated setting $T_{1/2eff}$ ~42 h, $T_{1/2rep}$= 2.8 h, α/β= 2.5 Gy, and $\alpha cortex$= 0.06 Gy-1. Renal failure is supposed to occur when reaching an sf of 20 per cent.

to be predictive for severe renal toxicity, so high absorbed doses (perhaps higher than 2.26 Gy/GBq, as considered in Figure 2.2) were probably associated with the patients more affected.

The rationale of using several cycles stands on the different repair capability and radiosensitivity between the renal tissue and the tumours, which should spare normal tissues more than tumours. This does not necessarily apply to all RNTs, but seems to be the case of PRRT, often addressed to slowly proliferating tumours, such as well differentiated NETs. In principle, increasing fractionation gives two useful options: a lower activity/cycle provides lower renal damage. Alternatively, higher cumulative activities can be injected with higher fractionation for a same damage and potential improved response. However, changes in the biokinetics during therapy such as tumour mass and/or uptake and critical organ function, may occur and shift the ground. Cycles seem to be a powerful tool especially in ^{90}Y-PRRT, while negligible incidence of renal injury is observed in patients treated with ^{177}Lu-peptides therapies, at least with the clinical protocols applied to date [50–56]. In addition, a possible reason signing a different outcome to the kidneys after ^{177}Lu-peptides therapies are the particle range and the peptide localization, occurring preferably in the proximal tubuli (radioresistant cells), versus the glomeruli (radiosensitive cells). The short range of the ^{177}Lu-peptides β-particles might irradiate more selectively the tubuli, while the long range of the ^{90}Y-peptides β-particles may increase the irradiation of the glomeruli, with consequent higher toxicity. Still, this is to be proven in clinical studies. The impact of the activity distribution at the macro- and microscopical levels remains to be deepened [57–59]. SPECT and PET images of patients undergoing PRRT suggest a non-uniform activity distribution in the kidneys with a preferential accumulation in the outer structure. However, a clear distinction between cortex and outer medulla is impeded by intrinsic limited resolutions. Unfortunately, data from ex-vivo autoradiography in humans regarding the activity distribution of radio-labelled somatostatin analogues are contradicting and not conclusive. The first detailed information was derived from a patient administered with ^{111}In-Octreotide [58]. The results showed inhomogeneous activity distribution, with about 70 per cent of activity localized in the cortex, and almost all of the remaining in the medulla, with much higher concentration in the outer part, progressively lowering to the inner medulla. On the contrary, ex-vivo autoradiographs from a patient treated with ^{90}Y/^{111}In-DOTATOC showed the radioactivity uniformly distributed in the cortical and medullar structures, without significant gradient. A possible explanation for these differences relies on the effect of amino acid protectors, used only for therapy, which interfere with the natural localization of peptides.

The controversy between two studies demand more investigation and dosimetry in a microscopic scale to improve the accuracy of dosimetric results and dose response relationship. In any case, the data allowed to extrapolate DVH for the same peptide labelled with ^{177}Lu or ^{90}Y, that could, in principle, represent general models ready to be applied depending on the situation. In case of uniform activity distributions, the trends are quite similar for ^{90}Y and ^{177}Lu, while in case of non-uniform activity distribution, the DHV curve for ^{177}Lu shows a larger dose non-uniformity [48].

The prediction of severe toxicity after PRRT has improved by taking into consideration the clinical risk factors. In a retrospective observation of patients treated with ^{90}Y-DOTATOC, a 28 Gy BED threshold to the kidneys was found in patients with risk factors as compared to the 40 Gy BED in patients without risk factors.

2.5.4 RED MARROW

Red marrow toxicity data come mostly from treatment with ^{131}I for thyroid carcinoma and ^{131}I-metaiodiobenzylguanidine (MIBG) therapy.

In many studies red marrow dosimetry is approached with great caution, and the treatments are usually associated with the absence of radiation toxicity, suggesting that an increase of tumour control may be obtained by increasing the injected activity on a patient-specific dosimetry basis. The use of dosimetric Specific Operative Procedures is basic to improving the radiobiological model through the standardization of data acquisition and analysis [60] because, in many studies red marrow dose–toxicity correlation is still poor. The blood-based approach may provide a reasonable estimate of red marrow dose as long as there is no specific uptake in red marrow or bone due to the presence of free radionuclides, disease, or retention of activity due to metabolism by the reticulo-endothelial system. The activity in the whole body should be deduced by using a dual-headed gamma camera. From the dosimetric point of view, an additional red marrow formula has been introduced by Traino and colleagues [61] introducing a non-linear scaling of the S-values according to the patient's weight. Recently, an image-based methodology, using a region of interest on the L2-L4 lumbar vertebrae, seems to better predict haematological toxicity compared with blood-based methods [62, 63] in radioimmunotherapy of NLH.

To avoid hypoplasia, a maximum absorbed dose of 2 Gy to the blood (considered a surrogate of red marrow) based on pioneering work of Benua and colleagues [37] for radioiodine treatment of differentiated thyroid cancer is generally accepted. A more recent work has adopted a higher limit of 3 Gy to the red marrow [64].

Nevertheless, even if this limit is not exceeded after a single administration, the risk of the patient developing a different end point – that is, the myelodysplastic syndrome after many administrations – cannot be excluded completely. An accurate estimation of the absorbed dose to the bone marrow will help find an adequate dosage. In the ^{131}I treatment of thyroid cancer, failure after conventional repeated fixed activity administrations seems to be a hopeless situation. Individualized high activity administrations – keeping the blood below 2 Gy (i.e. Maximal Safe Dose) – are expected to improve the outcome of patients with differentiated thyroid cancer resistant to fixed activity therapy. However, the latent side effects of large cumulative doses could be important. In the study of Lee and colleagues [65], an efficacy of 47 per cent (partial or complete remission) has been reported for patients who had not responded to a repeated fixed activity approach. Sixty-two percent of patients experienced transient cytopenia, while three patients did not fully recover.

This suggests that a better understanding of a radiobiological model could be helpful to avoid unnecessary repeated treatments and tailor therapeutic regimes.

Verburg and colleagues [66] sought to evaluate the safety and effectiveness of treating advanced DTC with high ^{131}I activities chosen primarily based on the results of dosimetry following the EANM SOP [67]. After 6 of 13 treatment courses in 6 out of 10 patients, short-term side effects of ^{131}I therapy – namely nausea, vomiting or transient sialadenitis – were observed. Leukocyte and platelet counts dropped significantly in the first few weeks after ^{131}I treatment but returned to pre-treatment levels within 3 months post-therapy. Authors conclude that in high-activity ^{131}I therapy for advanced DTC based on pre-therapeutic blood dosimetry has proved safe and well tolerated.

A novel approach for quantifying the number of radiation-induced DNA DSBs after radioiodine-therapy was introduced by Lassmann and colleagues [67]. Two markers for this DSB formation are gamma-H2AX and the damage sensor 53BP1. In 26 thyroid cancer patients, the authors studied the temporal behaviour of the number of radiation-induced gamma-H2AX and 53BP1 foci. The number of excess radiation-induced foci/nucleus per absorbed dose rate increased with time, potentially indicating a slower rate of DNA repair or, alternatively, a higher de novo rate of focus formation. The authors concluded that radiation-induced γ-H2AX and 53BP1 nuclear foci are useful markers for quantifying DSBs after radioiodine therapy.

In patients who underwent ^{131}I-MIBG treatment of pheochromocytoma, other authors reported a similar improved efficacy and a reduction of the total number of therapeutic administrations necessary for cure, with a moderate increase of toxicity, using intermediate activity rather than low-activity regimes of therapy. These authors also suggested an increase of activity per cycle without reaching myeloablative levels [68].

The toxicity of radiolabelled MoAb therapy of tumours is related to the radionuclide and on the kind of antibodies used. Most of the results are available from clinical treatment and preclinical studies using ^{131}I-labelled MoAb, which emits β-particles with a range of approximately 1 mm, sufficient to irradiate tumour cells not directly in the crossfire [69]. However, this range is also sufficient to irradiate most of the blood-forming cells of the bone marrow. Moreover, the high-energy photon that permits patient imaging gives rise to nonspecific and undesirable irradiation of the whole body. ^{125}I-Iodine represents an attractive alternative strategy, but microdosimetric studies are suitable to fully describe the dose-effect relationship [70].

2.6   BYSTANDER AND ABSCOPAL EFFECTS

Radiation-induced bystander or abscopal effects are biologic responses in cells that were not traversed by an ionizing radiation track and, thus, not subject to direct-energy deposition; that is, the responses occur in nonirradiated cells. The abscopal and the bystander are considered non-targeted *effects* because refer to radiation responses in areas separate from the irradiated tissue and are presumably mediated by secreted soluble factors. Generally, the bystander effect takes place in the neighbours of irradiated cells via cell-to-cell gap junctions while the abscopal is mediated by the secretion or shedding of soluble factors (i.e. nonirradiated cells receive secreted signals from irradiated cells).

Radiation-induced abscopal effect has been reported in literature since the 1940s [71, 72] and clastogenic factors in plasma from radiotherapy patients were first observed in the 1950s [73–75].

Radiatio- induced bystander/abscopal effects have been extensively documented over time, highlighting both the potential detrimental (e.g., radiation-induced secondary tumors) [76–78] and potentially beneficial (e.g., radioprotection) effects [79–81]. When a bystander effect is factored in, the actual radiobiologic response will be greater or less than that predicted by dosimetric estimates alone. Unfortunately, the abscopal effect is a rarely observed outcome of radiotherapy wherein there is a reduction in metastatic disease burden outside of the targeted treatment area.

The detrimental bystander effect potentially affects our risk assessment and therapeutic efficacy after the administration of therapeutic radiopharmaceuticals to patients.

Several studies have demonstrated that bystander effects are induced by high linear energy transfer (LET) [71, 82] – but not those induced by low LET. In addition, the bystander/abscopal effects depend on delivered dose [83] and radiation quality [84].

The assessment of possible bystander effects is more difficult when they are due to the decay of internally administered radionuclides than when they are due to external beam radiotherapy irradiation because many of the radionuclides emit photons, electrons, and alpha particles, with ranges much greater than the mammalian cell diameter (~10 mm) [85]. Several studies have investigated the bystander effect of unencapsulated therapeutic radionuclides [84, 86–89].

Several papers have discussed the involvement of oxidative metabolites and gap-junction intercellular communication in radiation-induced bystander effects [90], while others have emphasized the transfer of genetic instability from irradiated cells to neighbouring unirradiated ones [91, 92]. Some investigators have also identified secreted factors, including transforming growth factor–b1 [93] and interleukin (IL)-8 [94], that mediate bystander effects in vitro but do not require the existence of oxidative metabolites or gap junctions [94]. Other studies, examined the ability of medium from cultures in which cells were prelabelled with ^{123}I, ^{131}I, or ^{211}At to inhibit [88] or stimulate [89] cell proliferation in vitro (i.e. clonogenic survival).

Other in vitro studies have shown bystander effects for both beta-particle and Auger-electron emitters [86].

With renewed interest in therapy with α-particle emitters, these results support the use of 223RaCl2 as an adjuvant treatment for select patients at early stages of breast cancer. Radiation-induced bystander effects have been reported to play an important role for sterilizing disseminated tumour cells, to 223RaCl2, and that the response depends on injected activity [95].

An emerging challenge is how best to combine radiotherapy with immunotherapy because there is substantial evidence to suggest that ionizing radiation boosts the tumour-targeting immune response and potentially improves the patient outcome. Likely due to an "in situ vaccine" effect of radiotherapy, the question of whether the abscopal effect may be augmented by immunotherapy is under exploration [96, 97]. Several ongoing clinical trials have been designed to exploit this phenomenon [98] and might provide the first clues as to whether this approach holds promise.

Other authors found that nuclear factor kappa B (NF-κB) is essential for triggering the self-sustained production of reactive oxygen and nitrogen species that are involved in both direct and abscopal effects, thus making the bystander response similar to inflammation [99].

Validation of a role in vivo for biological bystander effects in systemic radionuclide therapy would greatly impact the way we would assess therapeutic response to radionuclide therapy, the design of clinical trials of novel treatments with radiopharmaceuticals, and risk estimates for both therapeutic and diagnostic radiopharmaceuticals [100]. More details on abscopal/bystander effects using radionuclides are summarized in [85, 101] comprising beta- and alpha-particles and Auger electrons used in tumour radiotherapy and diagnostics. Unfortunately, separation of the direct effect of radionuclide decay from crossfire and bystander effects in clinical targeted radionuclide therapy is impossible because of the lack of methods to assess whether, and to what extent, bystander effect is involved in the human organism.

2.7 CONCLUSION

In radiobiology there are many unanswered questions that present an opportunity for research. The future use of BED/EQX needs to be based on new technology SPET/CT or PET/CT. The next challenge is to relate the metric, 3D absorbed dose, to clinical data describing TCP or NTCP. Because of the modest amount of clinical data for RNT, we use more-established and readily available clinical response data from EBRT to estimate the radiation toxicity incidence. The challenge is to develop and assess these concepts with actual RNT data. In order to do this, accurate, patient-specific dose estimates should greatly enhance the reliability of this process. In conclusion, the reliability and utility of common radiobiological models will depend on the availability of more dosimetric and clinical data [27, 102]. All physicians and physicists are called on to contribute to this knowledge.

REFERENCES

[1] H. R. Withers, "The four R's of Radiobiology," *Advances in Radiation Biology*, vol. 5, pp. 241–47, 1975.

[2] H. R. Withers, "Biological basis of radiation therapy for cancer," *Lancet*, vol. 339, no. 8786, pp. 156–59, 1992, doi: 10.1016/0140-6736(92)90218-r.

[3] J. F. Fowler, "Radiobiological aspects of low dose rates in radioimmunotherapy," *Int J Radiat Oncol Biol Phys*, vol. 18, no. 5, pp. 1261–69, 1990, doi: 10.1016/0360-3016(90)90467-x.

[4]   R. G. Dale, "Dose-rate effects in targeted radiotherapy," *Phys Med Biol*, vol. 41, no. 10, pp. 1871–84, 1996, doi: 10.1088/0031-9155/41/10/001.

[5]   J. A. O'Donoghue, "Optimal therapeutic strategies for radioimmunotherapy," *Recent Results Cancer Res*, vol. 141, pp. 77–99, 1996.

[6]   A. I. Kassis and S. J. Adelstein, "Radiobiologic principles in radionuclide therapy," *J Nucl Med*, vol. 46 Suppl 1, pp. 4s-12s, 2005.

[7]   R. W. Howell, S. M. Goddu, and D. V. Rao, "Proliferation and the advantage of longer-lived radionuclides in radioimmunotherapy," *Med Phys*, vol. 25, no. 1, pp. 37–42, 1998, doi: 10.1118/1.598171.

[8]   V. K. Langmuir, J. F. Fowler, S. J. Knox, B. W. Wessels, R. M. Sutherland, and J. Y. Wong, "Radiobiology of radiolabeled antibody therapy as applied to tumor dosimetry," *Med Phys*, vol. 20, no. 2 Pt 2, pp. 601–10, 1993, doi: 10.1118/1.597055.

[9]   R. K. Bodey, G. D. Flux, and P. M. Evans, "Combining dosimetry for targeted radionuclide and external beam therapies using the biologically effective dose," *Cancer Biother Radiopharm*, vol. 18, no. 1, pp. 89–97, 2003, doi: 10.1089/108497803321269368.

[10] W. T. Millar, "Application of the linear-quadratic model with incomplete repair to radionuclide directed therapy," *Br J Radiol*, vol. 64, no. 759, pp. 242–51, 1991, doi: 10.1259/0007-1285-64-759-242.

[11] A. Jackson, R. K. Ten Haken, J. M. Robertson, M. L. Kessler, G. J. Kutcher, and T. S. Lawrence, "Analysis of clinical complication data for radiation hepatitis using a parallel architecture model," *Int J Radiat Oncol Biol Phys*, vol. 31, no. 4, pp. 883–91, 1995, doi: 10.1016/0360-3016(94)00471-4.

[12] L. Strigari, M. D'Andrea, C. L. Maini, R. Sciuto, and M. Benassi, "Biological optimization of heterogeneous dose distributions in systemic radiotherapy," *Med Phys*, vol. 33, no. 6, pp. 1857–66, 2006, doi: 10.1118/1.2198189.

[13] S. M. Bentzen *et al.*, "Bioeffect modeling and equieffective dose concepts in radiation oncology – terminology, quantities and units," *Radiother Oncol*, vol. 105, no. 2, pp. 266–68, 2012, doi: 10.1016/j.radonc.2012.10.006.

[14] H. R. Withers, H. D. Thames, Jr., and L. J. Peters, "A new isoeffect curve for change in dose per fraction," *Radiother Oncol*, vol. 1, no. 2, pp. 187–91, 1983, doi: 10.1016/s0167-8140(83)80021-8.

[15] R. F. Hobbs, R. W. Howell, H. Song, S. Baechler, and G. Sgouros, "Redefining relative biological effectiveness in the context of the EQDX formalism: Implications for alpha-particle emitter therapy," *Radiat Res*, 2013, doi: 10.1667/rr1343.1.

[16] J. A. O'Donoghue, "Implications of nonuniform tumor doses for radioimmunotherapy," *J Nucl Med*, vol. 40, no. 8, pp. 1337–41, 1999.

[17] L. C. Jones and P. W. Hoban, "Treatment plan comparison using equivalent uniform biologically effective dose (EUBED)," *Phys Med Biol*, vol. 45, no. 1, pp. 159–70, 2000, doi: 10.1088/0031-9155/45/1/311.

[18] A. Niemierko, "Reporting and analyzing dose distributions: A concept of equivalent uniform dose," *Med Phys*, vol. 24, no. 1, pp. 103–10, 1997, doi: 10.1118/1.598063.

[19] R. F. Hobbs *et al.*, "124I PET-based 3D-RD dosimetry for a pediatric thyroid cancer patient: real-time treatment planning and methodologic comparison," *J Nucl Med*, vol. 50, no. 11, pp. 1844–47, 2009, doi: 10.2967/jnumed.109.066738.

[20] R. F. Hobbs *et al.*, "Radiobiologic optimization of combination radiopharmaceutical therapy applied to myeloablative treatment of non-Hodgkin lymphoma," *J Nucl Med*, vol. 54, no. 9, pp. 1535–42, 2013, doi: 10.2967/jnumed.112.117952.

[21] C. Chiesa *et al.*, "Absorbed dose and biologically effective dose in patients with high-risk non-Hodgkin's lymphoma treated with high-activity myeloablative 90Y-ibritumomab tiuxetan (Zevalin)," *Eur J Nucl Med Mol Imaging*, vol. 36, no. 11, pp. 1745–57, 2009, doi: 10.1007/s00259-009-1141-x.

[22] M. Pacilio *et al.*, "A theoretical dose-escalation study based on biological effective dose in radioimmunotherapy with (90)Y-ibritumomab tiuxetan (Zevalin)," *Eur J Nucl Med Mol Imaging*, vol. 37, no. 5, pp. 862–73, 2010, doi: 10.1007/s00259-009-1333-4.

[23] L. Strigari, M. Benassi, C. Chiesa, M. Cremonesi, L. Bodei, and M. D'Andrea, "Dosimetry in nuclear medicine therapy: radiobiology application and results," *Q J Nucl Med Mol Imaging*, vol. 55, no. 2, pp. 205–21, 2011.

[24] D. Wigg, *Applied Radiobiology and Bioeffect Planning*. Madison: WI: Medical Physics Publishing, 2001, p. 268.

[25] C. Burman, G. J. Kutcher, B. Emami, and M. Goitein, "Fitting of normal tissue tolerance data to an analytic function," *Int J Radiat Oncol Biol Phys*, vol. 21, no. 1, pp. 123–35, 1991, doi: 10.1016/0360-3016(91)90172-z.

[26] S. J. Knox and R. F. Meredith, "Clinical radioimmunotherapy," *Semin Radiat Oncol*, vol. 10, no. 2, pp. 73–93, 2000, doi: 10.1016/s1053-4296(00)80045-4.

[27] L. Strigari *et al.*, "The evidence base for the use of internal dosimetry in the clinical practice of molecular radiotherapy," *Eur J Nucl Med Mol Imaging*, vol. 41, no. 10, pp. 1976–88, 2014, doi: 10.1007/s00259-014-2824-5.

[28] L. A. Dawson, R. K. Ten Haken, and T. S. Lawrence, "Partial irradiation of the liver," *Semin Radiat Oncol*, vol. 11, no. 3, pp. 240–46, 2001, doi: 10.1053/srao.2001.23485.

[29] L. A. Dawson and R. K. Ten Haken, "Partial volume tolerance of the liver to radiation," *Semin Radiat Oncol*, vol. 15, no. 4, pp. 279–83, 2005, doi: 10.1016/j.semradonc.2005.04.005.

[30] B. Emami *et al.*, "Tolerance of normal tissue to therapeutic irradiation," *Int J Radiat Oncol Biol Phys*, vol. 21, no. 1, pp. 109–22, 1991, doi: 10.1016/0360-3016(91)90171-y.

[31] J. C. Cheng *et al.*, "Biologic susceptibility of hepatocellular carcinoma patients treated with radiotherapy to radiation-induced liver disease," *Int J Radiat Oncol Biol Phys*, vol. 60, no. 5, pp. 1502–09, 2004, doi: 10.1016/j.ijrobp.2004.05.048.

[32] L. Strigari *et al.*, "Efficacy and toxicity related to treatment of hepatocellular carcinoma with 90Y-SIR spheres: radiobiologic considerations," *J Nucl Med*, vol. 51, no. 9, pp. 1377–85, 2010, doi: 10.2967/jnumed.110.075861.

[33] C. Chiesa *et al.*, "Radioembolization of hepatocarcinoma with (90)Y glass microspheres: development of an individualized treatment planning strategy based on dosimetry and radiobiology," *Eur J Nucl Med Mol Imaging*, vol. 42, no. 11, pp. 1718–38, 2015, doi: 10.1007/s00259-015-3068-8.

[34] S. Walrand, M. Hesse, F. Jamar, and R. Lhommel, "A hepatic dose-toxicity model opening the way toward individualized radioembolization planning," *J Nucl Med*, vol. 55, no. 8, pp. 1317–22, 2014, doi: 10.2967/jnumed.113.135301.

[35] M. Cremonesi *et al.*, "Radioembolization of hepatic lesions from a radiobiology and dosimetric perspective," *Frontiers in Oncology*, vol. 4, p. 210, 2014, doi: 10.3389/fonc.2014.00210.

[36] C. Allimant *et al.*, "Tumor Targeting and Three-Dimensional Voxel-Based Dosimetry to Predict Tumor Response, Toxicity, and Survival after Yttrium-90 Resin Microsphere Radioembolization in Hepatocellular Carcinoma," *J Vasc Interv Radiol*, vol. 29, no. 12, pp. 1662–1670.e4, 2018, doi: 10.1016/j.jvir.2018.07.006.

[37] R. S. Benua, N. R. Cicale, M. Sonenberg, and R. W. Rawson, "The relation of radioiodine dosimetry to results and complications in the treatment of metastatic thyroid cancer," *Am J Roentgenol Radium Ther Nucl Med*, vol. 87, pp. 171–82, 1962.

[38] H. Song *et al.*, "Lung dosimetry for radioiodine treatment planning in the case of diffuse lung metastases," *J Nucl Med*, vol. 47, no. 12, pp. 1985–94, 2006.

[39] O. W. Press *et al.*, "Radiolabeled-antibody therapy of B-cell lymphoma with autologous bone marrow support," *N Engl J Med*, vol. 329, no. 17, pp. 1219–24, 1993, doi: 10.1056/nejm199310213291702.

[40] T. W. Leung *et al.*, "Radiation pneumonitis after selective internal radiation treatment with intraarterial 90yttrium-microspheres for inoperable hepatic tumors," *Int J Radiat Oncol Biol Phys*, vol. 33, no. 4, pp. 919–24, 1995, doi: 10.1016/0360-3016(95)00039-3.

[41] R. Salem *et al.*, "Incidence of radiation pneumonitis after hepatic intra-arterial radiotherapy with yttrium-90 microspheres assuming uniform lung distribution," *Am J Clin Oncol*, vol. 31, no. 5, pp. 431–38, 2008, doi: 10.1097/COC.0b013e318168ef65.

[42] L. A. Dawson *et al.*, "Radiation-associated kidney injury," *Int J Radiat Oncol Biol Phys*, vol. 76, no. 3 Suppl, pp. S108–15, 2010, doi: 10.1016/j.ijrobp.2009.02.089.

[43] J. R. Cassady, "Clinical radiation nephropathy," *Int J Radiat Oncol Biol Phys*, vol. 31, no. 5, pp. 1249–56, 1995, doi: 10.1016/0360-3016(94)00428-n.

[44] R. Barone *et al.*, "Patient-specific dosimetry in predicting renal toxicity with (90)Y-DOTATOC: relevance of kidney volume and dose rate in finding a dose-effect relationship," *J Nucl Med*, vol. 46 Suppl 1, pp. 99s–106s, 2005.

[45] B. W. Wessels *et al.*, "MIRD pamphlet No. 20: the effect of model assumptions on kidney dosimetry and response – implications for radionuclide therapy," *J Nucl Med*, vol. 49, no. 11, pp. 1884–99, 2008, doi: 10.2967/jnumed.108.053173.

[46] S. Baechler, R. F. Hobbs, A. R. Prideaux, R. L. Wahl, and G. Sgouros, "Extension of the biological effective dose to the MIRD schema and possible implications in radionuclide therapy dosimetry," *Med Phys*, vol. 35, no. 3, pp. 1123–34, 2008, doi: 10.1118/1.2836421.

[47] M. Cremonesi *et al.*, "Dosimetry for treatment with radiolabelled somatostatin analogues. A review," *Q J Nucl Med Mol Imaging*, vol. 54, no. 1, pp. 37–51, 2010.

[48] A. Sarnelli *et al.*, "Therapeutic schemes in 177Lu and 90Y-PRRT: radiobiological considerations," *Q J Nucl Med Mol Imaging*, vol. 61, no. 2, pp. 216–31, 2017, doi: 10.23736/S1824-4785.16.02744-8.

[49] A. Imhof *et al.*, "Response, survival, and long-term toxicity after therapy with the radiolabeled somatostatin analogue [90Y-DOTA]-TOC in metastasized neuroendocrine cancers," *Journal of Clinical Oncology: Official Journal of the American Society of Clinical Oncology*, vol. 29, no. 17, pp. 2416–23, 2011, doi: 10.1200/jco.2010.33.7873.

[50] M. Cremonesi *et al.*, "Correlation of dose with toxicity and tumour response to (90)Y- and (177)Lu-PRRT provides the basis for optimization through individualized treatment planning," *Eur J Nucl Med Mol Imaging*, vol. 45, no. 13, pp. 2426–41, 2018, doi: 10.1007/s00259-018-4044-x.

[51] L. Bodei *et al.*, "Long-term tolerability of PRRT in 807 patients with neuroendocrine tumours: the value and limitations of clinical factors," *Eur J Nucl Med Mol Imaging*, vol. 42, no. 1, pp. 5–19, 2015, doi: 10.1007/s00259-014-2893-5.

[52] H. Bergsma *et al.*, "Nephrotoxicity after PRRT with (177)Lu-DOTA-octreotate," *Eur J Nucl Med Mol Imaging*, vol. 43, no. 10, pp. 1802–11, 2016, doi: 10.1007/s00259-016-3382-9.

[53] A. Sundlov *et al.*, "Individualised (177)Lu-DOTATATE treatment of neuroendocrine tumours based on kidney dosimetry," *Eur J Nucl Med Mol Imaging*, vol. 44, no. 9, pp. 1480–89, 2017, doi: 10.1007/s00259-017-3678-4.

[54] U. Garske-Roman *et al.*, "Prospective observational study of (177)Lu-DOTA-octreotate therapy in 200 patients with advanced metastasized neuroendocrine tumours (NETs): feasibility and impact of a dosimetry-guided study protocol on outcome and toxicity," *Eur J Nucl Med Mol Imaging*, vol. 45, no. 6, pp. 970–88, 2018, doi: 10.1007/s00259-018-3945-z.

[55] M. Del Prete *et al.*, "Personalized (177)Lu-octreotate peptide receptor radionuclide therapy of neuroendocrine tumours: initial results from the P-PRRT trial," *Eur J Nucl Med Mol Imaging*, vol. 46, no. 3, pp. 728–42, 2019, doi: 10.1007/s00259-018-4209-7.

[56] S. Rudisile *et al.*, "Salvage PRRT with (177)Lu-DOTA-octreotate in extensively pretreated patients with metastatic neuroendocrine tumor (NET): dosimetry, toxicity, efficacy, and survival," *BMC Cancer*, vol. 19, no. 1, p. 788, 2019, doi: 10.1186/s12885-019-6000-y.

[57] M. Konijnenberg, "From imaging to dosimetry and biological effects," *Q J Nucl Med Mol Imaging*, vol. 55, no. 1, pp. 44–56, 2011.

[58] M. Konijnenberg, M. Melis, R. Valkema, E. Krenning, and M. de Jong, "Radiation dose distribution in human kidneys by octreotides in peptide receptor radionuclide therapy," *J Nucl Med*, vol. 48, pp. 134–42, 2007, PMID: 17204710.

[59] M. W. Konijnenberg and M. de Jong, "Preclinical animal research on therapy dosimetry with dual isotopes," *Eur J Nucl Med Mol Imaging*, vol. 38 Suppl 1, pp. S19–27, 2011, doi: 10.1007/s00259-011-1774-4.

[60] M. Lassmann, H. Hanscheid, C. Chiesa, C. Hindorf, G. Flux, and M. Luster, "EANM Dosimetry Committee series on standard operational procedures for pre-therapeutic dosimetry I: Blood and bone marrow dosimetry in differentiated thyroid cancer therapy," *Eur J Nucl Med Mol Imaging*, vol. 35, no. 7, pp. 1405–12, 2008, doi: 10.1007/s00259-008-0761-x.

[61] A. C. Traino, M. Ferrari, M. Cremonesi, and M. G. Stabin, "Influence of total-body mass on the scaling of S-factors for patient-specific, blood-based red-marrow dosimetry," *Phys Med Biol*, vol. 52, no. 17, pp. 5231–48, 2007, doi: 10.1088/0031-9155/52/17/009.

[62] S. Shen *et al.*, "Improved prediction of myelotoxicity using a patient-specific imaging dose estimate for non-marrow-targeting (90)Y-antibody therapy," *J Nucl Med*, vol. 43, no. 9, pp. 1245–53, 2002.

[63] L. Ferrer *et al.*, "Three methods assessing red marrow dosimetry in lymphoma patients treated with radioimmunotherapy," *Cancer*, vol. 116, no. 4 Suppl, pp. 1093–100, 2010, doi: 10.1002/cncr.24797.

[64] R. Dorn, J. Kopp, H. Vogt, P. Heidenreich, R. G. Carroll, and S. A. Gulec, "Dosimetry-guided radioactive iodine treatment in patients with metastatic differentiated thyroid cancer: largest safe dose using a risk-adapted approach," *J Nucl Med*, vol. 44, no. 3, pp. 451–56, 2003.

[65] J. J. Lee *et al.*, "Maximal safe dose of I-131 after failure of standard fixed dose therapy in patients with differentiated thyroid carcinoma," *Ann Nucl Med*, vol. 22, no. 9, pp. 727–34, 2008, doi: 10.1007/s12149-007-0179-8.

[66] F. A. Verburg *et al.*, "Dosimetry-guided high-activity (131)I therapy in patients with advanced differentiated thyroid carcinoma: initial experience," *Eur J Nucl Med Mol Imaging*, vol. 37, no. 5, pp. 896–903, 2010, doi: 10.1007/s00259-009-1303-x.

[67] M. Lassmann *et al.*, "In vivo formation of gamma-H2AX and 53BP1 DNA repair foci in blood cells after radioiodine therapy of differentiated thyroid cancer," *J Nucl Med*, vol. 51, no. 8, pp. 1318–25, 2010, doi: 10.2967/jnumed.109.071357.

[68] M. R. Castellani *et al.*, "(131)I-MIBG treatment of pheochromocytoma: low versus intermediate activity regimens of therapy," *Q J Nucl Med Mol Imaging*, vol. 54, no. 1, pp. 100–13, 2010.

[69] E. C. Barendswaard *et al.*, "131I radioimmunotherapy and fractionated external beam radiotherapy: comparative effectiveness in a human tumor xenograft," *J Nucl Med*, vol. 40, no. 10, pp. 1764–68, 1999.

[70] L. E. Feinendegen and R. D. Neumann, "Dosimetry and risk from low- versus high-LET radiation of Auger events and the role of nuclide carriers," *Int J Radiat Biol*, vol. 80, no. 11–12, pp. 813–22, 2004, doi: 10.1080/09553000400007698.

[71] E. J. Hall, "The bystander effect," *Health Phys*, vol. 85, no. 1, pp. 31–35, 2003, doi: 10.1097/00004032-200307000-00008.

[72] R. H. Mole, "Whole body irradiation; radiobiology or medicine?" *Br J Radiol*, vol. 26, no. 305, pp. 234–41, 1953, doi: 10.1259/0007-1285-26-305-234.

[73] C. Mothersill, A. Rusin, and C. Seymour, "Relevance of non-targeted effects for radiotherapy and diagnostic radiology; a historical and conceptual analysis of key players," *Cancers (Basel)*, vol. 11, no. 9, 2019, doi: 10.3390/cancers11091236.

[74] C. Mothersill and C. Seymour, "Radiation-induced bystander effects: Past history and future directions," *Radiat Res*, vol. 155, no. 6, pp. 759–67, 2001, doi: 10.1667/0033-7587(2001)155[0759:ribeph]2.0.co;2.

[75] W. B. Parsons, Jr., C. H. Watkins, G. L. Pease, and D. S. Childs, Jr., "Changes in sternal marrow following roentgen-ray therapy to the spleen in chronic granulocytic leukemia," *Cancer*, vol. 7, no. 1, pp. 179–89, 1954, doi: 10.1002/1097-0142(195401)7:1<179::aid-cncr2820070120>3.0.co;2-a.

[76] M. Mancuso et al., "Dose and spatial effects in long-distance radiation signaling in vivo: Implications for abscopal tumorigenesis," *Int J Radiat Oncol Biol Phys*, vol. 85, no. 3, pp. 813–9, 2013, doi: 10.1016/j.ijrobp.2012.07.2372.

[77] M. Mancuso et al., "Oncogenic radiation abscopal effects in vivo: interrogating mouse skin," *Int J Radiat Oncol Biol Phys*, vol. 86, no. 5, pp. 993–99, 2013, doi: 10.1016/j.ijrobp.2013.04.040.

[78] M. Mancuso et al., "The radiation bystander effect and its potential implications for human health," *Curr Mol Med*, vol. 12, no. 5, pp. 613–24, 2012, doi: 10.2174/156652412800620011.

[79] K. Camphausen et al., "Radiation abscopal antitumor effect is mediated through p53," *Cancer Res*, vol. 63, no. 8, pp. 1990–93, 2003.

[80] L. Strigari et al., "Abscopal effect of radiation therapy: Interplay between radiation dose and p53 status," *Int J Radiat Biol*, vol. 90, no. 3, pp. 248–55, 2014, doi: 10.3109/09553002.2014.874608.

[81] R. Marconi, S. Strolin, G. Bossi, and L. Strigari, "A meta-analysis of the abscopal effect in preclinical models: Is the biologically effective dose a relevant physical trigger?" *PLoS One,* vol. 12, no. 2, p. e0171559, 2017, doi: 10.1371/journal. pone.0171559.

[82] H. Zhou, G. Randers-Pehrson, C. A. Waldren, D. Vannais, E. J. Hall, and T. K. Hei, "Induction of a bystander mutagenic effect of alpha particles in mammalian cells," *Proc Natl Acad Sci U S A,* vol. 97, no. 5, pp. 2099–104, 2000, doi: 10.1073/ pnas.030420797.

[83] S. G. Sawant, W. Zheng, K. M. Hopkins, G. Randers-Pehrson, H. B. Lieberman, and E. J. Hall, "The radiation-induced bystander effect for clonogenic survival," *Radiat Res,* vol. 157, no. 4, pp. 361–64, 2002, doi: 10.1667/0033-7587(2002)157[0361:trib ef]2.0.co;2.

[84] M. Boyd, A. Sorensen, A. G. McCluskey, and R. J. Mairs, "Radiation quality-dependent bystander effects elicited by targeted radionuclides," *J Pharm Pharmacol,* vol. 60, no. 8, pp. 951–58, 2008, doi: 10.1211/jpp.60.8.0002.

[85] G. Sgouros, S. J. Knox, M. C. Joiner, W. F. Morgan, and A. I. Kassis, "MIRD continuing education: Bystander and low dose-rate effects: are these relevant to radionuclide therapy?" *J Nucl Med,* vol. 48, no. 10, pp. 1683–91, 2007, doi: 10.2967/ jnumed.105.028183.

[86] L. Y. Xue, N. J. Butler, G. M. Makrigiorgos, S. J. Adelstein, and A. I. Kassis, "Bystander effect produced by radiolabeled tumor cells in vivo," *Proc Natl Acad Sci U S A,* vol. 99, no. 21, pp. 13765–70, 2002, doi: 10.1073/pnas.182209699.

[87] R. W. Howell and A. Bishayee, "Bystander effects caused by nonuniform distributions of DNA-incorporated (125)I," *Micron,* vol. 33, no. 2, pp. 127–32, 2002, doi: 10.1016/s0968-4328(01)00007-5.

[88] M. Boyd *et al.*, "Radiation-induced biologic bystander effect elicited in vitro by targeted radiopharmaceuticals labeled with alpha-, beta-, and auger electron-emitting radionuclides," *J Nucl Med,* vol. 47, no. 6, pp. 1007–15, 2006.

[89] H. Kishikawa, K. Wang, S. J. Adelstein, and A. I. Kassis, "Inhibitory and stimulatory bystander effects are differentially induced by Iodine-125 and Iodine-123," *Radiat Res,* vol. 165, no. 6, pp. 688–94, 2006, doi: 10.1667/rr3567.1.

[90] J. B. Little, "Genomic instability and bystander effects: a historical perspective," *Oncogene,* vol. 22, no. 45, pp. 6978–87, 2003, doi: 10.1038/sj.onc.1206988.

[91] E. G. Wright, "Commentary on radiation-induced bystander effects," *Hum Exp Toxicol,* vol. 23, no. 2, pp. 91–94, 2004, doi: 10.1191/0960327104ht424oa.

[92] W. F. Morgan, "Is there a common mechanism underlying genomic instability, bystander effects and other nontargeted effects of exposure to ionizing radiation?" *Oncogene,* vol. 22, no. 45, pp. 7094–99, 2003, doi: 10.1038/sj.onc.1206992.

[93] R. Iyer, B. E. Lehnert, and R. Svensson, "Factors underlying the cell growth-related bystander responses to alpha particles," *Cancer Res,* vol. 60, no. 5, pp. 1290–98, 2000.

[94] P. K. Narayanan, K. E. LaRue, E. H. Goodwin, and B. E. Lehnert, "Alpha particles induce the production of interleukin-8 by human cells," *Radiat Res,* vol. 152, no. 1, pp. 57–63, 1999.

[95] C. N. Leung *et al.*, "Dose-dependent growth delay of breast cancer xenografts in the bone marrow of mice treated with (223) Ra: The role of bystander effects and their potential for Therapy," *J Nucl Med,* vol. 61, no. 1, pp. 89–95, 2020, doi: 10.2967/ jnumed.119.227835.

[96] A. Levy, C. Chargari, A. Marabelle, J. L. Perfettini, N. Magné, and E. Deutsch, "Can immunostimulatory agents enhance the abscopal effect of radiotherapy?" *Eur J Cancer,* vol. 62, pp. 36–45, 2016, doi: 10.1016/j.ejca.2016.03.067.

[97] S. Bockel, B. Durand, and E. Deutsch, "Combining radiation therapy and cancer immune therapies: From preclinical findings to clinical applications," *Cancer Radiother,* vol. 22, no. 6–7, pp. 567–80, 2018, doi: 10.1016/j.canrad.2018.07.136.

[98] N. Bloy *et al.*, "Trial Watch: Radioimmunotherapy for oncological indications," *Oncoimmunology,* vol. 3, no. 9, p. e954929, 2014, doi: 10.4161/21624011.2014.954929.

[99] J. P. Pouget, A. G. Georgakilas, and J. L. Ravanat, "Targeted and off-target (bystander and abscopal) effects of radiation therapy: Redox mechanisms and risk/benefit analysis," *Antioxid Redox Signal,* vol. 29, no. 15, pp. 1447–87, 2018, doi: 10.1089/ars.2017.7267.

[100] D. Murray and A. J. McEwan, "Radiobiology of systemic radiation therapy," *Cancer Biother Radiopharm,* vol. 22, no. 1, pp. 1–23, 2007, doi: 10.1089/cbr.2006.531.

[101] M. Widel, "Radionuclides in radiation-induced bystander effect; may it share in radionuclide therapy?" *Neoplasma,* vol. 64, no. 5, pp. 641–54, 2017, doi: 10.4149/neo_2017_501.

[102] M. Lassmann, L. Strigari, and M. Bardies, "Dosimetry is alive and well," *Cancer Biother Radiopharm,* vol. 25, no. 5, pp. 593–95, 2010, doi: 10.1089/cbr.2010.0874.

3 Diagnostic Dosimetry

Lennart Johansson[†] and Martin Andersson

CONTENTS

DOI: 10.1201/9780429489549-3

3.1   INTRODUCTION

The use of compounds labelled "radioactive" for medical diagnoses implies that the patient is exposed to ionizing radiation. This means that a nuclear medicine examination relates to a small risk for cancer. After considering the health of the patient, the benefit of the investigation must outweigh the risk from the exposure, otherwise the examination is not justified. The safety of the patient therefore requires some form of estimation of the risk, albeit it only very small.

Radioactive transformations taking place in the body's tissues release energy as photons and kinetic energy of emitted particles. When this energy is transferred to the tissues it is quantified as the absorbed dose, the absorbed energy per unit mass. The energy from ionizing radiation that the patient is exposed to is extremely small compared to other energy forms, for example, heating. The damage to the cell is attributed to the radiation's ability to ionize. At the absorbed dose level of interest this may cause damage to DNA, which can, even if the probability is very small, contribute to cancer development. Thus, even if a risk estimate today due to limited knowledge is very rough, a first and unavoidable step is to calculate, or at least estimate, the absorbed dose to exposed organs and perhaps also estimate the effective dose.

From a physical perspective, the absorbed dose is a measure of the damage caused by the exposure. Assessing the absorbed dose in the body's organs is thus a physical quantity of fundamental importance for the judgement of risk. Assessing the absorbed dose is a first step, and it has to be completed with also taking the biological perspective into account, considering the radiation sensitivity of different tissues for different energy and types of radiation.

Internal dosimetry deals with the task to assess the absorbed dose in the body and its organs as a result of radionuclide transformation in tissues. The absorbed dose in the different organs of the body cannot be measured *in vivo*, but rather has to be calculated based on available information about physical and biological parameters. To calculate the absorbed dose with high accuracy for individual patients undergoing a diagnostic nuclear medicine study is neither possible nor justified – estimating internal doses is thus "an art of approximation". This approach is justified by the fact that the individual variation of the biological parameters affecting the dose and the sensitivity to ionizing radiation is considerable. Use of radionuclides for diagnostic purposes will not lead to deterministic effects, therefore, only stochastic risk is to be considered. And the stochastic risk cannot be assessed for individual patients.

3.1.1   SHORT HISTORICAL REVIEW

The need for internal dosimetry for patients who were given radionuclides for diagnostic as well as for therapeutic purposes arose in the late 1940s when, especially ^{131}I was introduced as a radionuclide for thyroid diagnostics and treatments [1]. The classical method for dose estimation from photons was developed by Marinelli and colleagues and published in 1948 [2]. This method was modified and improved by Loevinger who introduced the gamma constant, Γ, and equates the absorbed dose rate dR at a point P at distance d from an infinitesimal volume element dV as a function

$$dR_{\gamma,p} = \frac{C\rho\Gamma e^{\mu_{eff}d}}{d^2} dV \tag{3.1}$$

C is the activity concentration and ρ is the density. This equation can be integrated over the entire volume.

An organization that has played a main role in promoting development of methods for internal dosimetry is the MIRD-committee of the Society of Nuclear Medicine [3]. The committee started in the 1960s and was for a long time active in producing data to be used for dose calculations. With the introduction of computers, Monte Carlo simulations were performed to calculate the fraction of absorbed energy, first in simple geometries, spheres and ellipsoids [4]. These "mathematical phantoms" were then also developed into human-like anthropomorphic shapes [5], defined with mathematical expressions. A list of the MIRD pamphlets is attached at the end of this chapter in Table 3.8.

Another organization that can be mentioned in this context is the International Commission on Radiological Protection (ICRP), founded in 1928 when the society began to understand that there is some kind of risk with ionizing radiation. The ICRP also developed a framework for estimating and handling the risk from the radiation. They have produced, compiled, and published physiological and biological data necessary for calculating the absorbed dose. They have also published a number of reports presenting absorbed dose to patients from radiopharmaceuticals. These reports started with *ICRP-17* [6], which is now obsolete. *ICRP-53* [7] may be somewhat old but is still useful. Since new radiopharmaceuticals have been developed also new reports were needed, including *ICRP-80* [8], *ICRP-106* [9] and *ICRP-128* [10], published on this subject.

3.1.2 Dose Tables and Computer Programs

Information about organ doses and effective doses for different substances and different types of examinations are often found in the literature, including ICRP publications. In most cases this is enough information for a routine clinical investigation. In addition to the tabulated dose data published by ICRP and MIRD for different radionuclides, data are found in the scientific literature and on different internet sites. The need for performing your own dose calculations in normal clinical routine is therefore rather small. Also, different more or less sophisticated dose viewers and dosage calculators for children are available, see for example, the European and North American home pages (EANM.org and SNMMI. org), or you can just look up the absorbed dose for a specific radiopharmaceutical on various sites. Other sophisticated computer programs worth mentioning are the programs OLINDA [11] and IDAC [12].

This chapter focuses on methods to calculate organ-absorbed doses and effective doses using basic data from the literature. It also includes how to estimate doses for exposure situations that do not fit in the common templates, such as pathological deviations. Note that the methods described here apply only to the use of radiopharmaceuticals for diagnostic purposes, not therapy. This is also the case for the computer programs mentioned above. Therapeutic nuclear medicine requires an individual dose estimation, with higher demands of accuracy in organ dose, which requires another, but similar, methodology based on individual parameters [13].

3.2 PURPOSE

The primary purpose of calculating or estimating an internal absorbed dose from medical diagnostics is radiation protection of the patient. However, as is the case for therapeutic applications of radionuclides, there might also arise situations when an individual calculation is justified.

In nuclear medicine, as with any medical procedure, the risk and benefit must be weighed. The absorbed dose is an essential parameter in the risk estimation. The dose estimate is an important tool for the justification and optimization of the diagnostic procedure, which means that information about the radiation dose is required to compare the use and the risk of the various alternative radiodiagnostic techniques. Diagnostic nuclear medicine is also called functional imaging, which make this imaging mode unique in many cases.

There is also an international interest in statistics in order to estimate the collective radiation exposure. In some countries there are articles in the regulations that require the hospital to inform the patient about the risk for cancer due to the radiation exposure from the administered radiopharmaceutical. This is due to the great uncertainties in converting from dose to risk. It is sufficiently accurate to base the information on an absorbed dose calculated to a reference person for the specific study.

3.3　RADIONUCLIDES IN DIAGNOSTIC NUCLEAR MEDICINE

^{99m}Tc is today, without rival, the most-used radionuclide for imaging with a gamma camera and SPECT. The properties of this radionuclide are as close as possible to the ideal for a diagnostic imaging radionuclide with a gamma camera. ^{99m}Tc has a well-balanced half-life and energy of the photons, no beta radiation giving unwanted absorbed dose and a relatively small number of electrons. For PET studies today ^{18}F dominates the usage in clinical routine. This is due to the availability, combined with the good characteristics of fluorodeoxyglucose (FDG).

The most recent comprehensive nuclear decay data tables suitable for internal dose calculations can be obtained from *ICRP-107* [14]. There is no printed version of the tables, but the software DECDATA distributed together with the report can be used to produce tables of nuclear decay data for the various radionuclides.

Table 3.1 displays only the most important dose characteristics for some common radionuclides. Tables with comprehensive data suitable for internal dose calculations have been published by ICRP [14] and MIRD [15]. Data may also be found at different internet sites. It is important to note that the mean energy for the beta particles has to be used. Alternatively, the full beta spectrum can be applied; this may be obtained from the program DECDATA.

In case a radionuclide with a non-stable daughter is used, the potential absorbed dose from the decay should be considered. If the absorbed dose cannot be disregarded, which is the case for some radionuclides in Table 3.1, it may be

TABLE 3.1

Decay Characteristics for Radionuclides Commonly Used in Nuclear Medicine Diagnostics [14]

Radionuclide	Half-life	Type, $E_{average}$ (yield)	Remarks
^{99m}Tc	6.015 h	γ 141 keV (0.891)	Daughter: ^{99}Tc (2.11E5 y), no significant dose contribution
^{18}F	109.8 min	β$^+$ 250 keV (0.967)	PET
		γ 511 keV (1.934)	
^{123}I	13.3 h	γ 159 keV (0.833)	c. 4% of the total energy is emitted as Auger electrons, (yield
		X 27 keV (0.715)	13.7).
		31 keV (0.155)	
^{131}I	8.02 d	β$^-$ 192 keV (0.895)	Gamma photons with E > 0.5 MeV present with a few per cent.
		96 keV (0.072)	
		γ 364 keV (0.817)	
^{111}In	2.805 d	γ 171 keV (0.907)	
		245 keV (0.941)	
		X 23 keV (0.689)	
^{68}Ga	76.71 min	β$^+$ 836 keV (0.877)	PET. Also gamma 1.08 MeV (0.032)
		γ 511 keV (1.778)	
^{11}C	20.39 min	β$^+$ 386 keV (0.998)	PET
		γ 511 keV (1.995)	
^{75}Se	119.78 d	γ 121 keV (0.172)	Auger and conversion electrons to be added
		136 keV (0.583)	
		265 keV (0.589)	
		280 keV (0.250)	
		401 KeV (0.115)	
		X 10.5 keV (0.480)	
^{13}N	9.965 min	β$^+$ 492 keV (0.998)	PET
		γ 511 keV (1.996)	
^{67}Ge	3.26 d	γ 93 keV (0.392)	
		185 keV (0.212)	
		300 keV (0.168)	
^{201}Tl	71.91 h	X 12 keV (0.106)	
		70 keV (0.737)	
		γ 0.167 keV (0.10)	
^{14}C	5700 y	β$^-$ 49 keV (1.00)	No imaging

Note: Only radiation with a yield exceeding 10 per cent is included, and only photons >10 keV.

assumed that the daughter follows the metabolism of the administered substance, unless other information is available. The long half-life of ^{99}Tc, the daughter of ^{99m}Tc, means that the activity of this radionuclide is practically zero, even if for some radiopharmaceuticals it is a disadvantage that the presence of this radionuclide will decrease the specific activity. About 1 per cent of the ^{131}I atoms decay to ^{131m}Xe, which has a half-life of 11.8 d. The small activity of xenon formed in vivo will to a high degree leave the body via the lungs before decay. The dose from ^{131m}Xe can therefore be ignored. Indium-111 and ^{123}I decay to metastable isotopes, ^{111m}Cd and ^{123m}Te, respectively. The yield of these is however very low, ~10^{-5}, thus these may be neglected. The other daughter from ^{123}I, ^{123}Te, has a very long half-life in the order of ~10^{14} years, which means the resulting activity is practically zero.

3.4 ABSORBED DOSE

When a nuclear transformation takes place in body tissues, the energy released will be deposited in the organ from which it originated, in some other tissue or outside the body. The absorbed dose, D, in a point is defined as the average energy imparted, $\bar{\varepsilon}$, from ionizing radiation per unit mass, m.

$$D = \frac{d\bar{\varepsilon}}{dm} \tag{3.2}$$

3.4.1 BASIC INTERNAL DOSIMETRY

To calculate the absorbed dose from internally deposited radionuclides, information is needed about the time-dependent radionuclide distribution and the resulting time-dependent radiation field. Together with different biological parameters, the physical parameters describing the emitted radiation are important for estimating the absorbed dose (Table 3.2).

Also, the chemical properties of the substance used – for example, the stability of the radioactive label – will influence the absorbed dose. The biological parameters are summed up and expressed as number of transformations taking place in various defined source regions, $\tilde{A}(r_S)$. This is a dimensionless quantity. It is meaningful to normalize this quantity to administered activity to obtain the "time integrated activity coefficient" (TIAC) $\tilde{a}(r_S)$, the unit is seconds or hours

$$\tilde{a}(r_S) = \frac{\tilde{A}(r_S)}{A_0} = \int_0^\infty A(t, r_S) dt \tag{3.3}$$

TABLE 3.2
Important Biological and Physical Parameters for Estimating the Absorbed Dose

Physical parameters	Biological parameters
Radionuclide properties, well known with high accuracy, no variations between individuals	Describes anatomical and physiological characteristics. Great individual variations. Calculations are performed for a reference man/woman and children of specific ages.
• Type and energy of radiation emitted	• *Anatomy:* Mass, density and shape for organs and body.
	• Elemental composition – influences the attenuation
• Half-life of the radionuclide	• *Physiology:* Metabolism. Retention and its variation in time for the radionuclide.
• Is progeny stable or radioactive? If it is unstable – will transformations of the progeny contribute to a significant degree to the energy emitted?	• Transportation and retention in the excretion organs, intestine and urinary bladder.

---

where $A(t, r_S)$ is the retention function in a source. For patients in nuclear medicine diagnostics, the emitted radiation is practically always composed of both photons and particles, and in this context beta-particles and electrons of different origin as Auger and conversion electrons. Alpha particles are used for therapy but will not be considered here. For radiation with a very short range, a good approximation is to assume that the energy is absorbed "on the spot", or at least in the same organ as the source. These types of radiation are called *non-penetrating*, while radiation with a typical range larger than, or comparable to, the organ dimensions is called *penetrating* radiation. This categorizing of the emitted radiation facilitates the estimation of the organ doses, even if it is not always required when modern data and computer programs are available.

3.4.2 Non-penetrating Radiation

Particles, and photons with an energy <10 keV, are handled as radiation for which the energy can with good approximation be absorbed on the spot. When considering an infinite medium containing a homogeneous distribution of a radionuclide, the energy absorbed per unit mass (the absorbed dose) equals the amount of energy emitted from the radionuclide per unit mass (equilibrium condition). Let $\tilde{A}$ be the total number of transformations per unit mass, then the absorbed dose, D, in becomes

$$D = \tilde{A}\sum_i Y_i \overline{E_i} \tag{3.4}$$

Y_i is the yield – that is the number of particles or photons with the mean energy $\overline{E}_i$ emitted per transformation. When considering the exposure of an organ, *absorbed dose* refers to the *mean* absorbed dose in the organ or tissue – that is, the energy absorbed in the tissue divided by its mass. Equation 3.4 is especially useful for calculating the dose delivered by beta particles, Auger electrons, and photons with low energy (< 10 keV). In comparison with most organs in the human body, the range of these radiations is short.

For non-penetrating radiation, the fraction of absorbed energy $\varphi = 1$ if the target organ is identical with the source organ. If the source and target organs are separated then $\varphi = 0$. Bremsstrahlung is usually neglected in this context. A special situation occurs when the wall of an organ is the target, while the source is located the content, the absorbed dose to the inner surface of the wall is then approximately half of that to the content. A point on the surface is irradiated in a 2π geometry. As an approximation it may be assumed that this can be taken as the mean dose to the wall. For thin walls and high energy this underestimates the average dose, while it is overestimated for lower-energy particles and thicker walls. Even if data on absorbed fraction of energy are available for non-penetrating radiations, this has for long time been a common method to calculate absorbed dose to walls of the gastrointestinal tract and the urinary bladder.

Example 1: Consider a body of random shape with a mass of 200 g, which is filled with 1 MBq ^{32}P. Phosphorus-32 is a pure beta-emitter and the mean energy of the beta particles is 0.695 MeV [14]. 1 MeV≈1.602 × 10^{-13} J. The absorbed dose rate at a point inside the body is then 1 × 10^6 Bq × 0.695 MeV × 1.6021 × 10^{-13} J/ MeV / 0.2 kg = 5.57 × 10^{-7} Gy/s.

3.4.3 Absorbed Fraction of Energy

For radiation whose range is of the same order or larger than the dimension of the organ where the radionuclide is located, one has to account for loss of energy to the outside of the organ.

$$D < \tilde{A}\sum_i Y_i \overline{E_i} \tag{3.5}$$

When radionuclides emitting photons – that is, penetrating radiation – are taken up in different organs of the body, radiation emitted in one organ will give an absorbed dose in the studied organ and also in neighbouring organs. Let the fraction of energy absorbed in a target region r_T from radiation originating in a source region r_s be $\varphi_{r_T \leftarrow r_s}$, then the absorbed dose in target region r_T then becomes

$$D_{r_T} = \sum_{r_s}\tilde{A}_{r_s}\sum_i Y_i E_i \, \varphi_{r_T \leftarrow r_s}(E_i)\frac{1}{m_{r_T}} \tag{3.6}$$

$\tilde{A}_{r_s}$ is the total number of transformations in the source region, and E_i is the energy of the photons or the particles. The target may of course be identical with the source. Often the absorbed fraction is combined with the mass of the target organ, and then the so-called specific absorbed fraction (SAF), ϕ, is obtained. The equation for dose calculation can now be written.

$$D_{r_T} = \sum_{r_s} \tilde{A}_{r_s} \sum_i Y_i E_i \Phi_{r_T \leftarrow r_s}(E_i)$$ (3.7)

The MIRD committee of the Society of Nuclear Medicine produced and published in 1969 tables of absorbed fractions of energy for a number of important source and target organs [5]. This publication was replaced in 1978 with a revised version [5], tabulating specific absorbed fractions instead. At that time these organs were represented mathematically – that is, by describing limiting surface with two-dimensional equations. The absorbed fractions were calculated using Monte Carlo techniques [16].

When using a table of absorbed fractions, watch out – is it specific absorbed fractions or not? If it is, what is the unit? g^{-1} or kg^{-1}?

A closer look at Equation 3.8 reveals that much work can be avoided if data that are specific to the radionuclide and the phantom are brought together in one factor. Such a dose factor is called the S-value (or S-coefficient):

$$S_{r_T \leftarrow r_s} = \sum_i Y_i E_i \Phi_{r_T \leftarrow r_s}(E_i)$$ (3.8)

Using tabulated data for this factor, the absorbed dose in an organ r_T is easily calculated as the sum of the dose contribution from all source organs,

$$D_{r_T} = \sum_s \tilde{A}_{r_s} \times S_{r_T \leftarrow r_s}$$ (3.9)

S-factors were published by MIRD in 1975 [17] based on a slightly modified version of the earlier defined mathematical phantom. These tables, one per radionuclide, became (albeit a less accurate phantom) for a long time the "gold standard" for internal dosimetry. The unit of the S-value is Gy/decay, but it may often for convenience be tabulated in mGy/MBq-h, that is, per 3.6×10^9 decays. In MIRD pamphlet No. 11 [17] the data are given in rad/μCi-h which may be converted to mGy/MBq-h by multiplication with 270.27.

In 2016 the specific absorbed fractions calculated on the new ICRP/ICRU [18, 19] adult voxel phantom was published and is now, in combination with radionuclide decay data in *ICRP-107* [14], supposed to be used for dose calculations for radiation protection, particularly for the calculation of the effective dose.

3.4.4 In Practise

Using absorbed fractions or specific absorbed fractions for dose calculations of all organs of interest is a laborious and tedious task, particularly for radionuclides with many different energies of particles and photons. When S-values are available for calculating the absorbed dose it is straightforward, applying the TIACs for each source organ.

If no S-values are available Equation 3.9 may be applied, provided that absorbed fraction are found, or at least some reasonable approximation. A first and fundamental step for internal dose calculations is to differentiate between what is considered as "non-penetrating radiation", NP, and "penetrating radiation". Radiation has a range considerably shorter than the dimension of most organs in the body. Then Equation 3.9 above is valid, or at least a very good approximation of the absorbed dose. This comprises particles such as beta (including positrons), Auger- and conversional electrons, and also photons with low energy (< 10 keV). For radionuclides emitting beta radiation a first rough approximation of absorbed dose can obtained in this way. For example, for ^{131}I in the thyroid, with a mass of 23.4 g (including blood) the absorbed dose per transformation is 1.31×10^{-12} Gy/decay from particle radiation only. If all radiation is included the dose factor is 1.63×10^{-12} Gy/decay [14, 19]. This approximation will thus underestimate the dose only by 20 per cent and equals approximately the uncertainty in the dose calculation as a whole.

For a structure of limited size, a radionuclide emitting "penetrating radiation", that is, photons with energy > 10 keV, a fraction of the emitted energy will leave the structure and be absorbed somewhere else. This will lead to an overestimation of the absorbed dose. The overestimations will depend on the photon energy and yield, that is, the fraction of energy deposited elsewhere.

When considering in this context the exposure of an organ "absorbed dose", always refers to the *mean* absorbed dose in the organ or tissue, that is, the energy absorbed in the tissue divided by its mass.

Example 2: Uptake of a technetium and fluoride-labelled substance in the salivary glands. The salivary glands are not included in MIRD *Pamphlet No. 11.*

According to reference values given in *ICRP-89*, the salivary glands comprise three sets of pairs, with total masses for adult male of 89 g.

^{18}F decays with beta radiation and annihilation photons, because ^{18}F is the annihilation yield 2 × electron yield or $0.9673 \times 2 = 1.9346$ per nuclear transition (nt) with an annihilation energy of 0.511 MeV. The absorbed fraction for 0.511 MeV from source salivary glands to target salivary glands of the ICRP adult male is 0.0368. The absorbed dose for this case is 1.9346 1/nt × 0.511 MeV × 1.6021 × 10^{-13} J/MeV × 0.0368 /0.089 kg = 6.55 × 10^{-14} Gy/decay.

^{18}F decays with pure beta+ decay, with a yield per nuclear transition of 0.97 and an energy of 0.252 MeV results in a mean energy of 0.250 MeV per decay. Assuming total self-dose electron energy of ^{18}F decay in salivary gland 0.250 MeV × 1.6021 × 10^{-13} J/MeV / 0.089 kg = 4.50 × 10^{-13} Gy per decay.

The corresponding calculation with the ICRP internal computational framework is 4.17 × 10^{-13} Gy per decay, where the electron energy is Monte Carlo–simulated based on the whole ^{18}F beta spectrum.

The result of this simple approach deviates only 8 per cent from the result of the more complicated methods for estimating the electron absorbed dose to the salivary gland.

Example 3: The thyroid has a mass of 40 g instead of normal 20 g. What is an approximative thyroid dose to this patient from ^{131}I?

If all radiation is included, the ^{131}I thyroid dose factor is 1.63 × 10^{-12} Gy/decay for a thyroid tissue of 20 g. An approximate patient dose for a 40 g thyroid, assuming equal changes of blood, would be 20 g /40 g × 1.63 × 10^{-12} Gy/decay = 0.815 × 10^{-12} Gy/decay.

Example 4: A patient has only one kidney. What dose will be expected from an investigation with MAG3?

In *ICRP-128* [10] the absorbed dose per unit activity administered for ^{99m}Tc labelled MAG3 to an adult patient with two normal functional kidneys is 3.4 × 10^{-3} mGy/MBq. Of this absorbed dose is 3.2 × 10^{-3} mGy/MBq from the kidneys itself and 0.2 × 10^{-3} mGy/MBq from surrounding tissues, for example, urinary bladder.

Assuming that the same amount of MAG3 decays in the patient's one kidney as in the two kidneys case. This will result in a two times higher absorbed dose, as the same amount of decays will occur but only on half the kidney volume (or mass). For the external dose contribution, the result will be unchanged as both the deposit energy (J) and organ mass (kg) is reduced with a factor of two.

The absorbed kidney dose for a patient with one kidney is 2 × 3.2 × 10^{-3} mGy/MBq + 0.2 × 10^{-3} mGy/MBq = 6.6 × 10^{-3} mGy/MBq.

3.5   BIOKINETIC AND DOSIMETRIC MODELS

Biokinetic models are used to describe the radionuclide distributions and their variation in time. The biokinetic model describes in mathematical terms the uptake and turnover of a substance in an organ or the body. For each compound used in nuclear medicine, such models have been produced and published in the literature.

A dosimetric model describes in general terms, with mathematical equations or specified voxels, anatomical features for which knowledge is required in order to calculate or simulate how and where the energy is transported and absorbed from a radionuclide source.

The distribution of the radionuclide in the body can be obtained from the biokinetic models, which are used to calculate the total number of disintegrations taking place at different sites. This is obtained by calculating the area under the time-activity curve, which is integrating the curve for a fixed time, for nuclear medicine substances from zero to infinity. The result is termed "cumulated activity", or the "time-integrated activity", and if it is normalized to the administered activity, this defines the "time-integrated activity coefficient" (TIAC). An older term for this is "residence time". The source is usually located in one or several organs defined as a "source organs".

In diagnostic nuclear medicine the absorbed dose is primarily estimated for a standard or reference man or women [20]. This applies both to the physical, anatomical model of the patient (described elsewhere) as well as to the biokinetic model describing the metabolism of the substance in question. The uptake and retention of the radionuclide in the body and its organs may be described in different ways, by a flow scheme or by mathematical equations. Those models are the basis for calculating the total number of decays taking place in different parts or regions in the body (source regions).

In addition to the biokinetic models for organs, there are a number of general biological models. Models for the gastrointestinal tract and the urinary bladder have been designed for describing the intake or excretion of the activity in general terms, primarily for occupational internal dosimetry but they may also be used in revised form for nuclear medicine patients. Other models are primarily designed to handle dosimetric problems requiring assumptions in a similar manner for different substances.

- Model for the alimentary tract [21].
- Lung model [22, 23] primarily designed for occupational (or environmental) dosimetry. Aerosols given for diagnostic purposes are administered in a different way, and the model is thus of limited relevance.
- Model for excretion of a radionuclide via the kidney bladder. Designed for nuclear medicine [10].
- Model describing the passage of activity taken up in the liver and excreted via the gall bladder and intestine. Designed for nuclear medicine [10].
- Model describing the transportation of activity given intrathecally. A nuclear medicine procedure [7].
- A default model to be applied for activity taken up in the skeleton, to establish a defaults activity distribution between bone volume and surface deposition in cortical and trabecular bone [10, 20].
- Model for very short-lived radionuclides given intravenously. Nuclear medicine only [24].
- Model for lacrimal gland dosimetry. For radiopharmaceuticals taken up in the lacrimal glands [25].

Usually, the models are designed to describe the physiology and anatomy in a normal person, that is, a person free from disease, which is typical for the patients undergoing the described nuclear medicine study. Variations due to typical pathological conditions may be accounted for in different ways (see section 8).

3.5.1 Configuration of a Biokinetic Model

There are in principally two different ways of designing and presenting biokinetic models.

- Compartment models, including all organs of interest as an entity.
- A descriptive model for each organ. Fractional uptakes and biological half-times derived directly from measurements. This is sometimes called a "net model".

A compartment model divides the body into several pools of activity between which the radionuclides are exchanged. The flow between the pools usually follows first-order kinetics. This description of how the activity flows in the body may be made more physiologically realistic, provided the configuration, that is, how the boxes and arrows are arranged, is realistic. A complex flow pattern will, however, give rise to differential equations, which may be almost impossible to solve analytically. A dedicated computer program may be required. It is useful also to facilitate the calculation of the total number of transformations. An example of such a program, which often has been used for biokinetics of radiopharmaceuticals, is SAAM II [26].

A descriptive model is an empirical model where the time dependence of the observed activity in an organ is fitted to a proper equation, almost always a sum of exponentials. This retention equation is easily utilized for the calculation.

The total number of transformations $\tilde{A}$, in a source, r_s, is calculated as

$$\tilde{A}_{r_s} = A_0 \int_0^\infty q(t) e^{-\lambda_{phys}} dt \tag{3.10}$$

Where $q(t)$ is the retention function, λ_{phys} is the physical decay constant, and A_0 is the administered activity.

3.5.1.1 Descriptive Biokinetic Models

A descriptive model is obtained by fitting measured data to obtain a retention curve described with a mathematical equation. The retention curve for an organ or volume is obtained from quantitative measurements with a gamma-camera or a PET (see Volume 1 Chapters 13 and 18). Many biological or physiological processes follow a first-order kinetics, that is, it can be described with an exponential function or a linear combination of exponential functions, in practice no more than three exponential functions are needed. The obtained parameters are therefore often interpreted as biological half-times attributable to the retention of the substance in the specific organ. Usually one or two, in practice the resolution of the observed data does not allow for more than three exponetial functions. For dose calculation, the physical half-life also has to be considered. The half-life $T_{\frac{1}{2}}$ is obtained from the transfer factor λ as

$$T_{\frac{1}{2}} = \ln(2)/\lambda \tag{3.11}$$

The transfer factor represents the probability per unit time that the radionuclide will decay. If both biological excretion and physical transformation is considered, the effective transfer factor is $\lambda_{eff} = \lambda_{bio} + \lambda_{phys}$ from which it follows that the effective half-time can be calculated as

$$\frac{1}{T_{eff}} = \frac{1}{T_{bio}} + \frac{1}{T_{phys}} \tag{3.12}$$

and

$$T_{eff} = \frac{T_{bio} \times T_{phys}}{T_{bio} + T_{phys}} \tag{3.13}$$

For descriptive models it is common to set the initial content in the organs to a certain fraction of the administered activity, F_S. This is often an approximation that is good enough, since the uptake from the blood is fast in comparison with the biological half-times. Consider a simple case when the retention function can be described by a linear combination of two exponentials, and initial value is F_S, immediate uptake in the source organ is assumed, the activity in the source organ A_S is

$$A_S(t) = A_0 \times F_S \left(a_1 e^{(-\lambda_1 t)} + a_2 e^{(-\lambda_2 t)} \right) \tag{3.14}$$

where λ is the effective transfer factor and the factors a_1 and a_2 represent the fraction for the respective half-times. Integrating this expression yields the time-integrated activity coefficients (TIAC), $\tilde{a}_S$

$$\tilde{a}_S = \frac{1}{A_0} \int_0^\infty A_S(t)\,dt = F_S \left(a_1 \frac{T_{\frac{1}{2},1}}{\ln(2)} + a_2 \frac{T_{\frac{1}{2},2}}{\ln(2)} \right) \tag{3.15}$$

$T_{\frac{1}{2}}$ is the effective half-time. This coefficient has also been termed the relative cumulated activity or, in earlier MIRD terminology, the residence time. For calculating TIAC for an organ, S, which has a delayed uptake of activity from the blood, and n biological half-times, the flow of activity is described by

$$\frac{dA_S(t)}{dt} = A_0 \times F_S \left[\lambda_u A_b(t) - \sum_{i=1}^n a_i (\lambda_i + \lambda_p) A_S(t) \right] \tag{3.16}$$

$A_b(t)$ is the activity in the blood, λ_u is the uptake transfer rate from the blood, and λ_p is the physical decay constant. With $A_b(0)=A_0$ and $A_S(0)=0$ the solution becomes

$$A_S(t) = A_0 \times F_S \sum_{i=1}^1 \left[\frac{\lambda_u}{\lambda_i - \lambda_u} \left(e^{-(\lambda_i + \lambda_p)t} - e^{-(\lambda_u + \lambda_p)t} \right) \right] \tag{3.17}$$

Integrating this equation yields the time-integrated activity coefficient, using half-times, T, instead of transfer coefficients.

$$\tilde{a}_S = F_S \times \sum_{i=1}^{n} \left[\frac{T_i}{T_i - T_u} \left(\frac{T_{i,eff}}{T_{b,eff} - T_{i,eff}} \right) \right] \tag{3.18}$$

In Figure 3.1 curves are shown for both immediate uptake and delayed uptake and the same single elimination rate. For the curves in Figure 3.1 the physical half-life is for ^{99m}Tc ($T_{\frac{1}{2}}$ = 6.015 h) with a single elimination rate of 8 hours and for the delay uptake of 30 min and a fractional uptake of $F_S = 0.15$. The differences in TIAC between immediate uptake and delayed uptake is 5 per cent, meaning that for fast uptake ($T_i \ll T_u$), this is an acceptable assumption.

3.5.1.2 Compartment Models

A compartment model describes the flow of radionuclides between different pools of activity. A compartment is characterized by uniform kinetic behaviour. These compartments may be interpreted as biochemical mechanisms transferring the radionuclide from one state to another or from one organ to another. Thus, it is important to be aware that a compartment is not equal to an organ. One organ may contain several compartments, and one compartment may also be comprised of several organs. Also, it is the flow of the radioactive marker that is to be described, not the marquee itself. Thus, for example, release of free pertechnetate from a radiopharmaceutical is a flow of radioactivity between two compartments.

With a few exceptions, the flow of activity between the pools in a compartment model follows a first-order kinetics. That is the flow rate is proportional to the activity content in the pool from where the activity comes. This "proportionality constant", called "transfer coefficient", is here denoted $\lambda_{k,l}$ for the transfer from compartment k to compartment l. Note that in pharmacological literature it is usually standard to use a reversed order ($\lambda_{l,k}$). The transfer factors may be age-dependent, while the configuration of the model is not. An example of a compartment model used for iodide given orally is found in Figure 3.2. The biokinetic model of iodide have two different subsystems, one for inorganic and another of organic, iodide. As seen in Figure 3.2 for, liver, thyroid and kidneys are the correct organ representation of a two-compartment system to separate the transfer rates and compartments into two separate boxes inside an organ box, instead of including all transfer rates in one single compartment box.

The time-varying activity, A(k,t) in a single compartment, k, in a system of n compartments is the solution of:

$$\frac{dA(k,t)}{dt} = \sum_{\substack{l=1 \\ l \neq k}}^{n} A(l,t)\lambda_{l,k} - A(k,t)\sum_{\substack{l=1 \\ l \neq k}}^{n} \lambda_{k,l} \tag{3.19}$$

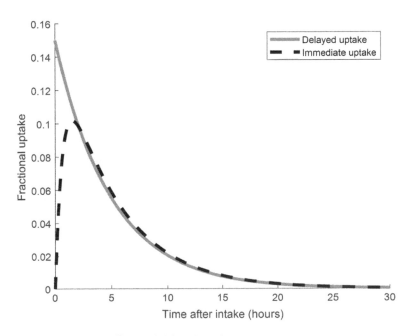

FIGURE 3.1 Retention curves of both immediate and delayed uptake.

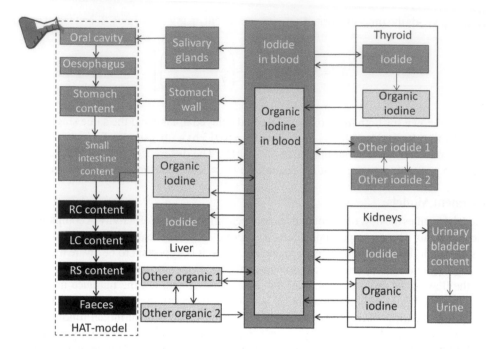

FIGURE 3.2 The ICRP compartment model for orally administered iodide. The transport of inorganic iodide in the body is marked with dark gray compartments, the organic iodine transfer is marked with light gray compartments, the black compartments is the generic human alimentary tract (HAT) model. The white boxes are just for the organs including both inorganic iodide and organic iodine.

This system of differential equations is preferably solved with numerical methods. The total number of decays is obtained by integrating the solution, which also may be performed numerically. When performing a numerical iterative integration, the integration has to account both for the fast and the slow transfer rates in the model. This means that immediately after the injection, a short integration time step is preferable to account for the fast transfer. After a while the distribution will be dependent on the slow transfer rates and, in this case, it will be better to change to a longer integration step, until only an insignificant amount of activity remains in the body.

One configuration of compartments for which an analytical solution can be easily found is a chain of catenary compartments. This is a model case – for example, for the previous representation of the ICRP gastrointestinal tract [27]. The activity $A(i,t)$ in the i :th compartment due to an intake in the first compartment at $t = 0$, can be written:

$$
\begin{aligned}
\frac{da_i(t)}{dt} &= \dot{I}_i(t) - \lambda_i a_i(t) & i &= 1 \\
\frac{da_i(t)}{dt} &= I_i(t) + \lambda_{(i-1,i)} a_{(i-1,i)}(t) - \lambda_i a_i(t) & i &= 2 \,\text{to}\, n
\end{aligned}
\tag{3.20}
$$

Where a_i is the activity in compartment i at time t , $\dot{I}_i$ is the rate of intake of activity outside the system into compartment i at time t . $\lambda_{(i-1,i)}$ is the rate constant for transfer of radionuclides from compartment $i-1$ to compartment i and λ_i is the rate constant for loss or excretion of radionuclides from compartment i . The biokinetic model describing the passage of a substance through the gastrointestinal tract has this configuration. The total number of decays in the different parts of the volume can thus often be analytically calculated.

In general, a biokinetic model describes the distribution of a radionuclide after it reaches the systemic circulation and its excretion from the human body instead of assuming an instant organ uptake of the administered activity as is done in the descriptive model described above. This makes the systemic biokinetic compartments models more complex and time-consuming to create than descriptive models. ICRP have also defined standardized biokinetic models to help create compartmental models if there is a lack of data. For example, measurement of activity in samples of faeces are preferable, but faeces collection is often considered unpractical. But all models should strive to be based on real measurements if it is possible and to use ICRP standardized models when needed.

3.5.1.3 Dosimetry Model for the Skeleton

The skeleton s compiled by an intricate pattern of different cell types and tissues of different densities, a complex mixture of bone and marrow. The bone, which has a density of 2.2 kg/dm³ may be either cortical or trabecular. A bone consists of an outer shell, the cortex, with part or all of the inner space occupied by a network of fine bone spicules and lamellae called trabecular or spongy bone. In the shaft of the long bones, the cortex is thick. The end of the long bones and the vertebral bodies consist of trabecular bone structure with a thin cortical shell. The bone marrow fills the spaces in the trabecular structure.

For radiological protection two cell populations have been identified as relevant for stochastic biological effects. The hematopoietic stem cells, that is the active or red bone marrow, and the osteoprogenitor cells, which are assumed to be located along the surface of the bone trabeculae and Haversian canals, now identified as the endosteal bone surfaces. With the introduction of the new ICRP/ICRU voxel phantom, the thickness of the endosteal surfaces was defined to be 50 µm [18] instead of the earlier assumption, 10 µm. The marrow cavities are typically 100–1000 µm [28]; this varies between different bones. Remaining tissues: the mineral bone and the yellow marrow are not considered as radiosensitive. The change of definition of surface thickness had a great impact on the calculated doses for the skeleton. Earlier data seems to have strongly overestimated the dose to the surfaces for a source in cortical bone, when the source is in trabecular bone, the dose is similar.

The cortical bone is hard and compact, and it is estimated to constitute about 80 per cent of the total skeletal mass in adults. Regarding the endosteal surfaces, only 40 per cent of the mass is associated with the cortical bone [20]. Since bone is not a homogeneous tissue, non-penetrating radiation also will distribute its energy in different types of cells. The various structures of cortical and trabecular bone implies that the fractional distribution of energy, also from particles and low-energy photons, varies depending on the locations of the source. Since the marrow cavities are found in the trabecular bone, a surface distribution will result in a larger dose to the red marrow, an organ with a relatively high radiosensitivity, leading to a higher effective dose.

The absorbed fractions in the skeleton have been estimated based on Monte Carlo simulations on detailed models of the skeleton [29]. Based on these methods, S-values from bone tissues to red bone marrow and the bone surfaces have been derived [30, 31]. The distribution between cortical and trabecular bone is of interest since one often only knows whether the compound is a bone seeker or a volume seeker. It is then assumed that the activity is homogeneously distributed, either in the volume or on the surface. The given mass ratios of cortical and trabecular bone for adults, 15- and 10-year-old children are 80:20 for bone volume and 40:60 for bone surface [10]. For 5- and 1-year-old children the mass ratios of cortical and trabecular bone are 60:40 for bone volume and 30:70 for bone surface.

For dosimetry of the bone, a first task is to identify the location of the radionuclide source on the surfaces or homogeneously in the volume. It is on the surface of the bone, which is supplied with blood vessels, that the deposition first takes place. The compound will then slowly internalize. Consequently, the radionuclides with shorter half-lives may as default be considered as surface seeker, while those with a longer half-life are assumed to be distributed homogeneously in the bone volume. In ICRP-30 [27] it was stated that, if nothing else is known, radionuclides with a half-life < 15 days should be considered as surface seekers and those with longer half-lives as volume seekers.

ICRP 30: The first step towards a method for calculating the absorbed dose to the sensitive bone tissues was taken in the 1950s by Spiers at the University of Leeds [28]. This resulted in a recommended simple method to calculate the dose, using schematically derived absorbed fractions for non-penetrating radiation that were published in *ICRP-30* [27]. *ICRP-26* [32], which introduced the concept effective dose equivalent, the bone surface was included with its own weighting factor. At that time, of the published MIRD pamphlets [33], only total bone was included as a target and source. This report, which is focused on internal dosimetry for occupational exposure, was the first to address the problem of establishing a method to estimate the absorbed dose-to-bone surfaces, and to red marrow from surface or volume-deposited beta and alpha emitting radionuclides.

3.5.2 General Biological Models

3.5.2.1 Model for the Human Alimentary Tract

A biokinetic and dosimetric model of the gastrointestinal tract was first developed in the mid 1960s [34] and later adopted by the ICRP and published in *ICRP-30* [27]. This model was a catenary compartment model comprised of four compartments: stomach, small intestine, and two compartments for the colon, upper and lower large intestine. First-order kinetics were assumed, even if this is rather far from the physiological reality. The systematic error thus introduced is almost insignificant in comparison with the uncertainties, as well as the great individual variations, in the transit times. Using first-order kinetics facilitates considerably the calculation of the cumulated activity. When the model was updated [35] and published in *ICRP-100* [21], the first-order kinetics remained, even if models involving zero-order kinetics has meanwhile been proposed [36].

This new ICRP human alimentary tract (HAT)-model, shown in Figure 3.3, is much more complex, encompassing more organs and including age- and gender-dependent transfer coefficients. In ICRP terminology, the total uptake to blood from the HAT model is given as a sum of all region's fractions, $f_A = \sum_i f_i$ where f_i is the uptake from each separate compartment HAT-model. So far in nuclear medicine is $f_A = f_{SI}$, but the HAT-model is designed to allow blood uptake from all compartments in the gastrointestinal tract. The transfer rate from the stomach to blood can be calculated as

$$\lambda_{SI,b} = \frac{f_{ST} \times \lambda_{SI}}{f_{ST} - 1}, f_{ST} \neq 1 \tag{3.21}$$

With these equations the TIACs for the different sections of the alimentary tract can easily be calculated with a spreadsheet program. Note also that if the physical half-life is long in comparison to the total transit time, and if there is no uptake to blood $\tilde{a}_i = \lambda_i$. When the uptake to blood is 100 per cent, it follows from these formulas that the substance goes directly to the blood from the stomach without staying in the intestine. This is an unrealistic effect of the first-order kinetics assumption, but a more-sophisticated model may be applied if there is relevant information.

For most radiopharmaceuticals, however, the uptake in blood from the gastrointestinal tract can with few exceptions be assumed to take place only from the small intestine, and the short transfer time through the oesophagus can be neglected. A simplified model to use for most nuclear medicine models is thus comprised of the five catenary compartments in Figure 3.4. The age and gender dependent mean transit times λ^{-1} are presented in Table 3.3. Analytical equations for the number of transfers taking place in the different parts can then be derived for the different compartments, for oral intake as shown below:

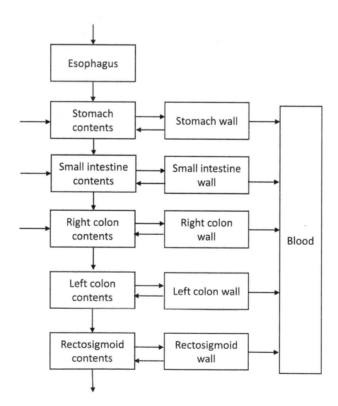

FIGURE 3.3 The human alimentary tract model.

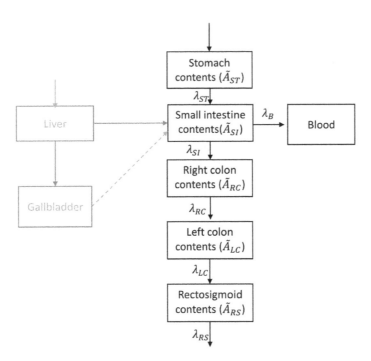

FIGURE 3.4   A simplified HAT-model for the gastrointestinal tract.

TABLE 3.3
HAT-Model, Transit Times

Organ	Adult male	Adult female	Age 5–15 years	Age 1 year
Stomach*	70 min	95 min	70 min	70 min
Small intestine	4 h	4 h	4 h	4 h
Right colon	12 h	16 h	11 h	10 h
Left colon	12 h	16 h	11 h	10 h
Sigmoideum	12 h	16 h	12 h	12 h

Note: * Total diet. For non-caloric liquids the transit time is 30 minutes for all. For caloric liquids it is 45 for all except adult females for which it is 60 minutes.

$$\tilde{A}_{ST} = \frac{1}{\lambda_{ST} + \lambda_p}$$

$$\tilde{A}_{SI} = \tilde{A}_{ST} \times \frac{\lambda_{ST}}{\lambda_{SI} + \lambda_b + \lambda_p}$$

$$\tilde{A}_{RC} = \tilde{A}_{SI} \times \frac{\lambda_{SI}}{\lambda_{RC} + \lambda_p}$$

$$\tilde{A}_{LC} = \tilde{A}_{RC} \times \frac{\lambda_{RC}}{\lambda_{LC} + \lambda_p}$$

$$\tilde{A}_{RS} = \tilde{A}_{LC} \times \frac{\lambda_{LC}}{\lambda_{RS} + \lambda_p}$$

(3.22)

Where λ_i is the transfer coefficient from compartment i to the next compartment. The transfer rate to blood from the small intestine is denoted λ_b and λ_p is the physical decay constant. The indices in these equations stand for: ST-stomach, SI-small intestine, b-biological uptake to blood, RC-right colon, LC-left colon, and RS-rectosigmoideum. $\tilde{A}_i$ is the time-integrated activity in compartment i.

3.5.2.2 Model for Urinary Bladder and Kidneys

The kidney is the major excretory organ for many radiopharmaceuticals and their metabolites. Radioactivity circulating in blood will thus locally irradiate this organ and particularly the urinary bladder, in which the substances excreted are collected and remain until the bladder is emptied. In contrary to uptakes in most other organs, where the activity is homogeneously distributed, the unique physiology of the kidneys leads to a non-uniform concentration of the radionuclides in the kidneys. In diagnostic nuclear medicine, where the principal interest is to estimate the mean dose, this property of the organ is of minor interest, but for therapy it means that there should be a wide margin between an estimated mean absorbed dose and the dose level where the risk for unwanted radiation effect is significant. Many radiopharmaceuticals are excreted with a short biological elimination half-time to the urine and may cause an absorbed dose to the bladder wall so large that this organ will dominate the effective dose, particularly the renography substances. There is thus a need to improve the accuracy in estimating the dose to the bladder wall. For nuclear medicine patients, the ICRP has hitherto calculated the absorbed dose using a constant voiding period of 3.5 hours for adults and children 10 years of older, for the 5-year-olds 3.0 hours is used and, for younger children, 2.0 hours [9]. A shortened time to first voiding will be a proper way to decrease the dose to bladder.

In former MIRD phantoms [5] as well as for the new ICRP/ICRU voxel phantom, the mass of the bladder volume is assumed to be a constant 200 g, and the shape spherical or near spherical. MIRD has assumed the surface dose of the volume as a substitute for the average dose to the wall. This overestimates the absorbed dose in comparison with the *ICRP-133* [19] typically a factor 2 to 3 for common diagnostic radiopharmaceuticals. For pure low-energy beta-emitters such as ^{14}C and ^{3}H the overestimation is larger up to 2 to 3 orders of magnitude, while the dose from a high-energy beta emitter such as ^{32}P is underestimated by a factor of five.

The kidneys have, as default, a mean transit time of 5 minutes. This will give a small, but sometimes significant, absorbed dose to the kidneys from the excretion process; the TIAC becomes

$$a_k = f_k \frac{1 - e\left(-\lambda_p \bar{T}_k\right)}{\lambda_p} \sum_i a_i \frac{\lambda_i}{\lambda_i + \lambda_p} \qquad (3.23)$$

3.5.2.3 Calculating the Cumulated Activity in Urinary Bladder

The cumulated activity in the urinary bladder can be calculated analytically, provided that the excretion to urine from an organ follows first-order kinetics. Let $A_1(t)$ be the activity at time t in an organ with a transfer factor to the urine λ_1. As a first approximation assume that the delay in the kidneys can be neglected, the activity in the urinary bladder with no voiding $A_u(t)$ can be obtained by solving the equation

$$\frac{dA_u(t)}{dt} = A_{(1,0)} \lambda_1 e(-\lambda_{e_1} t) - \lambda_p A_u(t) \qquad (3.24)$$

Where $A_{1,0}$ is the initial activity in the organ, λ_p is the physical decay constant, and $\lambda e_1 = \lambda_1 + \lambda p$ is the effective decay constant. Introducing a constant voiding interval and a fractional uptake a_1 in the organ the number of decays per activity unit, the TIAC is obtained as

$$\tilde{a}_u = a_1 \times \left[\frac{1}{1 - e^{(-\lambda_e t_v)}} \right] \times \left[\frac{1 - e^{-\lambda_e t_v}}{\lambda_p} - \frac{1 - e^{(-\lambda_e t_v)}}{\lambda_e} \right] \qquad (3.25)$$

This equation may be used to calculate the cumulated activity in the bladder. For radionuclides with a physical half-time that cannot be considered as very long in comparison with the mean transit time in the kidneys normally $T_k = 5$ minutes, the equation should be corrected by multiplying with $k = \exp(-\lambda_p \times \bar{T}_K)$. Together with the requirement that the initial bladder activity equals zero, the solution to Equation 3.23 is

$$A_u(t) = A_{(1,0)}\left(e^{(-\lambda_p t)} - e^{(-\lambda_e t)}\right) \qquad (3.26)$$

This equation is then integrated over the time interval $[0, t_v]$, where t_v is voiding interval.

$$\tilde{A}_{(u,1)} = \int_0^{t_v} A_u(t)dt = A_{(1,0)}\left(\frac{1 - e^{(-\lambda_p t_v)}}{\lambda_p} - \frac{1 - e^{(-\lambda_e t_v)}}{\lambda_e}\right) \qquad (3.27)$$

This is the total number of transformations bladder for the time interval. To obtain the total number of transformations in the bladder from activity distributed in the organ considered, one has to repeat the integration, adjusting the initial constant $A_{1,0}$ for physical decay and biological excretion:

$$\tilde{A}_u = \sum_{n=0}^{\infty}\left[\left(A_{1,0} \times e^{-\lambda_e \times n \times t_v}\right) \times \int_0^{t_v} A_u(t)dt\right] \qquad (3.28)$$

3.5.2.4 Dynamic Bladder Model

There are a number of approximations that have been done to calculate the dose to the urinary bladder wall from a source in the content. The most obvious one is to assume a constant volume and spherical shape of the bladder. Both the earlier MIRD phantoms as well as the ICRP/ICRU voxel phantom [18] assume a fixed urinary bladder with a fixed volume and shape. For occupational calculations the rate of elimination from the bladder is taken to be 12 d⁻¹. However, for diagnostic radiopharmaceuticals, which are designed to have a rapid excretion to the urinary bladder, the calculations are performed for a static urinary bladder with a constant voiding interval of 3.5 hours with complete activity emptying at each voiding [10]. For absorbed dose calculations to the wall of the bladder from non-penetrating in the content it has been assumed that this may be approximated with the surface dose, which is half the dose in the centre of the volume. This approximation will slightly overestimate the mean absorbed dose to the bladder. For therapy the dose to the inner surface of the wall is of interest, but in diagnostic nuclear medicine, for calculation of the effective dose it is important to use the average dose.

Instead of using static urinary bladder volumes and fixed time intervals, the calculations can be based on a dynamic bladder that changes with times and is based on biological parameters. MIRD has in one of the pamphlets published a dynamic bladder wall [37], where the parameters are inflow of urine and its variation over the day and night. Also, S-values for different filling rates were published [38].

A dynamic model should preferably include the following parameters:

- Excretion rate
- Urine production rate, for day and night
- Initial volume
- Voiding volume
- Residual volume

A common assumption is to keep the mass of the bladder wall constant, while the volume of the content varies with time, and thus also the $S_{(wall \leftarrow volume)}$-value will change depending on the thickness of the wall and the volume of the content. In the program IDAC version 2.2 [39]. There is a module that calculates the absorbed dose to the bladder wall based on a dynamic model given parameters as shown above.

3.5.2.5 Model for Excretion via the Gall Bladder

In nuclear medicine it is not uncommon that the labelled radionuclide is excreted via the liver and gall bladder to the intestine. The gall bladder is included as one of the 13 remaining organs included in the calculation of the effective dose according to the definition in *ICRP-103* [40]. The gall bladder wall and content are also organs identified in the ICRP/ICRU voxel phantom [19] (for internal dosimetry). In order to standardize the way of calculating the gall bladder dose, the ICRP has defined a "biokinetic and dosimetric" model [7, 10]. This model defines an emptying pattern for the gall bladder content, and it also defines a default fraction of the activity in the liver passing to the intestine via the gall bladder or directly to the small intestine. If nothing else is known it may be assumed the 35 per cent of the activity in the liver is transferred to the gall bladder, while the remaining 65 per cent goes directly to the intestine without passing the gall bladder. The gall bladder collects the substance [7, 10] and empties its content to the duodenum in connection with food intake [10]. For the purpose of dosimetry, ICRP has assumed that this takes place at 3, 9, and 24 hours after administration, transferring 75 per cent of the activity at the first two occasions while after 24 hours the emptying is complete (100%). Thereafter, it is assumed that no more transfer of activity to the intestine takes place via the gall bladder. This latter assumption is justified by the fact that the biological half-time for these substances normally is considerably smaller than 24 hours. As the voiding is complete radionuclides with long physical half-life will not contribute to the gall bladder dose.

The number of transformations in the gall bladder can be calculated by integrating Equation 3.27 in three steps, 0–3 hours, 3–9 hours, and 24 hours – infinity. This is similar to how the number of transformations in the different parts of the colon can be calculated. Activity in the gall bladder also leads to future decays in the intestine, in accordance with the ICRP alimentary tract model.

3.5.2.6 Intrathecal Model

Studies of the flow of the cerebrospinal fluid requires that a radiolabelled tracer is administered intrathecally in the fluid – for example, at cisternography. An anatomical model and flow model, depending upon the injection site, were presented in *ICRP-53*, with further details in Johansson and Nosslin [41]. Two sites of injection are considered, lumbar injection into cisterna terminalis caudalis or cisternal injection into the ventricles of the brain. This biological flow model may be used to estimate the transfer from different cerebrospinal regions to the blood. In addition to the flow model was an anatomical Monte Carlo–simulated model, based on different cylinders and spheres constructed and applied to the two regions to estimate absorbed fraction of energy. The anatomical models presented in *ICRP-53* have later been revised to more anatomically realistic models [42], also based on the 4D XCAT phantoms [43].

3.5.2.7 ICRP Model for the Respiratory Tract

The ICRP lung model has been designed to be used for the inhalation of aerosols. It is intended for occupational or environmental dosimetry, and the use for patients undergoing lung examinations is very limited. For inhalation of radioactive gases another methodology may be used. The model is described in detail in *ICRP-66* [22] with an accompanying supporting publication [44], and *ICRP-130*. In this model the respiratory tracts are divided into different compartments for the lungs and the bronchioles. The deposition pattern of the aerosol between the different compartments depends on the distribution of the aerosol size (AMAD) and is also affected by the physical activity of the exposed person, sleeping, light or heavy exercise, and so forth. After deposition, the activity will be either taken up in the body (blood, lymph) or it is cleared upwards in the in the airways and thereafter swallowed with the consequence that the gastrointestinal tract may be exposed and the activity is excreted this way unless it is absorbed to the blood on its way.

In nuclear medicine, lung studies may be performed either with an aerosol labelled with ^{99m}Tc [45] or the noble gases xenon radioisotopes and ^{81m}Kr; recently, positron emitters also have been used for this purpose [46]. Even if the aerosol used has a defined AMAD and the patient is resting during administration, the inhalation situation deviates significantly from what is an ICRP model (use of a mouthpiece, holding breath, rebreathing, and so forth), so trying to calculate the absorbed dose in that way will not be very successful.

Determining the size of the aerosol particles is important for the dosimetry, since smaller particles go deeper into the lungs when inhaled. For noble gases in the lungs, the dose is mainly due to radioactive transformations in the inhaled gas. For dosimetry of inhaled xenon, the reader is referred to ICRP publications that base their data on an old, but still relevant, studies by Goddard and Ackery [47] and a MIRD report by Atkins and colleagues [48]. For ^{81m}Kr there is also a MIRD report [48]. It is entirely dependent on breath-holding and rebreathing parameters, and activity concentration.

3.5.2.8 Model for Very Short-lived Radionuclides Given Intravenously

For radiopharmaceuticals that have a very short physical half-life (seconds up to a few minutes) for example, ^{82}Rb ($T_{1/2} =$ 1.3 min), the radionuclides will not reach a steady state in the circulating blood. Therefore, the relative blood volume of the different organs is not a representative method for modelling these radionuclides. Instead, the injected substances are assumed to be distributed by a model based on the relative blood flow to various tissues, as a proportion of cardiac output. Leggett and Williams [49] have tabulated blood flow data for most human tissues, and these values have also been adopted in *ICRP-89* [20]. The biokinetic distribution of ^{82}Rb chloride in *ICRP-128* [10] is modelled using the cardiac output values of Leggett and Williams [49].

3.5.2.9   Lacrimal Gland

With the introduction of compounds for PSMA-targeted PET agents, a need has arisen to calculate the dose to the lacrimal glands. An uptake of the substance has been observed in these glands, both with ^{68}Ga and ^{18}F labelled PSMA. These glands are not included as a target in any ICRP report; however, Monte Carlo-calculated S-values are found in the literature [25, 50, 51]. The lacrimal glands are not to be a radiosensitive organ for inducing cancer later in life [40]. However, depending on radionuclide and the amount of decays in the lacrimal glands, the absorbed dose to lens of the eye could be target organ of interest.

3.5.3   EFFECTIVE DOSE

In 1977 the ICRP first introduced the concept "Effective dose equivalent" [32]. The aim was to create a quantity that could be used for radiation protection of workers irrespective of variations of absorbed dose within the body. The limitation of the stochastic risk should be equal whether the irradiation of the body is uniform or non-uniform. To meet this condition, organ-weighting factors representing the proportion of the stochastic risk resulting from the organ to the total risk was derived. The name was later changed to "effective dose" and an updated set of weighting factors was introduced in 1990 [52]. A second revision was published in 2007 [40]. The effective dose equates the risk from an exposure to any part of the body to that of a uniform whole-body dose for a reference person, averaged between the two sexes:

$$E = \sum_T w_T H_T \tag{3.29}$$

H_T is the equivalent dose in tissue/organ T, averages between male and female. For all radionuclides used in nuclear medicine the radiation weighting factor is 1, thus H_T equals D_T, w_T is the so-called tissue-weighting factor.

Even if the initial intention was to calculate an effective dose only for workers the concept soon became used also for patients. It has been shown to be a useful tool, not only for prospective planning and regulation purposes, but also for optimization and justification of nuclear medicine examinations [53]. An important application is for comparison of different methods and possible imaging modalities and to indicate a risk with the examination, which also can serve as an approximate indicator for risk communications in general terms. However, to provide estimates or risk to individual patients goes beyond its intended applications [54, 55].

It may be worth noting that the ICRP calculated and published the effective dose equivalent for patients, or rather normal healthy persons undergoing different diagnostic nuclear medicine diagnostic examinations for the first time in *ICRP-53* [7] as a rough "index of harm". Results from calculation of the effective dose equivalent were published, even for children (using the same weighting factors) for lack of something better.

Stochastic effects are caused by both high and low doses, and are effects observed as a statistically detectable increase in the incidence of cancer or heritable disease occurring a long time after exposure. To estimate the biological effect from a disintegration, the mean absorbed dose is insufficient, on its own, for assessing detriment caused by ionizing radiation exposure, and two correction factors, the radiation weighting factor, w_R, and the tissue-weighting factor, w_T, are applied on the mean absorbed dose.

3.5.3.1   Radiation Weighting Factor

Radiation weighting factors, wR, have been specified in the definition of the protection quantities since *ICRP-60* [40]. They are factors by which the mean absorbed dose in any tissue or organ is multiplied to account for the detriment caused by the different types of radiation relative to photon radiation. The radiation weighting factors are defined largely to reflect the relative biological effectiveness (RBE) for stochastic effects of different types of radiation. There is no standard agreement on the reference radiation for RGB. However, the most common reference radiations are ^{60}Co- or ^{137}Cs-gamma rays or high-energy x rays, > 200 kV [56]. The RGB ratio gives a dose of a low-LET reference radiation to a dose of the radiation considered that gives an identical biological effect. The factors are dose, dose-rate dependent, and also on the biological endpoint of concern. The sex-averaged equivalent dose for tissue T is calculated as

$$H_T = \sum_R \frac{w_R D_{T,RRef.male} + w_R D_{T,RRef.female}}{2} \qquad (3.30)$$

$D_{T,RRef.male}$ and $D_{T,RRef.Female}$ are the mean absorbed dose in tissue T calculated for the ICRP male and female reference individuals for radiation type R. w_R is the radiation weighting factor and H_T is the sex-averaged equivalent dose for target tissue T.

For diagnostic nuclear medicine, only the radiation-weighting factors for photons and electrons are of concern. Photons and electrons are radiations with LET values of less than 10 keV/μm [40]. These radiations have always been given a radiation weighting of 1. The radiation weighting factors allow for including differences in the effect of various radiations causing stochastic effects.

In internal dosimetry, a single w_R value for all photons and electrons is a major simplification. It is important to note that this simplification is only sufficient for the intended application of assessing effective dose. For very low-energy electrons such as those from Auger electron emitters (like ^{51}Cr, ^{67}Ga, ^{99m}Tc, ^{111}In, and others) and bound to DNA, ICRP acknowledges that a larger radiation weighting factor may be appropriate, even if no specific value is recommended. Therefore, the equivalent dose is only an intermediate step in the calculation of effective doses. Exposure limits, constraints, and reference levels in relation to stochastic health effects are set in terms of effective dose. Equivalent dose has previously been used to specify limits for the avoidance of tissue reactions, but these are more appropriately set in terms of absorbed dose (Gy) [23].

3.5.3.2 Tissue-weighting Factor

The tissue-weighting factors are based on the result from extensive studies on survivors from Hiroshima and Nagasaki, together with other epidemiological studies. These data have been used to determine the risk/probability for fatal and non-fatal cancer. Also, a risk for hereditary effects is included in the effective dose concept. The development of the quantity effective dose has made it possible to compare the exposure from different radiation sources; it has also made a very significant contribution to radiological protection as it has enabled doses to be summed from whole and partial body exposure from external radiation of various types and from intakes of radionuclides. The tissue-weighting factors take into account the different relative radiosensitivities of the various organs and tissues in the human body.

The tissue-weighting factor is defined to reflect the relative contribution from the organ and tissue to the total detriment of stochastic effects, which is the total harm to health experienced by an exposed group and its descendants. The latest set of tissue-weighting factors, published in *ICRP-103* given in Table 3.4 are sex- and age- averaged values, and it is stressed that the application of these factors is restricted to the effective dose definition and not used for the assessment of individual risk.

Since the use initially was intended for radiation protection of workers, the tissue-weighting factor reflected the risk for adults 18–65 years of age. One has to be aware of the uncertainty in converting "effective dose" to risk, and in particular it is strongly recommended not to use the concept for individuals

3.5.3.3 Calculating the Effective Dose

In the *ICRP-103* [40], the method for calculating the effective dose is described. This requires the calculation of absorbed dose to 12 organs with specific weighting factors, see Table 3.4, and additionally 14 organs that constitutes

---

TABLE 3.4
Tissue-weighting Factors [40]

Tissue	w_T
Red bone marrow, Colon, Lung, Stomach wall	0.12
Breast, Remainder tissues*	
Gonads	0.08
Urinary bladder, Oesophagus, Liver, Thyroid	0.04
Endosteal bone, Brain, Salivary glands, Skin	0.01

Note: *Remainder tissues: Adrenals, Extrathocasic region, Gall bladder, Heart wall, Kidneys, Lymphatic nodes, Muscle, Oral mucosa, Pancreas, Prostate (male), Small intestine, Spleen, Thyroid, Uterus/cervix (female).

the remainder are given in a footnote. The weighting factor for the remainder is applied to the arithmetic average of the absorbed dose to the 13 organs for each sex. This means that a weighting factor $0.12/13 \approx 0.00923$ is applied to each of the organs listed.

The calculation has to be based on the standard anatomy described by the ICRP/ICRU reference voxel phantom for males and females. It may be noted that the ICRP/ICRU voxel phantoms and the biokinetic/dosimetric models presented by ICRP represents normal persons. The weighting factors are derived from cohorts of both men and women, they are thus averaged between the sexes. In the *ICRP-103* scheme, (1) Calculate the sex-specific dose to all the organs in Table 3.4, including remainder; use SAFs for male and female, and possible different biokinetics. (2) Sum the weighted absorbed doses for males and females separately using the same weighting factor (except prostate and uterus). (3) The average of these is the effective dose.

Example 5. Calculate the effective dose for 1 MBq oral administration of medium thyroid uptake of ^{131}I.

Absorbed doses are calculated with IDAC-Dose2.1 [12] using the biokinetic iodine model of Leggett [57]. Following Fig. 2, in *ICRP-103* [40] using the data in Table 3.5, the effective dose can be calculated as

$$E = \sum_T w_T H_T = \sum_T w_T \sum_R \frac{w_R D_{T,R\,Ref.male} + w_R D_{T,R\,Ref.female}}{2} = 16\,mSv$$

there $H_T^{Male} = \sum_R w_R D_{T,R\,Ref.male}$ and $w_R = 1$ for both electrons and photons.

TABLE 3.5
Dose Table for 1 MBq Oral Administration of Medium Thyroid Uptake of ^{131}I

Organ	H_T^{Male} [mGy]	H_T^{Female} [mGy]	H_T [mGy]	w_T	$H_T * w_T$
Red bone marrow	2.0E-01	2.4E 01	2.2E-01	0.12	2.6E-02
Colon wall	6.7E-02	6.4E-02	6.6E-02	0.12	7.9E-03
Lungs	2.9E-01	3.3E-01	3.1E-01	0.12	3.7E-02
Stomach wall	5.8E-01	5.9E-01	5.9E-01	0.12	7.0E-02
Breast	6.4E-02	1.4E-01	1.0E-01	0.12	1.2E-02
Remainder tissues*	3.7E-01	4.5E-01	4.1E-01	0.12	4.9E-02
Gonads	1.9E-03	5.9E-02	3.0E-02	0.08	2.4E-03
Urinary bladder wall	1.2E-01	1.3E-01	1.3E-01	0.04	5.0E-03
Oesophagus	2.2E+00	2.5E+00	2.4E+00	0.04	9.4E-02
Liver	1.4E-01	1.6E-01	1.3E-02	0.04	6.0E-03
Thyroid	3.6E+02	4.4E+02	2.4E+01	0.04	1.6E+01
Endosteum (bone surface)	1.0E-01	1.3E-01	1.2E-01	0.01	1.2E-03
Brain	5.9E-02	8.9E-02	7.4E-02	0.01	7.4E-04
Salivary glands	4.4E-01	6.9E-01	5.7E-01	0.01	5.7E-03
Skin	5.7E-02	7.2E-02	6.5E-02	0.01	6.5E-04
* arithmetic average of the organs given in Table 3.4.	Effective dose ($\sum H_T * w_T$)				= 1.6E+01 mSv

3.6 CHILDREN

3.6.1 BIOKINETIC DATA

To account for a usually faster metabolism in children, the age dependency of these models may be adjusted for by a shorter biological half-time. Since often the specific biokinetic data for children are not known, this may in many cases justify the use of adult biokinetic model as a basis for the calculation of absorbed dose for children. However general models for the urinary bladder and alimentary tract are age-dependent, and so is the dosimetric model for the skeleton (see sections 5.1.3, 5.2.1 and 5.2.2).

3.6.2 DOSIMETRY

The ICRP/ICRU phantoms for children are supposed to be used when calculating organ-absorbed doses for children of different ages for radiation protection purposes. SAFs for children of different ages has also been calculated based on former mathematical phantoms and published as Oak Ridge reports [58]. The effective dose is designed for adults only [40]. However, as an indication of risk it has been used also for children (see *ICRP-128*). The effective dose from a ^{99m}Tc labelled substance to a 15-year-old is about 30 per cent larger than for an adult. Assuming that the same biokinetic data and activities are used for 10-, 5-, and 1-year-olds, the effective dose is typically a factor of 2, 3, and 5 times higher, respectively, than for an adult male. The use of different risk coefficients for adults and pre-adults can make an effective dose a better instrument for the description of the relative radiation detriment of an examination than just the effective dose [59]. Even if the type and energy of radiation varies, similar data may also be taken as typical also for other radionuclide labels.

Children are more radiosensitive to radiation than adults, and administered activity should therefore be tailored to the patient's size or age. Both the SNMMI [60] and EANM [61] have for several radiopharmaceuticals weight-based recommended administered activity levels for paediatric examinations. Recommendations, which also have been harmonized between the two organizations [62, 63], are calculated based on a radiopharmaceutical specific baseline activity multiplied with a weight and class specific coefficient. However, there is always minimum recommended activity for each radiopharmaceutical. To facilitate the recommendations of weight-based administered activities, have both SNMMI and EANM pre-printed dose cards and also created dedicated online calculators that are easy to access and use [64, 65].

3.7 DOSE TO EMBRYO AND FOETUS

The unborn child is recognized as being sensitive to radiation, and special care is to be taken for pregnant women who need to be investigated with radiological methods. It is important that the clinic has routines to safely avoid exposing the foetus in a pregnant mother – that is, in advance, to ensure that women in fertile age are not pregnant and take proper measurements if this is the case. Often, other methods than nuclear medicine are preferred in those cases. Also, unless the uterus is located in the direct radiation field, ordinary X-ray is preferred from a radiation protection point of view.

However, if for medical reasons a nuclear medicine examination of a pregnant woman cannot wait, then special care should be taken to keep the foetus dose as low as possible. Accurate optimization of the imaging is important. A foetus will always be exposed from radiation originating in its mother's body. Many radiopharmaceuticals are excreted via the urine and, since the urinary bladder is close to the uterus external radiation, will contribute significantly to the dose to the foetus.

Fortunately, most radiopharmaceuticals are not actively taken up in the foetus due to the placenta barrier. However, radiopharmaceuticals composed of relatively small molecules may transfer the placenta barrier and thus enter the body of the unborn child. This is the case for the simple ionic forms of radionuclides, for example, fluoride, pertechnetate, iodide, and so forth. [66]. Also, ^{18}F-FDG have been to cross the placenta barrier [67]. Of special interest in this case is iodine radionuclides, which can concentrate in the thyroid of the foetus and there cause an unacceptable local high dose, not only as a result of therapeutic activities, but also from diagnostic investigations [68]. Giving ^{131}I to a pregnant woman may cause severe deterministic effects on the foetal thyroid.

3.7.1 CALCULATION

In its publications, ICRP has considered the absorbed dose to the embryo to be similar to the dose to the uterus. At this stage the embryo weight is less than 10 g and closely associated with the tissue of the uterus [69]. The absorbed dose to the foetuses from radioactive substances without placental transfer is also expected to be in the same range as the dose to the uterus. For radiopharmaceuticals with placental transfer as a first approximation, can use absorbed dose to organs and tissues of the mother. For substances in their ionic form, a comprehensive compilation of doses to the embryo and foetuses is found in *ICRP-88* [69].

S-values and/or absorbed fractions for foetuses at different gestation ages may be found in the literature [70–73]. Those have generally been produced with Monte Carlo methods based on various human-like phantoms. These phantoms provide the possibility to create more realistic absorbed dose calculations based on specific radiopharmaceutical data. The ICRP are also currently working with the revision of *ICRP-88*, which can provide new biokinetic data to be included in the calculations.

3.7.2 Dose to Breast-fed Infants

One has to pay particular attention to lactating patients who undergo a nuclear medicine investigation. Activity given as a radiopharmaceutical to a breast-feeding mother will for some radionuclides be to a significant degree excreted in the breast milk, causing exposure to the baby unless countermeasures are taken. As many radiopharmaceuticals are secreted in breast milk, it is safest to assume that, unless there are other data to the contrary, that at least some activity will be found in the breast milk when the radiopharmaceutical is given to a lactating female. Particularly substances for which free pertechnetate or iodide is released during the metabolism may show a high uptake in the breast milk. The fraction of excreted activity has been studied by several authors [74] and, also, the ICRP has given recommendations in this matter [10]. For calculation it is usually assumed that the radionuclide is in an ionic form. It should also be noted that the uptake from the intestine in newborns may be higher than in adults. For dose to the infant, see section 6.2 for children.

Reference data on foetal doses in occupational radiation protection are given in *ICRP-95* [75]. Absorbed dose estimates and recommendations regarding radiological protection of foetuses of occupationally exposed women are also available [76].

3.8 ESTIMATION OF DOSES FOR ORGANS SIGNIFICANTLY DEVIATING FROM "REFERENCE MAN"

In nuclear medicine diagnostic studies, it is obvious that for some investigations a large portion of the patients suffer from some disease that includes abnormal functioning of a specific organ. The biokinetics and also the size/mass of the organ might have been affected. The substances and studies are designed to discover these abnormalities. Even if deviations from normal individuals is accounted for in the calculation of the effective dose, it may still be of interest to get an estimation of the absorbed organ dose. Since the same abnormality will probably be found for a larger number of patients, absorbed doses for some common deviations from normal organ mass and uptake have been included in ICRP nuclear medicine publications [7, 10]. Examples of such pathological variations are:

- Impaired renal function, or renal blockage, for patients undergoing renography or any study where a large fraction of the activity will be rapidly excreted in the urine.
- Diffuse parenchymal liver disease will affect biokinetics and mass of liver and spleen.

Data for "standard pathological" states are presented, for example, in the *ICRP-53* [7] and *ICRP-128* [10]. When uptake or excretion rates are affected, an alternative set of TIACs may be calculated. If the organ mass deviates significantly, a first approximation is to estimate the organ dose considering only self-irradiation of the non-penetrating radiation. This is acceptable since the requirement for accuracy in the in those cases is comparatively low due to large individual variations.

Example 6: Administration of large colloids (100–1000 nm). A diffuse parenchymal liver disease will lead to a decreased uptake in the liver, while the uptake in spleen and red marrow increases. While the mass of the red marrow remains unaffected, the illness will first increase the mass of liver 30 per cent, but as the disease advances the mass instead decreases to about 75 per cent of its normal value. The mass of the spleen, however, increases to more than double in size for advanced disease. How this affects the absorbed dose for ^{99m}Tc labelled large colloids is illustrated in Table 3.6. In Table 3.6 the absorbed dose to liver, spleen and red marrow for abnormal and normal mass of liver and spleen, respectively, has been calculated using IDACDose2.1 [12].

For a normal kidney, the mean transit time is typically 4 or 5 minutes. For an impaired renal function, the ICRP has assumed that it is 20 minutes, and that a fraction is also taken up in the liver. For the case of acute unilateral renal blockage,

TABLE 3.6
Absorbed Dose per Unit Activity mGy/MBq

Organ	Liver			Spleen			Red marrow		
Status	Mass (g)	Uuptake	Dose mGy/MBq	Mass (g)	Uptake	Dose mGy/MBq	Mass (g)	Uptake	Dose mGy/MBq
Normal	2360	0.70	0.060	228	0.10	0.61	1394	0.10	0.0093
Early to intermediate	3147	0.50	0.035	336	0.20	0.83	1394	0.15	0.012
Intermediate to advanced	1836	0.30	0.034	537	0.30	0.85	1394	0.25	0.017

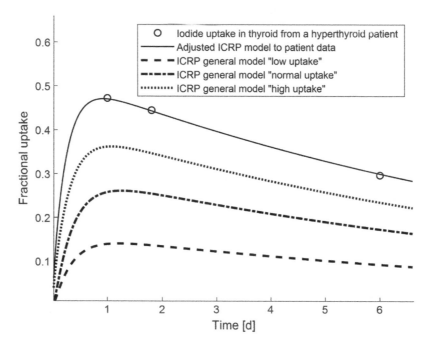

FIGURE 3.5 Radioactive [131]Iodide in thyroid. The three data points are measured fractional activity of ^{131}I of a Graves' patient. The four lines are three different values of thyroid uptake of inorganic iodide adjusted in the time-dependent ICRP biokinetic model.

i.e. sudden blockage in one of the tubes (ureters), ICRP assumes that half of the administered radiopharmaceutical is taken up by the blocked kidney and slowly transferred to the blood with a half-time of 5 days, and subsequently excreted by the other kidney, which is assumed to function normally.

Thyroid uptake of iodide is both dependent on the dietary intake of iodide and the levels of thyroid hormones thyroxine (T4) and triiodothyronine (T3). In patients with hyperthyroidism (overactive thyroid), these hormone levels will be increased. As a result of this condition, adjustment of thyroid uptake in the iodide compartment could be needed to better estimate the iodide uptake in both the thyroid and other organs and tissues. The ICRP have in its Publication 128 [10] three different uptake levels of iodide in thyroid from blood. Low 0.17 h^{-1}, normal 0.30 h^{-1} and high 0.48 h^{-1}. However, as shown in Figure 3.5, adjustments to, for example, measured fractional uptakes of a hyperthyroid patient, these three levels are not in this case representative of these measurements. Instead, an uptake rate of iodide from blood to thyroid of 0.675 h^{-1} would be more representative. For patients, the thyroid deviation might result in organ doses more than two times higher than those for a "normal" person [77]. Patient-specific dosimetry is thus needed, primarily for estimations of the absorbed dose to the thyroid but, also, to take into account the patient-specific absorbed dose to non-target organs.

3.8.1 Dose Estimations when the Radionuclide Is Known to be Heterogeneously Distributed in an Organ

3.8.1.1 Kidneys

Some radiopharmaceuticals are known to be taken up heterogeneously in normal organs. For example, DMSA is taken up in the kidney cortex. In MIRD Pamphlet No. 19, Bouchet and colleagues [78] present S-values useful for a more accurate absorbed dose estimation for the kidneys in these cases – particularly if there is an interest in maximum dose in the kidneys, which is the case in nuclear medicine therapy. The difference in the mean organ dose that is relevant for radiation protection purposes is insignificant for common diagnostic substances, even if the absorbed dose to the kidney cortex is about 30 per cent higher than the average.

3.8.1.2 Brain

There are substances designed for molecular imaging of different parts of the brain. Those compounds may often be labelled with ^{123}I or ^{18}F. Also, in this case, MIRD has published a set of S values [79]. Even if in these cases the mean absorbed dose to the brain also has to be calculated for the effective dose, the altered source configuration will affect the average dose to the whole organ to some degree. The effect is, however, rather small and normally any inhomogeneous distribution can be neglected for calculation of the effective dose. If the S-value for total brain as a source is used, this will underestimate the mean absorbed dose by approximately 10 per cent if the source is located in the caudate nuclei, a structure located in the centre of the brain. On the other hand, the dose in this small part will be 50–100 times higher than the average, depending on the radionuclide. The caudate nuclei have a mass of around 10 g compared to the brain, which is 1.5 kg. Fortunately, the substance is not concentrated entirely in this part of the brain, or otherwise it would have been an example of when the use of effective dose is less suitable.

Another inhomogeneity that, from a risk perspective, the distribution of the energy deposition within the cell is of interest. Auger electrons have a range in tissue of only a few nanometres – that is, the same order of magnitude as the DNA molecules, which reside in the cell nucleus, resulting in an inhomogeneous distribution of the absorbed energy within the cell, which will affect the biological effectiveness of the absorbed dose. This is of special importance, for example, for radionuclides emitting a significant amount of low-energy electrons, ^{123}I or ^{201}Tl. For estimating the absorbed dose in different parts of the cell, MIRD has calculated S-values that may be used [80].

3.9 COMPARISON INTERNAL DOSIMETRY FOR MEDICAL AND RADIATION PROTECTION PURPOSES

The procedure for dose calculations for occupational exposed workers or for the general public due to radioisotopes in the environment is in principle similar to that of nuclear medicine patients. However, two major differences are the route and mode of intake and the half-lives of common radionuclides of interest.

3.9.1 Radionuclides

As opposed to nuclear medicine, a larger number of radionuclides are relevant for occupational exposures in the nuclear industry, research, and other types of industrial applications. The principal difference is that the physical half-life of those are considerably longer than for radionuclides in nuclear medicine. In diagnostic nuclear medicine, with few exceptions, the half-life is short – often less than a day. The half-life for a number of radionuclides used in the working environment will often have half-lives of several years and since the biological elimination rate of those also often is slow in comparison with the compounds designed for medical use, this means that a slightly different biokinetic models might be needed.

3.9.2 Intake

In diagnostic nuclear medicine the radioactive substance is with few exceptions administered intravenously as bolus. The activity given to the nuclear medicine patient is controlled and very well known.

In a working environment, however, contamination may create a risk for oral intake, or intake via inhalation of an aerosol. Furthermore, unless the source of the intake is discovered and action taken, the intake may become chronic, that is, extended over a longer period. There are a number of unknown factors concerning the internally contaminated individual, which complicates the dose estimation.

- It may not always be clear what radionuclide the worker is contaminated with. Nuclide-specific measurements are then required.
- the amount of activity taken in is unknown or just roughly estimated based in information about handled activity. A better estimation could be obtained from urine and/or whole-body measurements or biological samples.
- uncertainties about the time when the intake took place.
- for a chronic intake, the rate as well as when it started is less known.
- It can also be problematic to determine the route of intake, whether it is inhalation or ingestion.

To estimate the inhaled or ingested activity repeated measurements on excreta and whole-body counting, together with knowledge or assumptions about the intake scenario and biokinetic models can be used.

3.9.3 Biokinetic Models

Biokinetic models intended for occupational dosimetry are found in different ICRP publications for different radionuclides in ionic form [23, 81–83] by applying a biokinetic model, provided that the radionuclide is known. If this is undoable, a rough estimate of the time of integrated activity may be obtained directly from data from the repeated measurements of the total body activity. New ICRP publications also include an electronic dose viewer.

The ICRP inhalation model and the human alimentary tract model are both primarily designed for radiation protection purposes. They are important since the activity often enters through them. ICRP has not designed any specific model for the bladder for occupationally exposed workers. In general, for dose calculations, a first-order kinetics is assumed for predicting the activity in the urinary bladder. The time-integrated activity obtained with a transfer coefficient of 12 d^{-1} is the same as with a voiding interval of 4 hours, if the physical and biological half-lives are long. The exponential model is thus justified since the half-life is very long in comparison with the voiding interval.

3.9.4 Dose Calculations

For a very long physical half-life, and if the biological half-time also is long, when calculating the time-integrated activity it is not realistic to integrate to infinity as for the nuclear medicine patient. The integration time is therefore limited to 50 years for adults or up to an age of 70 years for children. It should also be noted that the dose calculated are the committed dose equivalent and committed effective dose [23, 40]. Furthermore α-particles may be important if present – probably the most important type of radiation. The ICRP/ICRU phantoms are designed to be used for internal dosimetry for radiation protection purposes, irrespective of whether it is for workers or patients. Earlier, the MIRD phantom was often used, as was the *ORNL 5000 Report* [84], when the radionuclides of interest were not included in MIRD *Pamphlet No 11* [17].

A program designed for use in occupational dosimetry is Integrated Modules for Bioassay Analysis (IMBA), a Windows program suite designed for calculating internal occupational doses [85]. It is a commercially available computer program with inherent biokinetic models from earlier ICRP publications [86–88]. The program uses the MIRD mathematical phantom for dose calculations. It is especially useful when the calculation has to be based on data from contamination measurements of urine and biological samples. It also includes parameters necessary for calculating doses from inhalation.

3.9.5 Calculating Organ Doses Using *ICRP-133*

When the ICRP first introduced the concept of "effective dose equivalent" in 1977, the MIRD tables of S-values or absorbed fractions represented the standard method for internal dose calculations. In ICRP-26 a number of organs with weighting factors which at that time were not in the MIRD tables were included – for example, breast and bone surfaces. Different approximative methods thus had to be used to assess the effective dose equivalent [8]. Also, after the revision of the weighing factors in 1990 [52] some approximations still were necessary – for example, to use the thyroid dose as a substitute for the thymus [8].

In 2007, when the ICRP [40] made a second revision on the weighting factors, this was later accompanied by data on specific absorbed fractions to be used for the calculations. These data, which were published in *ICRP-133* [19], was based on a new revised voxel phantom representing an adult male and female described in *ICRP-110* [18]. The

SAF-values in *ICRP-133* [19] are not printed out, but are published digitally as accompanying data files. Phantoms and data for children phantoms of different ages are published in *ICRP-143* [89], and the corresponding SAF values will be published later. The data are supposed to be used together with physical decay data available in *ICRP-107* [14]. Also, the data in *ICRP-107* and *ICRP-110* are available in digital form.

The ICRP/ICRU voxel phantom comprises 43 source regions and 79 target regions. Virtually all organs of interest in radiation protection and diagnostic radiology are accounted for. To make the phantom as versatile as possible, the number of regions exceeds what is normally relevant for dose calculation in diagnostic nuclear medicine. However, in practise, utilizing the SAF data in *ICRP-133* [19] is a rather heavy and comprehensive procedure, and it is hardly done manually, depending on radionuclide and number of organs of interest. Using a spread sheet software, it is possible to extract the most important data from the tables and to estimate the organ-absorbed dose to an accuracy good enough for many applications. A more detailed description of the electronic SAF-files is found in the printed text in *ICRP-133* [19] or the accompanying "readme-file". There is also software [12] freely available on the internet that may be used for calculating organ-absorbed doses and effective dose based on the data in *ICRP-133*.

Besides the use of voxel phantoms instead of a mathematical phantom there are a number of other important differences to consider when using these ICRP tables.

- Specific absorbed fractions are also published for electrons, alpha particles, and neutrons. It can be noted that the SAF > 0 for most organs for electrons even when the targets are well separated from the source: this is due to bremsstrahlung. The dose from bremsstrahlung is small, however, and usually may be neglected.
- The mass of the target organs that are based on the anatomical and physiological data given in *ICRP-89* [20] are in *ICRP-133* [19], both including and excluding blood content. The SAFs are calculated using the mass *including* blood. Earlier published MIRD reports, MIRD *Pamphlet No. 10* [90] and MIRD *Pamphlet No. 5* revised [91], base their data on the organ masses *excluding* blood. Thus, absorbed organ doses calculated based on the *ICRP-133* are slightly lower than doses calculated with these data.
- Blood is included as a source organ.
- There is no organ named "total body", neither as a source nor a target. To calculate the absorbed dose to or from "other tissues" and "total body", a mass weighted average of the SAFs for the remaining organs connected to the circulating blood can be used.
- The target organs' extrathoracic region – lung, colon, and lymphatic nodes – are composed of different defined target regions. To calculate the dose to these organs, specified weighted fractions of the doses to these regions are added; see Table 3.3 in *ICRP-133* [19].
- *ICRP-107* includes the spectral distributions of beta particles [19]. For a more accurate dose calculation these may be used for dose calculations together with the specific absorbed fractions for electrons. Normally, applying the mean energy and total yield will be accurate enough.

To calculate organ doses: For a more detailed description see the mentioned ICRP publications.

(1) Produce .rad and .bet files with the program DECDATA, which accompanies *ICRP-107*. The .bet file is the beta spectrum.
(2) The SAF files accompanying *ICRP-133* can be opened with a spread sheet program.
(3) The first line in the table is a headline containing the energies in MeV, for which the SAFs have been calculated
(4) Identify the lines for the different target–source organ combinations you are interested in.
(5) The SAF for a specific energy may be obtained by interpolating: logarithmic interpolation is usually good enough.

3.10 UNCERTAINTIES

There are uncertainties associated with all aspect of estimations of internal doses to nuclear medicine patients.

The total uncertainty in the estimated dose depends on the uncertainties in the input parameter values. The physical parameters, half-life, energy, and yield – together with the attenuation coefficients for the tissue components involved – are well known for all used radionuclides, and the small uncertainties in these parameters are of minor significance for the total uncertainty [92, 93]. Factors influencing uncertainty in the internal dose calculation are given in Table 3.7.

A major component of the uncertainty arises from great uncertainties in the parameters of the biokinetic model, which relies heavily on the availability of reliable data obtained from measurements [95]. For the calculation of organ

TABLE 3.7
Factors Influencing Uncertainty in the Internal Dose Calculation

Parameter	Factors influencing uncertainty
Physical half-life	Is well known with high accuracy. Radionuclides with short physical half-life may dominate the effective half-life of the substance; this leads to a better accuracy
Yield of photons	No significant contribution to the general uncertainty
Yield of particles	Well known. An exception is the yield of Auger electrons for some radionuclides, which may also be influenced by the chemical binding that involves the radioactive isotope. Since the energy is low this will contribute to the absorbed dose to a non-significant degree. Uncertainty in the risk due to inhomogeneous distribution within the cell nucleus in connection with very short range.
Energy of photons	Well known. Neglectable uncertainty
Energy of particles	Well known. However, if the mean energy of beta particles is used instead of the spectrum, this may introduce a small error, for small organs, or organs with walls.
Mass of organs	If the organ deviates from the reference organ this will be a considerable source of uncertainty. It also depends on whether the uptake is independent of organ mass or not. The dose rate due to self-irradiation by non-penetrating particles or photons is directly proportional to the activity concentration. Target organ masses are included in the specific absorbed fractions and S-values.
S-values, absorbed fractions	For organs with a longer distance between, there may be a significant statistical error in the result of the dose calculation.
Fractional distribution. Uptake	A major contributor to the uncertainty in organ dose
Transfer coefficients, biological elimination rate	Together with the fractional uptakes these parameters dominate source of uncertainty in dose to many organs in the calculated absorbed dose. (±30% for the reference person) [94].

dose to a reference person, it has been estimated that the uncertainty in the radionuclide uptake distribution and retention is ±30 per cent and, for the earlier used anthropomorphic mathematical phantom, the random errors for organ shape and geometry were estimated at ±40 per cent [54]. The recently introduced ICRP/ICRU voxel phantom should have reduced this error, but probably only to a minor degree.

The effective dose calculated according to *ICRP-103* is by definition not subject to uncertainty. This is because the biokinetic models and dose data have been calculated using the ICRP/ICRU reference phantoms representing reference persons and using reference-parameter values. Even if a biokinetic model is a rough mathematical approximation of complex biological and physiological processes, those parameter values are by definition fixed numbers without uncertainties. The results of these calculations are intended for regulatory purposes.

Inter- and intra-individual biological variability contributes to the uncertainty of the model outputs. An important source of uncertainty is the limited knowledge of the processes and the lack of data for identifying the models and quantifying their characteristic parameters. Those uncertainties must be taken into account when the absorbed dose is to be assessed individually for some reason – for example, as a parameter for epidemiological studies.

Since, by definition of the effective dose, all organ doses are to be calculated for the ICRP/ICRU phantom and not for the real patient, the anatomical model does not contribute to the total uncertainty.

However, if there is an interest in the organ dose to a specific patient, the individual variability of the anatomy is of great importance. The organ mass will play a dominant role in this case; additionally, the organ mass may also affect the result when assessing biokinetic parameters. In a radiotherapeutic situation, this must be handled in some way, but in diagnostics only the individual variability of the biokinetic – that is uptake and retention of the substance – can be considered.

In total, estimates of absorbed dose to different organs will not generally deviate by more than a factor of three from the actual absorbed dose in patients. The deviation is less for substances with short-lived radionuclides such as ^{99m}Tc. The effective dose is less sensitive than organ doses to variations in the distribution pattern and may vary by a factor of two [54, 96].

3.10.1 Uncertainties in Utilizing the Effective Dose as a Measure of Risk

The effective dose was designed as a tool for estimating risk for the exposed population group. Considerable uncertainties are inherent in the derived weighting factors [40, 54]. The risk coefficient which is derived from epidemiological data of the atomic bomb survivors and other exposed population groups, is developed for normal adults. The age distribution of patients undergoing medical procedures differs considerably from that of the general population, which introduces a systematic error if effective dose is used for risk estimations for different groups of patients. Furthermore, partial or very heterogeneous exposure of organs, which may be the case for many patients, is another source of uncertainty and problematic for the assessment and interpretation of the effective dose. A similar problem occurs when one organ, for example, the thyroid or the urinary bladder, obtains a much higher dose than rest of the body.

3.11 THYROID DOSIMETRY, IODIDE AND PERTECHNETATE

3.11.1 Iodide

The dosimetry of internalized radioactive iodine in its ionic form, iodide, is of interest for occupationally exposed workers, for environmental exposure, and for nuclear medicine diagnosis as well as therapy. This was the first radionuclide intentionally given to a human for medical reasons [97]. Initially ^{128}I ($T_{1/2}$ 25 min), which had been produced with neutron activation, was used for animal experiments to study thyroid uptake but later in the 1940s, ^{131}I was available from Oak Ridge, and the first thyroid uptake measurements in humans and treatment took place [98].

Radioactive iodine constituted a strong incentive to develop methods to calculate the absorbed dose in the thyroid after administration of a radioactive compound. It was early understood that the small mass of the thyroid, together with a seemingly high uptake, would lead to a high absorbed dose. For this reason, a simple anatomical model was used by Evans [99]. This geometrical model enabled an analytical calculation of the energy imparted in the thyroid from particles and photons together with the assumption that 50 per cent of the activity was located in the thyroid with an effective half-life of 5 days. A more sophisticated, but still simple, model had been published by Riggs in 1952 [100] and adopted by ICRP for occupational exposures. [23, 86]

ICRP models for occupational exposures are in general focused on long-lived isotopes, the earlier iodide model is therefore not appropriate to use for ^{123}I, since a too-slow uptake in the thyroid is assumed [101]. The iodide model in ICRP-53 [7] is a simple mono-exponential model with a delayed thyroid uptake designed for dose estimation of the medically used isotopes of iodine. Inorganic iodide that enters the blood is taken up in the thyroid, where it is used for synthesis of hormones. Thus, organically bound iodine is excreted from the thyroid to the blood and distributed in other organs. In a compartment model this chemical form occupies compartments other than the inorganic iodine.

The present biokinetic model for iodide used in nuclear medicine [10] is similar to that for occupationally exposed workers [82], and they are both based on a compartment model by Leggett [57] (see Figure 3.2). The fraction taken up in thyroid depends strongly on the daily dietary intake of stable iodine and therefore, as a consequence, the "normal uptake" varies between different regions of the world [102]. Dose tables therefore vary with which fractional uptake might be assumed for the region in question. In the MIRD publications on iodide dosimetry [103, 104] a normal uptake was set to 15 per cent, which is typical for North America, a region with a relatively high dietary intake of iodine. *ICRP-53* gives dose data for uptakes between 5 and 55 per cent. In the recent nuclear medicine model, three transfer factors to thyroid from inorganic iodine in blood are given – low, medium, and high uptake – corresponding respectively to a fractional uptake of ^{131}I of approximately 16, 26, and 36 per cent after 24 hours [10]. This is accomplished by adjusting the transfer factor from inorganic iodine to the thyroid, 0.30 h^{-1} for the medium uptake, which also is adopted for occupational exposure; a high uptake is obtained with a transfer factor of 0.48 h^{-1} and, for low uptake, a factor of 0.17 h^{-1} is used. With this model, the uptake in the thyroid peaks at about 26 hours, a shorter half-life as, for ^{123}I, the peak comes after about 12 hours with an uptake of 12 per cent. The fractional uptakes given in per cent in ICRP Publication 128 [10] is the fraction that sooner or later is taken up in the thyroid and not the 24 h uptake as in the previous model in ICRP Publication 53 [7]. A 35 per cent uptage in ICRP-128 corresponds to a 26 per cent uptake at 24 h. Figure 3.6 shows the fractional uptake of thyroid retention curves for the intravenous administration of ^{131}I, ^{123}I, and stable iodide.

When substances labelled with radioactive iodine are given to a patient, free iodide is released as a result of metabolism. In order to obstruct unnecessarily high thyroid doses, the uptake in the thyroid can be blocked by administrating

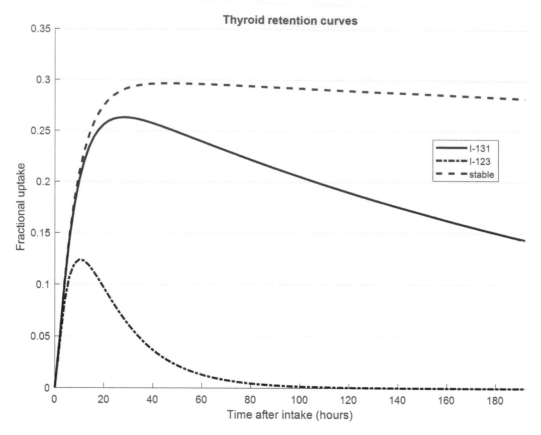

FIGURE 3.6   Fractional uptake in thyroid of intravenously administered ^{131}I, ^{123}I and stable iodide.

stable iodide to the patient. The model for a blocked thyroid may be obtained by setting the transfer factor to organic iodine from inorganic iodide to zero. This leads to a thyroid uptake of only inorganic iodide. This renders a quick uptake of inorganic iodine of only 3.5 per cent after some minutes, falling to < 0.5 per cent by 24 hours. To calculate the total absorbed dose from this substance, the biokinetic model for blocked thyroid should be connected to that of the substance, without the "organic compartments". To calculate the amount of activity released as free iodide – and use this as a starting point for an additional dose calculation – is an acceptable approximation, since the thyroid uptake is fast.

3.11.2 Pertechnetate

Similar to iodine-labelled substances, pertechnetate is released during the metabolism of many technetium-labelled substances. Pertechnetate is also present in the thyroid, but to a much lesser extent than iodide. ICRP has assigned an uptake of 2 per cent in the thyroid. Its physical half-life is shorter, and the biological elimination rate much faster than for iodide. Next to the walls of the gastro-intestinal tract, however, the thyroid receives the highest dose from an intravenous injection of pertechnetate.

A blocking agent, usually potassium perchlorate $KClO_4$, may be given to the patient for the purpose of reducing the dose to the thyroid. For intravenously administered pertechnetate the "normal uptake" in the thyroid is 2 per cent, and with a complete blockage the uptake is set to zero, this will reduce the absorbed dose to the thyroid with a factor of approximately 10. The *ICRP-128* model [10] assumes an immediate uptake in all organs except the intestinal wall. It is accurate enough to calculate the dose contribution from the released free pertechnetate as a fraction of the absorbed dose from the blocked or unblocked pertechnetate model.

3.12 IN MEMORIAM: LENNART JOHANSSON 1951–2020

During the development of this chapter, Professor Lennart Johansson unexpectedly passed away at his home in Umeå, Sweden. Lennart had long-term expertise in this field and was a member of ICRP Task Group 36 on radiopharmaceutical dosimetry since its start in 1981. Lennart was an esteemed researcher and teacher in radiation dosimetry, with applications for patients, professionals, and the general public. He combined deep knowledge in his field with wisdom, kindness, and humility in his contacts with colleagues and in relation to his work.

TABLE 3.8
MIRD Pamphlets, Published by the Society of Nuclear Medicine

No.	Title	Year	Vol:page
1	A revised scheme for calculating the absorbed dose from biologically distributed radionuclides*	1976	-
2	Energy deposition in water by photons from point isotropic sources	1968	Suppl 1
3	Absorbed fractions for photon dosimetry	1968	Suppl 1
4	Radionuclide decay schemes and nuclear parameters for use in radiation dose estimation	1969	Suppl 2
5	Estimates of absorbed fractions for monoenergetic photon sources uniformly distributed in various organ of a heterogeneous phantom. *Revised version published in 1978*	1969	Suppl 3
6	Radionuclide decay schemes and nuclear parameters for use in radiation dose estimation. Part 2	1970	Suppl 4
7	Distribution of absorbed dose around point sources of electrons and beta particles in water and other media	1971	Suppl 5
8	Absorbed fractions for small volumes containing photon-emitting radioactivity	1971	Suppl 5
9	Radiation dose to humans from 75Se-L-selenomethionine	1972	Suppl 6
10	Radionuclide decay schemes and nuclear parameters for use in radiation dose estimation**	1975	-
11	"S," Absorbed dose per unit cumulated activity for selected radionuclides and organs	1975	-
12	Kinetic models for absorbed dose calculations	1977	-
13	Specific absorbed fractions for photon sources uniformly distributed in the heart chambers and heart wall of a heterogeneous phantom	1981	22:65–71
14	A dynamic urinary bladder model for radiation dose calculations. Task Group of the MIRD Committee, Society of Nuclear Medicine. *Revised*	1999	40:102S-23S
15	Radionuclide S values in a revised dosimetric model of the adult head and brain.	1999	40:62S-101S
16	Techniques for quantitative radiopharmaceutical biodistribution data acquisition and analysis for use in human radiation dose estimates.	1999	40:37S-61S
17	The dosimetry of nonuniform activity distributions – Radionuclide S values at the voxel level.	1999	40:11S-36S
18	Administered cumulated activity for ventilation studies.	2001	42:520–6
19	Absorbed fractions and radionuclide S values for six age-dependent multiregion models of the kidney	2003	44:1113–47
20	The effect of model assumptions on kidney dosimetry and response – implications for radionuclide therapy.	2008	49:1884–99
21	A generalized schema for radiopharmaceutical dosimetry – standardization of nomenclature	2009	50:477–84
22	Radiobiology and dosimetry of α-particle emitters for targeted radionuclide therapy (abridged)	2010	51:211–328
23	Quantitative SPECT for patient-specific 3-dimensional dosimetry in internal radionuclide therapy	2012	53:1310–25
24	Guidelines for quantitative ^{131}I SPECT in dosimetry applications	2013	54:2128–8
25	MIRDcell V2.0 software tool for dosimetric analysis of biologic response of multicellular populations.	2014	55:1557–64
26	Joint EANM/MIRD guidelines for Quantitative Lu-177 SPECT applied for dosimetry of radiopharmaceutical therapy.	2016	57:151–62

Notes: * Superseded by: *MIRD Primer for Absorbed Dose Calculations, revised (1991)*
** Eckerman, K. F. and Endo A.: *MIRD: Radionuclide Data and Decay Schemes. 2nd edition.*

REFERENCES

[1] D. Nosske, S. Mattsson, and L. Johansson, "Dosimetry in nuclear medicine diagnosis and therapy," in *Medical Radiological Physics*. A. Kaul, Ed.: Springer-Verlag Berlin and Heidelberg, 2012.

[2] L. D. Marinelli, E. H. Quimby, and G. J. Hine, "Dosage determination with radioactive isotopes; practical considerations in therapy and protection," *Am J Roentgenol Radium Ther*, vol. 59, no. 2, pp. 260–81, 1948.

[3] R. Loevinger, T. F. Budinger, and E. E. Watson, *MIRD Primer for Absorbed Dose Calculations*. Revised Edition, 1991.

[4] W. H. Ellett, A. B. Callahan, and G. L. Brownell, "Gamma Ray dosimetry of internal emitters. Monte Carlo calculations of absorbed dose from point sources," *Br J Radiol*, vol. 37, pp. 45–52, 1964, doi: 10.1259/0007-1285-37-433-45.

[5] W. Snyder, M. Ford, and G. Warner. *MIRD Pamphlet No 5: Estimates of specific absorbed fractions for photon sources uniformly distributed in various organs of a heterogeneous phantom*. (1978). Society of Nuclear Medicine. New York.

[6] ICRP, *Protection of the Patient in Radionuclide Investigations*, ICRP Publication 17, *Ann ICRP*, 1971.

[7] ICRP, *Radiation Dose to Patients from Radiopharmaceuticals*, ICRP Publication 53, *Ann ICRP*, 18 (1–4), 1988.

[8] ICRP, *Radiation Dose to Patients from Radiopharmaceuticals Addendum 2 to 53*, ICRP Publication 80, *Ann ICRP*, 28 (3), 1998.

[9] ICRP, *Radiation Dose to Patients from Radiopharmaceuticals – Addendum 3 to 53*, ICRP Publication 106, *Ann ICRP*, 38 (1–2), 2008.

[10] ICRP, *Radiation Dose to Patients from Radiopharmaceuticals: A Compendium of Current Information Related to Frequently Used Substances*, ICRP Publication 128, *Ann ICRP*, 44 (2S), 2015.

[11] M. G. Stabin and J. A. Siegel, "RADAR Dose Estimate Report: A Compendium of Radiopharmaceutical Dose Estimates Based on OLINDA/EXM Version 2.0," *J Nucl Med*, vol. 59, no. 1, pp. 154–60, 2018, doi: 10.2967/jnumed.117.196261.

[12] M. Andersson, L. Johansson, K. Eckerman, and S. Mattsson, "IDAC-Dose 2.1, an internal dosimetry program for diagnostic nuclear medicine based on the ICRP adult reference voxel phantoms," *EJNMMI Res*, vol. 7, no. 1, p. 88, 2017, doi: 10.1186/s13550-017-0339-3.

[13] ICRP, *Radiological Protection in Therapy with Radiopharmaceuticals*, ICRP Publication 140, *Ann ICRP* 48 (4), 2019.

[14] ICRP, *Nuclear Decay Data for Dosimetric Calculations*, ICRP Publication 107, *Ann ICRP* 38 (3), 2008.

[15] K. Eckerman and A. Endo, *MIRD: Radionuclide Data and Decay Schemes, 2nd Edition*. 2008.

[16] D. E. Raeside, "Monte Carlo Principles and Applications," *Phys. Med. Biol.*, vol. 21, pp. 181–97, 1976.

[17] W. Snyder, M. Ford, G. Warner, and S. Watson. *MIRD Pamphlet No 11: "S," absorbed dose per unit cumulated activity for selected radionuclides and organs*. (1975). Society of Nuclear Medicine. New York.

[18] ICRP, *Adult Reference Computational Phantoms*, ICRP Publication 110, *Ann ICRP*, 39 (2), 2009.

[19] ICRP, *The ICRP Computational Framework for Internal Dose Assessment for Reference Adults: Specific Absorbed Fractions*, ICRP Publication 133, *Ann ICRP*, 45 (2), 2016.

[20] ICRP, *Basic Anatomical & Physiological Data for Use in Radiological Protection – Reference Values*, ICRP Publication 89, *Ann ICRP*, 32 (3–4), 2002.

[21] ICRP, *Human Alimentary Tract Model for Radiological Protection*, ICRP Publication 100, *Ann ICRP*, 36 (1–2), 2006.

[22] ICRP, *Human Respiratory Tract Model for Radiological Protection*, ICRP Publication 66, *Ann ICRP*, 24 (1–3), 1994.

[23] ICRP, *Occupational Intakes of Radionuclides Part 1*, ICRP Publication 130, *Ann ICRP*, 44 (2), 2015.

[24] R. W. Leggett and L. R. Williams, "A proposed blood circulation model for Reference Man," *Health Phys*, vol. 69, no. 2, pp. 187–201, 1995, doi: 10.1097/00004032-199508000-00003.

[25] K. Sandgren *et al.*, Radiation dosimetry of [(68)Ga]PSMA-11 in low-risk prostate cancer patients. *EJNMMI Phys*, vol. 6, no. 1, p. 2, 2019, doi: 10.1186/s40658-018-0239-2.

[26] P. H. Barrett *et al.*, "SAAM II: Simulation, Analysis, and Modeling Software for tracer and pharmacokinetic studies," *Metabolism*, vol. 47, no. 4, pp. 484–92, 1998, doi: 10.1016/s0026-0495(98)90064-6.

[27] ICRP, *Limits for Intakes of Radionuclides by Workers*, ICRP Publication 30 (Part 1), *Ann ICRP*, 2 (2–4), 1979.

[28] F. W. Spiers and G. W. Reed, "Radiation and the Structure of Bone," *Postgrad Med J*, vol. 40, pp. 149–51, 1964, doi: 10.1136/pgmj.40.461.149.

[29] L. G. Bouchet and W. E. Bolch, "A three-dimensional transport model for determining absorbed fractions of energy for electrons within cortical bone," *J Nucl Med*, vol. 40, no. 12, pp. 2115–24, 1999.

[30] K. F. Eckerman and M. G. Stabin, "Electron absorbed fractions and dose conversion factors for marrow and bone by skeletal regions," *Health Phys*, vol. 78, no. 2, pp. 199–214, 2000, doi: 10.1097/00004032-200002000-00009.

[31] L. G. Bouchet, W. E. Bolch, R. W. Howell, and D. V. Rao, "S values for radionuclides localized within the skeleton," *J Nucl Med*, vol. 41, no. 1, pp. 189–212, 2000.

[32] ICRP, *Recommendations of the ICRP*, ICRP Publication 26, *Ann ICRP*, 1 (3), 1977.

[33] R. Adams, *MIRD Pamphlet No 10: Radionuclide Decay Schemes and Nuclear Parameters for Use in Radiation-Dose Estimation (1975)*. Superseded by MIRD Decay Schemes 2nd Edition. (1975). Society of Nuclear Medicine. New York.

[34] I. S. Eve, "A review of the physiology of the gastrointestinal tract in relation to radiation doses from radioactive materials," *Health Phys*, vol. 12, no. 2, pp. 131–61, 1966, doi: 10.1097/00004032-196602000-00002.

[35] R. Leggett, J. Harrison, and A. Phipps, "Reliability of the ICRP'S dose coefficients for members of the public: IV. Basis of the human alimentary tract model and uncertainties in model predictions," *Radiat Prot Dosimetry,* vol. 123, no. 2, pp. 156–70, 2007, doi: 10.1093/rpd/ncl104.

[36] J. B. Stubbs, "Results from a New Mathematical Model of Gastrointestinal Transit that Incorporates Age and Gender-Dependent Physiological Parameters," *Radiation Protection Dosimetry,* vol. 41, no. 2–4, pp. 63–69, 1992, doi: 10.1093/oxfordjournals.rpd.a081231.

[37] S. R. Thomas, M. G. Stabin, C. Chen, and R. C. Samaratunga, "MIRD Pamphlet No. 14: A dynamic urinary bladder model for radiation dose calculations," *J Nucl Med,* vol. 33, pp. 783–802, 1992.

[38] M. Andersson, D. Minarik, L. Johansson, S. Mattsson, and S. Leide-Svegborn, "Improved estimates of the radiation absorbed dose to the urinary bladder wall," *Phys Med Biol,* vol. 59, no. 9, pp. 2173–82, 2014, doi: 10.1088/0031-9155/59/9/2173.

[39] M. Andersson, S. Mattsson, and L. Johansson, "Dynamic absorbed dose calculations to the urinary bladder wall for the ICRP compartmental models of iodide and technetium," *EJNMMI,* vol. 46, no. 1, pp. 281–82, 2019.

[40] ICRP, *The 2007 Recommendations of the International Commission on Radiological Protection,* ICRP Publication 103, *Ann ICRP* (2–4), 2007.

[41] L. Johansson and B. Nosslin, "Dosimetry of intrathecally administered radiopharmaceuticals," in *Proceedings from the fifth international radIopharmaceutical dosimetry symposium CONF-910529,* Oak Ridge, TN, E. E. Watson and A. T. Schlafke-Stelson, Eds., 1991.

[42] J. Y. Hesterman, S. D. Kost, R. W. Holt, H. Dobson, A. Verma, and P. D. Mozley, "Three-Dimensional Dosimetry for Radiation Safety Estimates from Intrathecal Administration," *J Nucl Med,* vol. 58, no. 10, pp. 1672–78, 2017, doi: 10.2967/jnumed.117.190611.

[43] W. P. Segars, G. Sturgeon, S. Mendonca, J. Grimes, and B. M. W. Tsui, "4D XCAT phantom for multimodality imaging research," *Med Phys,* vol. 37, pp. 4902–15, 2010.

[44] ICRP, *Guide for the practical application of the ICRP human respiratory tract model.* Supporting Guidance 3, *Ann ICRP,* 32 (1–2), 2002.

[45] M. Bajc *et al.,* "EANM guideline for ventilation/perfusion single-photon emission computed tomography (SPECT) for diagnosis of pulmonary embolism and beyond," *Eur J Nucl Med Mol Imaging,* 2019, doi: 10.1007/s00259-019-04450-0.

[46] P. Y. Le Roux, R. J. Hicks, S. Siva, and M. S. Hofman, "PET/CT Lung Ventilation and Perfusion Scanning using Galligas and Gallium-68-MAA," *Semin Nucl Med,* vol. 49, no. 1, pp. 71–81, 2019, doi: 10.1053/j.semnuclmed.2018.10.013.

[47] B. A. Goddard and D. M. Ackery, "Xenon-133, 127Xe, and 125Xe for lung function investigations: a dosimetric comparison," *J Nucl Med,* vol. 16, no. 8, pp. 780–86, 1975.

[48] H. L. Atkins *et al.,* "Estimates of radiation absorbed doses from radioxenons in lung imaging," *J Nucl Med,* vol. 21, no. 5, pp. 459–65, 1980.

[49] R. W. Leggett, K. F. Eckerman, and L. R. Williams, "A blood circulation model for reference man," in *Proceedings from the sixth international radiopharmaceutical dosimetry symposium CONF-960536.* Gatlinburg, TN (United States), 7–10 May 1996.

[50] D. Plyku *et al.,* "Combined model-based and patient-specific dosimetry for (18)F-DCFPyL, a PSMA-targeted PET agent," *Eur J Nucl Med Mol Imaging,* vol. 45, no. 6, pp. 989–98, 2018, doi: 10.1007/s00259-018-3939-x.

[51] E. Demirci *et al.,* "Estimation of the organ absorbed doses and effective dose from 68Ga-PSMA-11 PET scan," *Radiat Prot Dosimetry,* vol. 182, no. 4, pp. 518–24, 2018, doi: 10.1093/rpd/ncy111.

[52] ICRP, *1990 Recommendations of the International Commission on Radiological Protection,* ICRP Publication, *Ann ICRP,* 60 (Users Edition), 1991.

[53] H. G. Menzel and J. Harrison, Effective dose: A radiation protection quantity, *Ann ICRP,* vol. 41, no. 3–4, pp. 117–23, 2012, doi: 10.1016/j.icrp.2012.06.022.

[54] C. J. Martin, "Effective dose: practice, purpose and pitfalls for nuclear medicine," *J Radiol Prot,* vol. 31, no. 2, pp. 205–19, 2011, doi: 10.1088/0952-4746/31/2/001.

[55] J. Harrison and P. O. Lopez, Use of effective dose in medicine, *Ann ICRP,* vol. 44, no. 1 Suppl, pp. 221–28, 2015, doi: 10.1177/0146645315576096.

[56] ICRP, *Relative biological effectiveness (RBE), quality factor (Q), and radiation weighting factor (wR),* ICRP Publication 92, *Ann ICRP,* 33 (4), 2003.

[57] R. W. Leggett, "A physiological systems model for iodine for use in radiation protection," *Radiat Res,* vol. 174, no. 4, pp. 496–516, 2010, doi: 10.1667/rr2243.1.

[58] M. Cristy and K. F. Eckerman, *Specific Absorbed Fractions of Energy at Various Ages from Internal Photon Sources.* Report ORNL/TM-8381/V1-V7, Oak Ridge National Laboratory, Oak Ridge, TN, 1987,

[59] S. Mattsson, "Need for Individual Cancer Risk Estimates in X-Ray and Nuclear Medicine Imaging," *Radiat Prot Dosimetry,* vol. 169, no. 1–4, pp. 11–6, 2016, doi: 10.1093/rpd/ncw034.

[60] S. T. Treves, M. J. Gelfand, F. H. Fahey, and M. T. Parisi, "2016 Update of the North American Consensus Guidelines for Pediatric Administered Radiopharmaceutical Activities," *J Nucl Med,* vol. 57, no. 12, pp. 15N–18N, 2016.

[61] F. Jacobs *et al.*, "Optimised tracer-dependent dosage cards to obtain weight-independent effective doses," *Eur J Nucl Med Mol Imaging,* vol. 32, no. 5, pp. 581–88, 2005, doi: 10.1007/s00259-004-1708-5.

[62] S. T. Treves and M. Lassmann, "International guidelines for pediatric radiopharmaceutical administered activities," *J Nucl Med,* vol. 55, no. 6, pp. 869–70, 2014, doi: 10.2967/jnumed.114.139980.

[63] M. Lassmann and S. T. Treves, "Pediatric Radiopharmaceutical Administration: Harmonization of the 2007 EANM Paediatric Dosage Card (Version 1.5.2008) and the 2010 North American Consensus guideline," *Eur J Nucl Med Mol Imaging,* vol. 41, no. 8, p. 1636, 2014, doi: 10.1007/s00259-014-2817-4.

[64] Society of Nuclear Medicine & Molecular Imaging. "SNMMI Pediatric Injected Activity Tool (Version 1.04.2016)." www.snmmi.org/ClinicalPractice/PediatricTool.aspx?ItemNumber=11216&navItemNumber=11219%22. SNMMI Dose Optimization Task Force.

[65] European Association of Nuclear Medicine. "EANM Dosage Calculator," https://www.eanm.org/publications/dosage-calculator/Paediatric and Dosimetry Committees of the EANM, 2020.

[66] J. R. Russell, M. G. Stabin, and R. B. Sparks, "Placental transfer of radiopharmaceuticals and dosimetry in pregnancy," *Health Phys,* vol. 73, no. 5, pp. 747–55, 1997, doi: 10.1097/00004032-199711000-00002.

[67] P. Zanotti-Fregonara *et al.*, "New Fetal Dose Estimates from 18F-FDG Administered During Pregnancy: Standardization of Dose Calculations and Estimations with Voxel-Based Anthropomorphic Phantoms," *J Nucl Med,* vol. 57, no. 11, pp. 1760–63, 2016, doi: 10.2967/jnumed.116.173294.

[68] R. K. Millard, M. Saunders, A. M. Palmer, and A. W. Preece, "Approximate distribution of dose among foetal organs for radioiodine uptake via placenta transfer," *Phys Med Biol,* vol. 46, no. 11, pp. 2773–83, 2001, doi: 10.1088/0031-9155/46/11/302.

[69] ICRP, *Doses to the Embryo and Fetus from Intakes of Radionuclides by the Mother,* ICRP Publication 88, *Ann ICRP,* 31 (1–3), 2001.

[70] T. Xie and H. Zaidi, "Fetal and maternal absorbed dose estimates for positron-emitting molecular imaging probes," *J Nucl Med,* vol. 55, no. 9, pp. 1459–66, 2014, doi: 10.2967/jnumed.114.141309.

[71] C. Y. Shi, X. G. Xu, and M. G. Stabin, "SAF values for internal photon emitters calculated for the RPI-P pregnant-female models using Monte Carlo methods," *Med Phys,* vol. 35, no. 7, pp. 3215–24, 2008, doi: 10.1118/1.2936414.

[72] M. G. Stabin, X. G. Xu, M. A. Emmons, W. P. Segars, C. Shi, and M. J. Fernald, "RADAR reference adult, pediatric, and pregnant female phantom series for internal and external dosimetry," *J Nucl Med,* vol. 53, no. 11, pp. 1807–13, 2012, doi: 10.2967/jnumed.112.106138.

[73] M. Stabin, E. Watson, M. Cristy, et al. *"Mathematical Models and Specific Absorbed Fractions of Photon Energy in the Nonpregnant Adult Female and at the End of Each Trimester of Pregnancy."* Oak Ridge, TN: Oak Ridge National Laboratory; ORNL report ORNL/TM-12907, 1995.

[74] S. Leide-Svegborn, L. Ahlgren, L. Johansson, and S. Mattsson, "Excretion of radionuclides in human breast milk after nuclear medicine examinations. Biokinetic and dosimetric data and recommendations on breastfeeding interruption," *Eur J Nucl Med Mol Imaging,* vol. 43, no. 5, pp. 808–21, 2016, doi: 10.1007/s00259-015-3286-0.

[75] ICRP, *Doses to Infants from Ingestion of Radionuclides in Mothers' Milk,* ICRP Publication 95, *Ann ICRP,* 34 (3–4), 2004.

[76] A. Almén and S. Mattsson, "Radiological protection of foetuses and breast-fed children of occupationally exposed women in nuclear medicine – Challenges for hospitals," *Phys Med,* vol. 43, pp. 172–77, 2017, doi: 10.1016/j.ejmp.2017.08.010.

[77] M. Andersson and S. Mattsson, "Improved Patient Dosimetry at Radioiodine Therapy by Combining the ICRP Compartment Model and the EANM Pre-Therapeutic Standard Procedure for Benign Thyroid Diseases," *Front Endocrinol (Lausanne),* vol. 12, p. 634955, 2021, doi: 10.3389/fendo.2021.634955.

[78] L. G. Bouchet *et al.*, "MIRD Pamphlet No 19: absorbed fractions and radionuclide S values for six age-dependent multiregion models of the kidney," *J Nucl Med,* vol. 44, pp. 1113–47, 2003.

[79] L. G. Bouchet, W. E. Bolch, D. A. Weber, H. Atkins, and J. W. Poston, "MIRD Pamphlet No. 15: Radionuclide S Values in a Revised Dosimetric Model of the Adult head and Brain," *J Nucl Med,* vol. 40, pp. 62S-101S, 1999.

[80] R. W. Howell, "The Mird Schema - From Organ to Cellular Dimensions," *J Nucl Med,* vol. 35, pp. 531–33, 1994.

[81] ICRP, *Occupational Intakes of Radionuclides Part 4,* ICRP Publication 141, *Ann ICRP,* 48 (2/3), 2019.

[82] ICRP, *Occupational Intakes of Radionuclides Part 3,* ICRP Publication 137, *Ann ICRP,* 46 (3/4), 2017.

[83] ICRP, *Occupational Intakes of Radionuclides Part 2,* ICRP Publication 134, *Ann ICRP,* 45 (3/4), 2016.

[84] W. S. Snyder, M. R. Warner, G. G. Watson "Tabulation of Dose Equivalent per Microcurie-Day for Source and Target Organs of an Adult for Various Radionuclides". Oak Ridge, TN: Oak Ridge National Laboratory; ORNL/TM-5000, 1974.

[85] A. Birchall *et al.*, "IMBA Professional Plus: A flexible approach to internal dosimetry," *Radiat Prot Dosimetry,* vol. 125, no. 1–4, pp. 194–7, 2007, doi: 10.1093/rpd/ncl171.

[86] ICRP, *Age-dependent Doses to Members of the Public from Intake of Radionuclides – Part 1,* ICRP Publication 56, *Ann ICRP,* 20 (2), 1990.

[87] ICRP, *Age-dependent Doses to Members of the Public from Intake of Radionuclides - Part 2,* ICRP Publication 67, *Ann ICRP,* 23 (3–4), 1993.

[88] ICRP, *Dose Coefficients for Intakes of Radionuclides by Workers,* ICRP Publication 68, *Ann ICRP,* 24 (4), 1994.

[89] ICRP, *Paediatric Reference Computational Phantoms,* ICRP Publication 143, *Ann ICRP,* 49 (1), 2020.

[90] L. T. Dillman. *MIRD Pamphlet No 5: Revised: Estimates of Absorbed Fractions for Photon Sources Uniformly Distributed in Various Organs of a Heterogeneous Phantom* (1975). Society of Nuclear Medicine. New York.

[91] W. Snyder, M. Ford, and G. Warner. *MIRD Pamphlet No 5: Revised: Estimates of Absorbed Fractions for Photon Sources Uniformly Distributed in Various Organs of a Heterogeneous Phantom* (1978). Society of Nuclear Medicine. New York.

[92] M. G. Stabin, "Uncertainties in internal dose calculations for radiopharmaceuticals," *J Nucl Med,* vol. 49, no. 5, pp. 853–60, 2008, doi: 10.2967/jnumed.107.048132.

[93] B. Breustedt, A. Giussani, and D. Noßke, "Internal dose assessments – Concepts, models and uncertainties," *Radiation Measurements,* vol. 115, pp. 49–54, 2018, doi: 10.1016/j.radmeas.2018.06.013.

[94] C. J. Martin, "Effective dose: how should it be applied to medical exposures?" *Br J Radiol,* vol. 80, no. 956, pp. 639–47, 2007, doi: 10.1259/bjr/25922439.

[95] K. Norrgren, S. L. Svegborn, J. Areberg, and S. Mattsson, "Accuracy of the quantification of organ activity from planar gamma camera images," *Cancer Biother Radiopharm,* vol. 18, no. 1, pp. 125–31, 2003, doi: 10.1089/108497803321269403.

[96] P. B. Zanzonico, "Internal radionuclide radiation dosimetry: A review of basic concepts and recent developments," *J Nucl Med,* vol. 41, pp. 297–308, 2000.

[97] D. V. Becker and C. T. Sawin, "Radioiodine and thyroid disease: the beginning," *Semin Nucl Med,* vol. 26, no. 3, pp. 155–64, 1996, doi: 10.1016/s0001-2998(96)80020-1.

[98] S. Mattsson, L. Johansson, H. Jönsson, and B. Nosslin, "Radioactive iodine in thyroid medicine-How it started in Sweden and some of today's challenges," *Acta oncologica (Stockholm, Sweden),* vol. 45, pp. 1031–36, 2006, doi: 10.1080/02841860600635888.

[99] T. C. Evans, G. Clarke, and E. Sobel, "Increase in I131 uptake of thyroid after whole body roentgen irradiation," *Anat Rec,* vol. 99, no. 4, p. 577, 1947.

[100] D. S. Riggs, "Quantitative aspects of iodine metabolism in man," *Pharmacol Rev,* vol. 4, no. 3, pp. 284–370, 1952.

[101] L. Johansson, S. Leide-Svegborn, S. Mattsson, and B. Nosslin, "Biokinetics of iodide in man: refinement of current ICRP dosimetry models," *Cancer Biother Radiopharm,* vol. 18, no. 3, pp. 445–50, 2003, doi: 10.1089/108497803322285206.

[102] I. A. Zvonova, "Dietary intake of stable I and some aspects of radioiodine dosimetry," *Health Phys,* vol. 57, no. 3, pp. 471–75, 1989.

[103] "MIRD Dose Estimate Report 5: Summary of Current Radiation Dose Estimates to Humans from 123I, 124I, 125I, 126I, 130I, 131I, and 132I as Sodium Iodide," *J Nucl Med,* vol. 16, no. 9, pp. 857–60, 1975.

[104] M. Berman. *MIRD Pamphlet No 12: Kinetic Models for Absorbed Dose Calculations* (1977). Society of Nuclear Medicine. New York.

4 Time-activity Curves

Data, Models, Curve Fitting, and Model Selection

Gerhard Glatting

CONTENTS

4.1 INTRODUCTION

In diagnostic and therapeutic applications of Nuclear Medicine, the knowledge of the pharmacokinetics, that is, the change of the concentration of a radiopharmaceutical with time in the investigated patient's or animal's organs, is essential, as this is the basis for the adequate diagnosis and treatment of the patient.

Specifically, for dosimetry the number of decays in the considered organs or structures are an important input for the calculation of the absorbed doses. This number of decays requires the knowledge of pharmacokinetics, that is, the corresponding activity curve over time (Time-activity Curve, TAC). Based on the TAC the number of decays can be calculated by mathematically integrating the activity curve over time [1, 2]. However, since the activity can regularly only be measured for a few points in time, the complete pharmacokinetics for all points in time must be determined by interpolation between the measuring points and also extrapolation for times outside the measuring points [2, 3].

DOI: 10.1201/9780429489549-4

This interpolation can be performed, for example, using the trapezoidal rule until the last data point. For larger times, a decay with the physical half-life of the used radionuclide can be assumed [2]. Other options are to fit analytical functions, for example, an exponential function, or an appropriate compartmental model function, to the data. However, considerably different results are obtained for the approaches shown in Figure 4.1 [3], demonstrating the relevance of

- choosing an adequate method or function for this interpolation, and
- determining the uncertainty of the result (and thus the possibility of controlling this uncertainty).

The number and temporal sampling of the data together with the noise/uncertainty in the data determine the reliability, that is, the accuracy and precision of the calculated TACs and the time-integrated activities (TIAs) in a source region (Figure 4.1).

Based on the above, a general scheme for the determination of the TACs and the TIAs is shown in Figure 4.2. Data and Models are the input. This input is used to fit the chosen set of models to the data yielding the parameters of each model. Based on the fitting result, then the models most supported by the data can be chosen according to a model selection criterion. These models and their parameter values determine the TACs and, upon integration over time, the TIAs.

In science a result also needs to include a statement on its uncertainty [4]. Therefore, for both, the inputs and the processing steps, it is essential to consider the uncertainties adequately to obtain an accurate and precise result [5].

Clearly, the "garbage in – garbage out" principle applies to the scheme shown in Figure 4.2. However, in contrast to the usual definition that only data serve as input, here also models are an input. Consequently, the use of just "garbage" models will also lead to poor results.

The structure of this chapter is built along Figure 4.2, that is, first the typically available and measured *data* are presented, secondly different types of *mathematical models* used are introduced, thirdly, the *curve-fitting* method is described using both inputs. Fourthly, the *model selection* process is presented followed by the final step, the output of the *TACs and TIAs*, which are based on the selected models and the associated parameters.

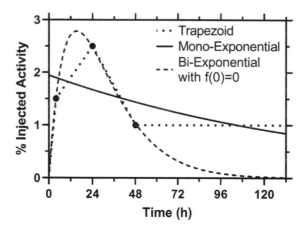

FIGURE 4.1 Schematic view demonstrating different methods for calculating the time-integrated activity in a source region. Assuming that the bi-exponential function corresponds to the actual pharmacokinetics, it becomes also clear that a later measurement of the last data point will substantially change the time-integrated activities obtained from the other functions.

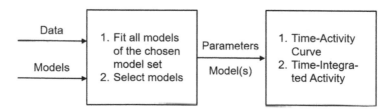

FIGURE 4.2 Scheme of the processes of determining a time-activity curve and its time-integrated activity (see text for explanation).

4.2 DATA

In this section, after a brief remark on data quality, the different types of input data used in determining TACs are discussed.

Generally, for all used data an essential prerequisite is that the data are *accurate*, that is, quantitatively correct with low bias, and *precise*, that is, with a relatively low noise. The wording "low bias" and "low noise" follows from the impossibility of zero bias and noise. Therefore, the uncertainties of the data always need to be controlled during the measurement and considered during the subsequent processing [4].

To determine TACs of an individual organ of interest, *individual data* are necessary [6]. Usually, measurements of the activity for a number of time points are used, but – as stated above – the uncertainty of the data also must be considered [7]. If measured, these uncertainties are also input data for the processing shown in Figure 4.2. Although it frequently happens that solely these activity data for a few time points or time intervals are used [2, 5], depending on the mathematical models used for the definition of the TACs (see Section 4.3, Mathematical Models), additional individual anatomical data like the whole-body or organ weights, the height, the age and/or the sex of the patient may also be used as input data. The same applies for individual physiological data which may have been measured before, like for example the blood flow to, or receptor density in, a specified tumour.

In addition to the above-mentioned individual data, a further type of input data are *population data*. These may be of the same type as individual data, that is, the typical activities and their uncertainty for some time points, or anatomical and physiological data. As these data represent the respective population, they all have an uncertainty measure, which reflects the distribution of the respective data in the population. Such data may be integrated into the TACs calculation as prior knowledge by mixed models [8] or within the Bayesian framework [9]. This prior knowledge may be obtained, for example, from an earlier pilot study with the same radiopharmaceutical applied to patients with the same disease.

Furthermore, the parameters of a possibly used error model (Section 4.3.2, Uncertainty Models) are input data.

Last, *start parameters* for the curve-fitting process also are input data. Although in the best case the result of the fitting process does not depend on the starting values, good starting parameters at least accelerate the convergence of the fitting algorithm. This acceleration becomes particularly relevant in the case of the existence of many local minima of the objective function of the fitting process.

4.2.1 NUMBER OF SAMPLING POINTS

The most important data to determine TACs of an individual organ of interest are measurements of the activity for a number of time points [2]. Each measurement contributes to patient load and diagnosis or treatment costs. Therefore, the number of measurements should be kept low. On the other hand, to ensure low bias and noise in the determination of the TACs, a high number of measurements is advantageous. Thus, the number of measurements used must find a balance between the requested accuracy and the costs (patient load and other resources). Note that, strictly speaking, the requested accuracy also can be defined in principle based on costs: The costs for the patient and for the health system depending on the accuracy of the determination of the TACs, as inaccurate TACs will result in less-effective treatment.

As the exact determination of the costs is ultimately too complex, often the following rules are used: A rule of thumb is that a minimum of 3 sampling points should be chosen per exponential [2, 10]. This presupposes the knowledge of the number of needed exponentials and their half-lives. Another rule, which is compatible with the case of 2 exponentials as it suggests 5 time points, proposes to use the following multiples of the effective, or – in case this is not known – of the physical half-life: 1/5, 1/3, 1, 3, and 5 [11].

A reduction of the number of needed measurements can be achieved using a priori information about the expected kinetics. Depending on the desired accuracy of the result (and the homogeneity of the patient group under investigation), the use of a priori information with an adequate mathematical model may allow for reducing the number of measurements dramatically [8, 12] and even may allow the prediction of the therapeutic biodistribution based on a single quantitative PET or SPECT measurement [13, 14].

4.2.2 TEMPORAL SAMPLING

In addition to the number of measured time points, the selection of the time points to be measured is also of great importance for the accuracy of the result. The example in Figure 4.3 demonstrates – for the ideal case of no measurement error! – a large error depending on the number and time points of the measurements. In this example, this is a consequence of using a wrong fit function. However, it is never possible to use the true fit function, as fit functions always

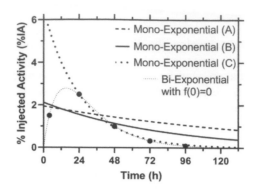

FIGURE 4.3 Different temporal sampling schemes and their influence on the time-integrated activity result. A mono-exponential was fitted to 3 data points as follows: (A) (4, 24, 48) h, (B) (4, 24, 72) h and (C) (24, 48, 96) h yielding the time-integrated activities 308.4%IA h, 164.1%IA h and 163.8%IA h, respectively. The assumed underlying truth is actually described by the shown bi-exponential with the true time-integrated activity = 116%IA h. Note that these large differences are obtained for assumed noise-free measurements.

are assumed to be simple functions compared to the true underlying time-activity curve. Therefore, optimal temporal sampling is a means of improving the accuracy of the TACs for a fixed number of measurements, that is, for approximately fixed costs.

The optimal sampling time points depend on the pharmacokinetics of the substance under investigation. There exists a vast literature on the topic using either sophisticated mathematical approaches [15–17] or just brute force [18, 19]. Since the availability of fast computer power, the latter has the advantage of mathematical simplicity and easy incorporation of constraints like working hours in the clinic [20].

4.3 MATHEMATICAL MODELS

A good definition of what a model is reads as follows: "A model is a construct invented by a researcher to summarize what is known and hypothesized about a system under study" [21]. Therefore, the model is built from different components and their interaction is defined. In a mathematical model the components and their interactions are described by mathematical equations. From this definition it follows immediately that a mathematical model contains information about the system under study. Therefore. it must be ensured that an adequate mathematical model is employed, because a wrong mathematical model – even when used together with valid data – will result in garbage output ("garbage in – garbage out" principle), as demonstrated in Figure 4.3.

On the other hand, mathematical modelling allows for integrating available a priori information by defining a specific model structure based, for example, on well-known anatomical and physiological properties like for example organ volumes and blood circulation. This additional general information contained in such "law-driven" models can help reducing the needed number of individual measurements.

In this section, first the models for describing the biokinetics of radiopharmaceuticals and, second, the different variance models for the input data are presented and discussed.

4.3.1 Pharmacokinetic Models

A pharmacokinetic model is a mathematical description of the distribution of a substance over time [22]. In the following these models are divided into 4 groups:

1. empirical,
2. analytical,
3. compartmental models, and
4. physiologically based pharmacokinetic (PBPK) whole-body compartmental models.

These models include more and more information and, especially the last group, contains detailed anatomical and physiological structures and parameters. As all these models contain assumptions about the underlying physiology – this could be as obscure as in the trapezoid "model" (Figure 4.1) – there is not always a clear separation line between the different groups.

4.3.1.1 Empirical Pharmacokinetic Models

The simplest empirical model is the trapezoidal rule (polygon approach or linear spline): The straight lines connecting the points can be already regarded as a model. (Note that the trapezoidal model is best applied to decay-corrected data. Therefore, the decay must be implemented when performing the integration to obtain the TIAs.) This polygon approach can be refined using splines of higher order, resulting in smoother interpolations between the data points. To what extent this interpolation reflects the true kinetic, however, remains unclear.

The following disadvantages therefore need to be considered:

1. If the measuring points are not optimally selected in respect to number and position, the numerical integration for the calculation of the TIAs leads to corresponding errors.
2. An assumption is needed for the time between injection of the radiopharmaceutical and the first measurement point. This can be, for example, the assumption that at the time of injection the activity in the organ under consideration is zero, or also that the activity then corresponds to a homogeneous activity distribution in the body. In any case, the first measurement time should not be chosen too late, so that the error due to this assumption remains small [2].
3. A corresponding assumption is required for the times after the last measurement. A conservative estimate assumes that the activity remains in the tissue and decays only by radioactive decay. However, this estimate is only conservative if there is no relevant redistribution of activity after the last measurement. The application of this conservative estimate for several organs generally leads to an overestimation of the total number of decayed nuclei and therefore contradicts the preservation of mass. A final measurement, for example, after at least 5 effective half-lives, is desirable [2, 11]. In this case, almost 97% of the radioactive nuclei have already decayed, and the error due to the assumption would be correspondingly small.

4.3.1.2 Analytical Pharmacokinetic Models

The extrapolation of the TACs for time ranges outside the measured values is an unsolved problem of the empirical models, which can be solved by fitting analytical functions to the data. In this case, the inherent assumption is that the TACs outside the measured time range behave according to the fitted functions.

Many biological processes are first-order kinetics, for example, describing the transfer of substances between different tissues. Such processes can be described by a sum of exponential functions [22]. This follows from the general solution of a linear differential equation system which describes the transport between n different tissues:

$$A(t) = e^{-\lambda_{phys} \cdot t} \cdot \sum_{i=1}^{n} A_i \cdot e^{-\lambda_i \cdot t} \tag{4.1}$$

The activity $A(t)$ is a function of time t with the $2n$ macro parameters A_i and $\lambda_i \geq 0$ [22]. The decay constant of the used radionuclide λ_{phys} should always be explicitly integrated in the model, because (1) better results are achieved [23, 24] and (2) a projection for other physical half-lives is easily possible. The number n of exponential functions for a fitting to a given data set can be determined automatically and user-independently by using a model selection procedure (Section 4.5, Model Selection).

A great advantage of using exponential functions is the simple calculation of the total number N of decays by integration from injection time zero to infinity:

$$N = \int_{0}^{\infty} \left(e^{-\lambda_{phys} \cdot t} \cdot \sum_{i=1}^{n} A_i \cdot e^{-\lambda_i \cdot t} \right) dt = \sum_{i=1}^{n} \frac{A_i}{\lambda_i + \lambda_{phys}} \tag{4.2}$$

Therefore, these functions are used most often [2, 9]. A principal disadvantage of these analytical models with sums of exponential functions is that biological processes often have non-linear components. Therefore, equations 4.1 and 4.2 represent only an approximation for the actual pharmacokinetics.

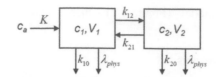

FIGURE 4.4 Two-compartment model. Activity is supplied via the arterial input function c_a (arterial activity concentration). Radioactive decay is integrated in the model with the "transfer rate" λ_{phys} (decay constant). c = activity concentrations, V = volumes, k_{ij} = transfer rates, K = arterial input.

4.3.1.3 Compartmental Pharmacokinetic Models

For a compartmental description of pharmacokinetics "a biological system is treated as an assortment of interconnected compartments consisting of an ensemble of identical chemical or physical units." [22]. These ensembles are located in specific anatomic spaces like an organ (or a tumour) or subspaces like the cytosol of all tumour cells. This combination of similarly behaving spaces and substances allow a simplified description of physiological processes [22, 25].

Thus, an organ/tumour is made up of a few compartments, for example, the tumour may consist of one compartment for the proportion of substance c_2 in all tumour cells, another compartment for substance c_2, for example, a metabolite in all tumour cells (Figure 4.4).

Between these compartments an exchange of substance c_1 or a transformation into substance c_2 takes place, which is described by the following system of linear differential equations (Figure 4.4):

$$\dot{c_1}(t) = -\left(k_{12} + k_{10} + \lambda_{phys}\right) \cdot c_1(t) + k_{21} \cdot c_2(t) + \mathrm{K} \cdot c_a(t) \tag{4.3}$$

$$\dot{c_2}(t) = +k_{12} \cdot c_1(t) - \left(k_{21} + k_{20} + \lambda_{phys}\right) \cdot c_2(t) \tag{4.4}$$

Although different substances may be "in the same space/volume," they have to be described by different compartments because they are chemically different substances. Each compartment is described by the amount of substance it contains and its volume. Physiologically based pharmacokinetic (PBPK) models are those compartment models whose structure corresponds to the actual anatomy and physiology (with approximations) [26]. The distinction between simply empirical compartment models without precise reference to physiological processes and more physiologically based pharmacokinetic models is not entirely clear, but PBPK models should include the blood flows between organs.

The kinetics of all compartments of compartment models with n compartments have the form of Equation 4.1, where the prefactors A_i are functions of the transfer rates between the compartments. Therefore, measuring the prefactors A_i of only one compartment does not allow for determining the exact structure of the compartment model. Consequently, the kinetics in individual organs cannot be determined from (even arbitrarily accurate) measurements of serum kinetics. Only the measurement of kinetics in different organs (e.g. by quantitative imaging) allows the determination of kinetics in the different organs.

In general, the mathematical description of the movement of an injected substance within such a compartment model is mathematically described by a non-linear differential equation system. The establishment of such a differential equation system should reflect the system physiology: However, usually only simple models (Figure 4.4) with very few compartments are investigated due to

1. the limited possibilities to generate data from all the single compartments – in a voxel there is a sum of all compartments measured – and because of
2. the often very small number of (time point) measurement data in total, and also
3. the measurement errors that occur.

Linear two-compartment models are most often used because they have a mathematically simple general analytical solution. Other linear models with more compartments as well as non-linear compartment models in general can be solved only numerically. However, efficient algorithms are available for this purpose in all common programming languages.

4.3.1.4 Whole-body Physiologically Based Pharmacokinetic Models

In contrast to the compartment models described above, whole-body PBPK models [27–29] not only cover the whole body (Figure 4.5), but also integrate a particularly high level of anatomical and physiological knowledge in their structure [30–32].

Additional previous knowledge can be integrated by determining universal transfer rates, like for example the association and dissociation constants of antibody-antigen or peptide-receptor complexes, which can be measured in vitro. Then such known transfer rates for certain populations or even individuals from previous measurements (for a specific substance or a substance with similar properties) do not need to be determined from the TACs. This enables the generation of personalized or individualized PBPK models [33–35] that would otherwise have far too many unknown parameters.

4.3.2 Uncertainty Models

In general, input (time-activity) data have an uncertainty [4]. If these uncertainties are known as absolute values, then these values are input data, too (Section 4.2, Data). If not, the uncertainties can be estimated from the data based on an (adequately) assumed model for the data variances.

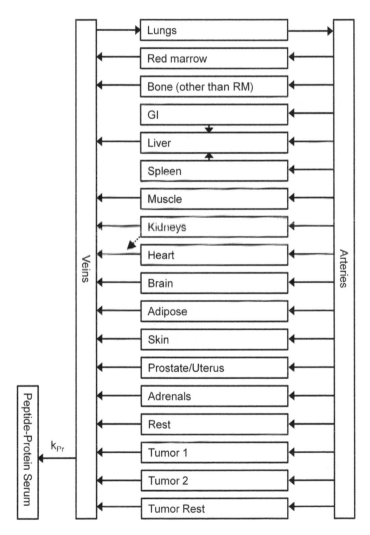

FIGURE 4.5 Whole-body physiologically based pharmacokinetic model (from supplemental data to ref. [32]). Only the basic structure is shown; the individual organs consist of different compartments as shown for example in Figure 4.4. The injection is given into the veins. In this model, excretion occurs only via the kidneys (arrow).

Based on prior knowledge about the data and their measurement, appropriate variance models can be designed. A general model for the variances σ_i^2 of datum i is [9, 36]:

$$\sigma_i^2 = v \cdot \vartheta_i^2 \tag{4.5}$$

$$\vartheta_i^2 = A + B \cdot y_i^C \tag{4.6}$$

$$\vartheta_i^2 = A + B \cdot \left(f\left(t_i\right)\right)^C \tag{4.7}$$

Parameters A, B and C allow for adapting different weightings, and v is the scaling factor of the variances of the data set, which can be treated as a fit parameter in curve fitting. The user may choose between data- (Equation 4.6) or model-based (Equation 4.7) weighting.

Specific settings for the parameters (A, B, C) are for example (0, 1, 1) for Poisson weighting, (0, 0.01, 2) for a fractional standard deviation of 10%, and simply (1, 0, 0) for a constant weighting.

4.4 CURVE FITTING

4.4.1 GENERAL IDEA BEHIND CURVE FITTING

"Given a set of observations one often wants to condense and summarize the data by fitting it to a 'model' that depends on adjustable parameters." [37]. The models could either be just convenient functions, like sums of exponentials [22], or based on detailed physiological knowledge [30, 38]. It can also be regarded as interpolation and extrapolation, which are constrained by the data and the model functions.

To impose that constraint, an objective function (OF) must be defined which measures the agreement between the data and the model. The model parameters then are adapted in such a way that the OF is minimal. Due to the inevitable noise in the data, the parameters will have an uncertainty which also must be specified. Lastly, it must be checked that the model actually fits the data (goodness-of-fit).

In the following, a general OF is first introduced; second, considerations before the fitting are discussed and, finally, quality criteria for fits are presented.

4.4.2 OBJECTIVE FUNCTION

The OF measures the agreement between the data and the used model. Many different OFs have been investigated and which type of OF is best may depend on the data [39]. Commonly, the OF is the logarithm of the product of the likelihood of the N observed data for the given function and that of the prior parameter distribution. The latter integrates a priori knowledge about the K adjustable parameters, which results from previous measurements. As the likelihoods are assumed to be normally distributed, for the logarithm of the likelihood P, we obtain

$$OF = -2\ln\left(P\right) = \sum_{i=1}^{N}\left\{\ln\left(2\pi\sigma_i^2\right) + \frac{\left[y_i - f\left(x_i\right)\right]^2}{\sigma_i^2}\right\} + \sum_{j=1}^{K}\left\{\ln\left(2\pi\omega_j^2\right) + \frac{\left[p_j - \bar{p}_j\right]^2}{\omega_j^2}\right\} \tag{4.8}$$

y_i, σ_i^2 and $f\left(x_i\right) = f\left(x_i; \{p_j\}\right)$ are the measured data point i, its variance and the corresponding function value. p_j is the value of the adjustable parameter j, $\bar{p}_j$ and ω_j^2 are its a priori known mean and variance values. Note the following interpretation for the second sum in Equation 4.8: This sum corresponds to K additional measurements which resulted in the values for $\bar{p}_j$ and ω_j^2. Thus, this "a priori" information could still be obtained after the y_i measurements in individual cases.

From the OF it becomes clear that not only quantitative accurate data (Section 4.2, Data) and a "good" model (Section 4.3, Mathematical Models) are needed, but also knowledge about the precision of the data, as the results for the parameters will depend on these [39]. If the precision is unknown, but a variance model for the used data is established (Section 4.3.2, Uncertainty Models), then a scaling factor may be used as an additional adjustable parameter. This, however, will increase the number of parameters, will strongly influence goodness-of-fit criteria like the χ^2 value, and must also be considered when selecting the best-fit function [40].

The inclusion of a priori knowledge is based on the Bayes theorem. It becomes particularly important for noisy measurements as then the OF often has many local minima due to the noise. Adding the Bayes terms ensures a better performance of the fitting process. Note that previous knowledge is included in Equation 4.8, not only due to the second sum with the Bayesian terms, but also by the chosen-fit function: The function contains structural information, as it reduces the space of possible curves into a set of curves defined by the parameters of that function. Therefore, the selection of a well-suited function is highly important.

4.4.3 CONSIDERATIONS BEFORE FITTING

There exist many software packages with the ability to fit a function to measurement data. Therefore, in the following we will discuss points that need to be decided before starting to minimize the OF.

After deciding on the data to be used, the uncertainty of the data must also be defined. Either measurement data are available for this purpose or an error model must be selected. If an error (or variance) model is selected – for example, the parameters A, B and C (Section 4.3.2, Uncertainty Models) are chosen – it must be decided whether the scaling factor is fixed or whether it should also be fitted. Model-based weighting (Equation 4.7) appears to have advantages over data-based weighting [39], but probably only for a well-chosen fit function. If the appropriate error model for the collected data is not known or not easy to determine, the fit can be made with different error models to check whether different error models lead to (significantly) different results. If the latter is the case, then more time must be invested in the search for the correct error model.

Next, a well-suited fit function (i.e. a model) must be found. The most commonly used functions are sums of exponential functions [2, 22]. The number of free parameters are often reduced by reasonable boundary conditions like $f(t = 0) = 0\ \%$ or $f(t = 0) = 100\ \%$ [9, 41], or by applying a (simple) compartmental model [9, 42]. In addition, it is advisable to factor out the decay of the radionuclide (as in Equation 4.1) for nuclear medicine applications [23, 24]. Note that the latter reduces the parameter domains for the macro-parameters $\lambda_i \geq 0$ compared to $\lambda_i + \lambda_{phys} \geq 0$ in case the decay of the radionuclide is not factored out.

Once the fit function is chosen, a decision should be made on the inclusion of Bayesian terms for a priori knowledge about some, or even all, of the parameters of this function (Equation 4.8). This information can be used to great advantage in nuclear medicine when the data are very noisy or there are only a few measurement points available. Note that – in principle – when using Bayesian information for all the fit parameters, it is possible to perform a fit even when only one data point is available ($N = 1$). Thus, for a first step towards individualization of treatment planning in nuclear medicine, a single measurement together with a priori obtained population data is possible [8, 12]. The same approach may enable voxel-based curve-fitting: The TACs of the whole organ can be fitted, and the parameters obtained can then be used as a priori "population" information to regularize the fitting at the voxel level, which is normally complicated by high noise.

Before starting the fit routine to minimize the OF, initial values must be set for the fit parameters. Depending on the initial values for the function parameters, the minimization algorithm may yield different results. This is a consequence of the possibly many local minima of the OF that is used to fit the model to the data, which in turn is a consequence of having only few data with large measurement errors in nuclear medicine therapy. Therefore, methods for quickly finding suitable initial values should be applied. For example, if a priori knowledge about the parameters is available, the mean values can be used. Or, if guessing is not an option, the whole parameter space can be sampled by random numbers or systematically to identify good starting values [9].

Finally, an adequate algorithm together with, for example, absolute/relative tolerance levels and step sizes, for the OF minimization need to be chosen [37]. The convergence of the algorithm should be ensured, and different starting values for the model parameters should be used to check whether the global minimum has been found. If necessary, procedures that search for the global minimum must be used [37].

4.4.4 QUALITY CRITERIA FOR FITS

The fit of a model or – more specifically – the model parameters to measurement data must meet certain quality criteria. The following procedure should be followed ([9], see also Table 1 there):

- Visual inspection of the graph of the function and the measurement data. Depending on the data, logarithmic or semi-logarithmic plots also should be checked.
- The value of the coefficient of determination R^2 should be close to 1.
- The parameter values should be plausible. If, for example, they stand for transfer rates between compartments, then they must all be positive, or, if they stand for physiological quantities, like the weight of a patient, then they should be within the physiologically possible range.

- The standard errors for the parameters shall be either precise or at least acceptable. A coefficient of variation < 25% is considered precise [31], and a coefficient of variation < 50% is considered acceptable [43].
- The elements of the correlation matrix should not be too large, and their absolute value should be less than 0.8 (for most parameters) [43].
- The weighted residuals should be randomly distributed. If they are systematically arranged around the zero line, the model will not capture all the information contained in the data.

In general, all these criteria must be met in order to accept the result of curve fitting.

Often also the χ^2 value is used as a goodness-of-fit measure with the following rule of thumb [37]:

$$\chi^2 = \sum_{i=1}^{N} \left\{ \frac{\left[y_i - f(x_i) \right]^2}{\sigma_i^2} \right\} \approx N - K \tag{4.8}$$

In case $\chi^2 \ll N - K$ then the assumed data variances are either too large or there is an over-fitting due to the use of too many fit parameters (i.e. a wrong model). Such a fit is therefore inadequate for extrapolations, for example, after the last measured data point in pharmacokinetic measurements and may even lead to wrong results for interpolations. If $\chi^2 \gg N - K$ either the assumed data variances are too small, or the model function is wrongly chosen. However, this rule of thumb is inaccurate for low $N - K$ values [37] and thus often not applicable in nuclear medicine.

4.5 MODEL SELECTION

The fit of mathematical models, that is, their parameters, to measured data is a common method to simplify the description of biological systems. However, it is often unclear which model or function best describes the data. This is particularly important if the model is to be used not only to describe the data but also to perform predictions. Therefore, different requirements apply for a model that is intended to calculate the area under a curve for dosimetry or for a model that is intended to allow a better understanding of the biological system and, for example, to predict the influence of a change in the amount of substance injected on the area under the curve.

The number of models to be considered is limited by various boundary conditions. The number of existing data points limits the number of possible model parameters, and noise in the data can lead to a further reduction of the determinable number of parameters. If a model already exists in the literature, it should be considered. Last, but not least, knowledge that is already available independently of the data collected should also be taken into account when selecting a model [44].

Various criteria for selecting the best model from a set of models for a given data set are described in the literature [44–47], for example, the F-test [48], the Akaike Information Criterion (AIC) [49], and the Bayes Information Criterion (BIC) [50].

In the following, we first focus on the corrected AIC (AICc), which is an extension of the AIC for a small number of data relative to the used number of parameters [44, 51]. Second, the model selection procedure is presented.

4.5.1 AKAIKE INFORMATION CRITERION

The AIC is an information theory measure that measures the information lost when the model under study is used instead of the true model [44, 49]. Akaike derived a relationship using log-likelihood that measures this measure without knowing the true model. In doing so, he assumed large amounts of data, an assumption that is practically impossible to fulfil, especially for pharmacokinetic patient data. For this reason, Hurvich and Tsai later proposed a corrected AIC (AICc), which contains a penalty term that depends on the size of the data set and the number of model parameters [51].

While the derivation of the AICc is complex, the calculation of the AIC and the AICc is straightforward:

$$AIC = -2\ln(P) + 2K \tag{4.9}$$

$$AICc = AIC + \frac{2K(K+1)}{N-K-1} \tag{4.10}$$

Where N is the number of data points, K is the number of fit parameters of the model and $-2\ln(P)$ the log-likelihood (Equation 4.8). If the scaling factor of the variances of the data (Equation 4.5) is fitted, then K must be replaced by $K+1$, as one additional parameter is fitted.

The value of the AICc for the examined data set has no meaning of its own, but only acquires this meaning when comparing different models on the basis of the same (!) data set (including the same uncertainty model): The model with the lowest AICc value is the model most supported by the data from the set of models examined [44]. Note, therefore, that – if only unsuitable models are compared – the AICc can only select a poor model as the best model. This underlines the great importance of the definition/selection of the models to be compared by the AICc: No "saving" should be made here, because otherwise the result will be unsatisfactory despite the selection by means of the AICc. At this point, namely when determining the set of models/functions to be examined, previous knowledge must also be integrated – as far as possible – in order to select a model using AICc that is actually suitable for the planned application.

The Akaike weight w_i for each model i indicates the probability that this model is the best among the models studied [52]:

$$w_i = \frac{e^{-AICc_i/2}}{\sum_{r=1}^{R} e^{-AICc_r/2}},$$

(4.11)

where R is the number of compared candidate models. Note that the uncertainty of the Akaike weights can be determined using for example the Jackknife method for the data [40]. This is important for the evaluation of the certainty of the result.

4.5.2 Model Selection Procedure

The selection of the model for the description of the data consists of the following steps [9]:

1. Definition of candidate models (prior knowledge of the observer is integrated).
2. Fit of all candidate models to the measurement data. Prior knowledge can be integrated for example, by constraints for the parameters (e.g. positivity of transfer rates) or also in the form of Bayesian constraints.
3. Candidate models that do not meet the quality criteria according to Section 4.4.4, Quality Criteria for Fits (goodness-of-fit) are excluded as inappropriate models.
4. Calculation of the Akaike weights w_i (or other selection criteria).
5. Selection of the model most supported by the data (and the integrated prior knowledge in the OF).

If several models with weight $w_i > 0.01$ occur in the last step, then model averaging should be performed, whereby the weighting of the different models is carried out with the corresponding Akaike weights [44, 46].

4.6 TIME-ACTIVITY CURVES AND TIME-INTEGRATED ACTIVITY

The TACs and the therefrom-derived TIAs are main contributors to the dosimetric estimates in the MIRD scheme [2, 5]. Determining this quantity accurately and precisely is challenging as it includes choosing a well-suited set of fit functions, possibly integrating prior knowledge, applying an adequate uncertainty model, finding good initial parameter values for the fit procedure, and performing a model selection, as described in this chapter.

According to Figure 4.2 the TACs are defined by the parameters of the selected model(s) most supported by the data. The parameters have an uncertainty, which (in science) is an integral part of the result (and thus must be given [4]). Correspondingly, the TACs have an uncertainty and also the TACs-derived TIA values. The latter need to be calculated based on propagation of uncertainty for enabling an adequate judgment of the result [10].

If the result is not deemed sufficiently accurate and precise, all the contributors to the uncertainty of the result presented in the previous sections (Figure 4.2) need to be checked for possible improvement. Sensitivity analysis is a method to identify those parameters being the origin of the largest contribution to uncertainty [53, 54]. This makes it possible to carry out the improvement on the basis of the available resources in a targeted and resource-saving manner.

REFERENCES

[1] W. E. Bolch, K. F. Eckerman, G. Sgouros, and S. R. Thomas, "MIRD Pamphlet No. 21: A Generalized Schema for Radiopharmaceutical Dosimetry—Standardization of Nomenclature," *J Nucl Med,* vol. 50, no. 3, pp. 477–84, 2009.

[2] J. A. Siegel *et al.*, "MIRD pamphlet No. 16: Techniques for quantitative radiopharmaceutical biodistribution data acquisition and analysis for use in human radiation dose estimates," *J Nucl Med,* vol. 40, no. 2, pp. 37S-61S, 1999.

[3] M. Konijnenberg, "From imaging to dosimetry and biological effects," *Q J Nucl Med Mol Imaging,* vol. 55, no. 1, pp. 44–56, 2011.

[4] GUM, "Evaluation of measurement data: Guide to expression of uncertainty in measurement," 2008,

[5] R. W. Howell *et al.*, "The MIRD perspective 1999. Medical Internal Radiation Dose Committee," *J Nucl Med,* vol. 40, no. 1, pp. 3S-10S, 1999.

[6] M. Ljungberg and K. Sjögreen Gleisner, "Personalized Dosimetry for Radionuclide Therapy Using Molecular Imaging Tools," *Biomedicines,* vol. 4, no. 4, p. 25, 2016.

[7] J. I. Gear *et al.*, "EANM practical guidance on uncertainty analysis for molecular radiotherapy absorbed dose calculations," *Eur J Nucl Med Mol Imaging,* vol. 45, no. 13, pp. 2456–74, 2018, doi: 10.1007/s00259-018-4136-7.

[8] M. T. Madsen, Y. Menda, T. M. O'Dorisio, and M. S. O'Dorisio, "Technical Note: Single time point dose estimate for exponential clearance," *Med Phys,* vol. 45, no. 5, pp. 2318–24, 2018, doi: 10.1002/mp.12886.

[9] P. Kletting *et al.*, "Molecular radiotherapy: the NUKFIT software for calculating the time-integrated activity coefficient," *Med Phys,* vol. 40, no. 10, p. 102504, 2013, doi: 10.1118/1.4820367.

[10] M. Lassmann, C. Chiesa, G. Flux, M. Bardies, and E. D. Committee, "EANM Dosimetry Committee guidance document: Good practice of clinical dosimetry reporting," *Eur J Nucl Med Mol Imaging,* vol. 38, no. 1, pp. 192–200, 2011, doi: 10.1007/s00259-010-1549-3.

[11] S. J. Adelstein *et al.*, "Absorbed-dose specification in nuclear medicine," *Journal of the ICRU,* vol. 2, no. 1, pp. 1–110, 2002.

[12] C. Maass, J. P. Sachs, D. Hardiansyah, F. M. Mottaghy, P. Kletting, and G. Glatting, "Dependence of treatment planning accuracy in peptide receptor radionuclide therapy on the sampling schedule," *EJNMMI Res,* vol. 6, no. 1, p. 30, 2016, doi: 10.1186/s13550-016-0185-8.

[13] D. Hardiansyah *et al.*, "The role of patient-based treatment planning in peptide receptor radionuclide therapy," *Eur J Nucl Med Mol Imaging,* vol. 43, no. 5, pp. 871–80, 2016, doi: 10.1007/s00259-015-3248-6.

[14] H. Hänscheid and M. Lassmann, "Will SPECT/CT Cameras Soon Be Able to Display Absorbed Doses? Dosimetry from Single-Activity-Concentration Measurements," *J Nucl Med,* vol. 61, no. 7, pp. 1028–29, 2020, doi: 10.2967/jnumed.119.239970.

[15] D. Z. D'Argenio, "Optimal sampling times for pharmacokinetic experiments," *J Pharmacokinet Biopharm,* vol. 9, no. 6, pp. 739–56, 1981, doi: 10.1007/BF01070904.

[16] I. DiStefano, Joseph J., "Algorithms, software and sequential optimal sampling schedule designs for pharmacokinetic and physiologic experiments," *Mathematics and Computers in Simulation,* vol. XXIV, pp. 531–34, 1982.

[17] R. Kalicka and D. Bochen, "Properties of D-optimal Sampling Schedule for Compartmental Models," *Biocybernetics and Biomedical Engineering,* vol. 25, no. 1, pp. 23–36, 2005.

[18] A. Rinscheid, J. Lee, P. Kletting, A. J. Beer, and G. Glatting, "A simulation-based method to determine optimal sampling schedules for dosimetry in radioligand therapy," *Z. Med. Phys,* vol. 29, no. 4, pp. 314–25, 2019, doi: 10.1016/j.zemedi.2018.12.001.

[19] A. Rinscheid, P. Kletting, M. Eiber, A. J. Beer, and G. Glatting, "Technical Note: Optimal sampling schedules for kidney dosimetry based on the hybrid planar/SPECT method in ^{177}Lu-PSMA therapy," *Med Phys,* vol. 46, no. 12, pp. 5861–66, 2019, doi: 10.1002/mp.13846.

[20] A. Rinscheid, P. Kletting, M. Eiber, A. J. Beer, and G. Glatting, "Influence of sampling schedules on [^{177}Lu]Lu-PSMA dosimetry," *EJNMMI Phys,* vol. 7, no. 1, p. 41, 2020, doi: 10.1186/s40658-020-00311-0.

[21] C. Cobelli, D. Foster, and G. Toffolo, *Tracer Kinetics in Biomedical Research: From Data to Model.* New York: Kluwer Academic / Plenum Publishers, 2000.

[22] S. E. Strand, P. Zanzonico, and T. K. Johnson, "Pharmacokinetic modeling," *Med Phys,* vol. 20, no. 2 Pt 2, pp. 515–27, 1993, doi: 10.1118/1.597047.

[23] L. E. Williams *et al.*, "On the correction for radioactive decay in pharmacokinetic modeling," *Med Phys,* vol. 22, no. 10, pp. 1619–26, 1995, doi: 10.1118/1.597421.

[24] G. Glatting and S. N. Reske, "Treatment of radioactive decay in pharmacokinetic modeling: Influence on parameter estimation in cardiac ^{13}N-PET," *Med Phys,* vol. 26, no. 4, pp. 616–21, 1999, doi: 10.1118/1.598561.

[25] S. R. Cherry, J. A. Sorenson, and M. E. Phelps, *Physics in Nuclear Medicine.* Elsevier Health Sciences, 2012.

[26] G. Z. Ferl, F. P. Theil, and H. Wong, "Physiologically based pharmacokinetic models of small molecules and therapeutic antibodies: A mini-review on fundamental concepts and applications," *Biopharm Drug Dispos,* vol. 37, no. 2, pp. 75–92, 2016, doi: 10.1002/bdd.1994.

[27] I. Nestorov, "Whole body pharmacokinetic models," *Clin Pharmacokinet,* vol. 42, no. 10, pp. 883–908, 2003, doi: 10.2165/00003088-200342100-00002.

[28] I. Nestorov, "Whole-body physiologically based pharmacokinetic models," *Expert Opin Drug Metab Toxicol,* vol. 3, no. 2, pp. 235–49, 2007, doi: 10.1517/17425255.3.2.235.

[29] D. K. Shah and A. M. Betts, "Towards a platform PBPK model to characterize the plasma and tissue disposition of monoclonal antibodies in preclinical species and human," *J Pharmacokinet Pharmacodyn,* vol. 39, no. 1, pp. 67–86, 2012, doi: 10.1007/s10928-011-9232-2.

[30] L. Kuepfer *et al.*, "Applied Concepts in PBPK Modeling: How to Build a PBPK/PD Model," *CPT Pharmacometrics Syst. Pharmacol.,* vol. 5, no. 10, pp. 516–31, 2016, doi: 10.1002/psp4.12134.

[31] P. L. Bonate, *Pharmacokinetic-Pharmacodynamic Modeling and Simulation*, 2nd ed. New York: Springer, 2011.

[32] P. Kletting *et al.*, "Optimized Peptide Amount and Activity for ^{90}Y-Labeled DOTATATE Therapy," *J Nucl Med,* vol. 57, no. 4, pp. 503–8, 2016, doi: 10.2967/jnumed.115.164699.

[33] P. Kletting, D. Bunjes, S. N. Reske, and G. Glatting, "Improving anti-CD45 antibody radioimmunotherapy using a physiologically based pharmacokinetic model," *J Nucl Med,* vol. 50, no. 2, pp. 296–302, 2009, doi: 10.2967/jnumed.108.054189.

[34] P. Kletting *et al.*, "Investigating the Effect of Ligand Amount and Injected Therapeutic Activity: A Simulation Study for ^{177}Lu-Labeled PSMA-Targeting Peptides," *PLoS One,* vol. 11, no. 9, p. e0162303, 2016, doi: 10.1371/journal.pone.0162303.

[35] N. J. Begum, G. Glatting, H. J. Wester, M. Eiber, A. J. Beer, and P. Kletting, "The effect of ligand amount, affinity and internalization on PSMA-targeted imaging and therapy: A simulation study using a PBPK model," *Sci Rep,* vol. 9, no. 1, p. 20041, 2019, doi: 10.1038/s41598-019-56603-8.

[36] P. H. Barrett *et al.*, "SAAM II: Simulation, snalysis, and modeling software for tracer and pharmacokinetic studies," *Metabolism,* vol. 47, no. 4, pp. 484–92, 1998, doi: 10.1016/s0026-0495(98)90064-6.

[37] W. H. Press, S. A. Teukolsky, W. T. Vetterling, and B. P. Flannery, *Numerical Recipes in C: The Art of Scientific Computing*, 2nd ed. Cambridge University Press, 1992.

[38] L. D. Jiménez-Franco, G. Glatting, V. Prasad, W. A. Weber, A. J. Beer, and P. Kletting, "Effect of Tumor Perfusion and Receptor Density on Tumor Control Probability in ^{177}Lu-DOTATATE Therapy: An In Silico Analysis for Standard and Optimized Treatment," *J Nucl Med,* vol. 62, no. 1, pp. 92–98, 2021, doi: 10.2967/jnumed.120.245068.

[39] R. F. Muzic, Jr. and B. T. Christian, "Evaluation of objective functions for estimation of kinetic parameters," *Med Phys,* vol. 33, no. 2, pp. 342–53, 2006, doi: 10.1118/1.2135907.

[40] G. Glatting, P. Kletting, S. N. Reske, K. Hohl, and C. Ring, "Choosing the optimal fit function: comparison of the Akaike information criterion and the F-test," *Med Phys,* vol. 34, no. 11, pp. 4285–92, 2007, doi: 10.1118/1.2794176.

[41] G. Glatting *et al.*, "Internal radionuclide therapy: The ULMDOS software for treatment planning," *Medical Physics,* vol. 32, no. 7, Part1, pp. 2399–2405, 2005, doi: 10.1118/1.1945348.

[42] H. Hänscheid *et al.*, "EANM Dosimetry Committee series on standard operational procedures for pre-therapeutic dosimetry II. Dosimetry prior to radioiodine therapy of benign thyroid diseases," *Eur J Nucl Med Mol Imaging,* vol. 40, no. 7, pp. 1126–34, 2013, doi: 10.1007/s00259-013-2387-x.

[43] M. E. Wastney, B. H. Patterson, O. A. Linares, and P. C. Greif, *Investigating Biological Systems Using Modeling*. San Diego, CA: Academic Press, 1998, p. 400.

[44] K. P. Burnham and D. R. Anderson, *Model Selection and Multimodel Interference: A Practical Information-theoretic Approach*, 2nd ed. New York: Springer, 2002.

[45] T. M. Ludden, S. L. Beal, and L. B. Sheiner, "Comparison of the Akaike Information Criterion, the Schwarz Criterion and the F Test as Guides to Model Selection," *J. Pharmacokinet. Biopharm.,* vol. 22, no. 5, pp. 431–45, 1994.

[46] P. Kletting and G. Glatting, "Model selection and inference in pharmacokinetics: The corrected Akaike information criterion and the F-test," *Z. Med. Phys.,* vol. 19, no. 3, pp. 200–6, 2009.

[47] S. S. V. Golla *et al.*, "Model selection criteria for dynamic brain PET studies," *EJNMMI Phys,* journal article vol. 4, no. 1, p. 30, 2017, doi: 10.1186/s40658-017-0197-0.

[48] L. Sachs, *Angewandte Statistik: Anwendung statistischer Methoden*, 7. Auflage ed. Berlin: Springer-Verlag, 1992.

[49] H. Akaike, "Information theory and an extension of the maximum likelihood principle," in *Selected Papers of Hirotugu Akaike*, E. Parzen, G. Kitagawa, and K. Tanabe, Eds. New York: Springer, 1997, pp. 199–214.

[50] G. Schwarz, "Estimating the dimension of a model," *Ann. Statist.,* vol. 6, no. 2, pp. 461–64, 1978.

[51] C. M. Hurvich and C.-L. Tsai, "Regression and time series model selection in small samples," *Biometrika,* vol. 76, no. 2, pp. 297–307, 1989.

[52] M. J. Mazerolle, "Mouvements et reproduction des amphibiens en tourbières perturbées," Ph.D., Université Laval, Canada, 2004.

[53] A. Saltelli *et al.*, *Global Sensitivity Analysis: The Primer*. Chichester: John Wiley & Sons, 2008.

[54] D. Hardiansyah *et al.*, "Important pharmacokinetic parameters for individualization of ^{177}Lu-PSMA therapy: A global sensitivity analysis for a physiologically based pharmacokinetic model," *Med Phys,* vol. 48, no. 2, pp. 556–68, 2021, doi: 10.1002/mp.14622.

5 Tracer Kinetic Modelling and Its Use in PET Quantification

Mark Lubberink and Michel Koole

CONTENTS

5.1 INTRODUCTION

PET is an extremely powerful tool for measuring (patho-)physiology in vivo by studying the time-dependent behaviour of radiopharmaceuticals, and as such to *measure* biological processes. By measuring the distribution of the tracer over time, functional parameters can be estimated, such as for example perfusion, oxygen consumption, metabolism, internalization, receptor concentrations, transporter availability, enzyme activity, and so forth, depending on the tracer being used. Because of the high sensitivity of PET, the amount of radiopharmaceutical that has to be injected to measure a certain process is often so small that it has no pharmacological effects. In this case, we speak of the tracer principle: A process can be measured without disturbing it. The idea of labelling molecules with radioactive isotopes to be able to follow these inside the body, was first suggested in the 1920s by George de Hevesy [1, 2], who received the Nobel Prize in 1943 for his research. Quantitative measurement of physiological processes was actually what PET was mainly used for in its early years before ^{18}F-FDG (fluorodeoxyglucose), a PET analog for glucose, became a routine clinical investigation in the 1990s, and whole-body scans, instead of dynamic scans over a single bed position, became standard practice. However, the PET signal measured at one hour after injection, as is typically done for routine clinical PET scanning, is a combination of delivery to the tissue of interest (blood flow), non-specific uptake in the tumour (in the case of FDG, the presence of free, non-metabolised FDG in tissue), and specific signal (in the case of FDG, FDG-6-phosphate produced after the first step in its metabolism). Even in routine clinical practice, it can be beneficial to separate these three components and provide more specific information on either blood flow or specific binding. In many research questions it is mandatory to do so to obtain a correct answer to the question at hand. The standard approach to separate the PET signals in different components is to use a compartment model, which will be discussed in the next paragraph, together with some relevant examples.

5.2 COMPARTMENT MODELS

The use of compartment models is the standard approach for the analysis of PET tracer kinetics, with compartment models being established for PET measurements of blood flow [3], glucose consumption [4], and receptor ligand binding [5]. An excellent overview of the theory of compartment models can be found in [6]. Essentially, a compartment model uses different compartments to describe the exchange rate of tracer between plasma and tissue and between different binding states of the tracer in tissue. As such, the tissue compartments are not necessarily physical compartments, but can also describe the different states of a tracer such as free tracer, tracer bound to receptors, internalized tracer, and so forth. Figure 5.1A shows the simplest compartment model, a so-called single-tissue compartment model where $C_T(t)$ is the time course of the tracer concentration in the tissue of interest, the so-called time-activity curve (TAC), and $C_P(t)$ is the time course of the tracer concentration in plasma. The rate constants, denoted K_1 and k_2, describe the rate of transport from plasma to tissue, in mL per gram tissue per minute, and the clearance rate from tissue in min^{-1}. From these so-called micro-parameters, the volume of distribution V_T can be derived as the ratio of K_1 over k_2, which is considered a macro-parameter in pharmacokinetics and equals the ratios of tracer concentrations in tissue and plasma at equilibrium. If we assume steady state during the PET scan, such that K_1 and k_2 can be considered constant, and an instantaneous, homogeneous tracer distribution within each compartment, a single-tissue compartment model is described by the following differential equation:

$$\frac{dC_T(t)}{dt} = K_1 C_P(t) - k_2 C_T(t) \tag{5.1}$$

The corresponding operational equation is given by

$$C_T(t) = K_1 C_P(t) \otimes e^{-k_2 t} \tag{5.2}$$

With $\otimes$ representing the convolution operator.

If we draw a volume of interest (VOI) over the tissue of interest and project it on the time series of dynamic PET data, we can extract $C_{PET}(t)$ (Figure 5.2). However, since this VOI contains not only tissue but also a small amount of blood vessels, we cannot use $C_{PET}(t)$ as such but need to correct the PET signal for the small contribution of the blood pool. Therefore, a single-tissue compartment model is described by the following equation:

$$C_{PET}(t) = (1 - V_A) C_T(t) + V_A C_A(t) = (1 - V_A) K_1 C_P(t) \otimes e^{-k_2 t} + V_A C_A(t) \tag{5.3}$$

With $C_A(t)$ the time course of the activity concentration of tracer in blood and V_A the relative contribution of the blood pool to the PET signal. Given $C_P(t)$ and $C_A(t)$, this equation can be fitted to the dynamic PET data $C_{PET}(t)$ using non-linear regression (NLR) to estimate V_A, K_1, k_2, and, hence, V_T. Therefore, $C_A(t)$ and $C_P(t)$ which correspond

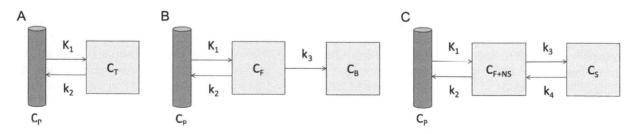

FIGURE 5.1 The three most commonly used compartment models in PET: (A) single-tissue, (B) irreversible two-tissue and (C) reversible two-tissue model.

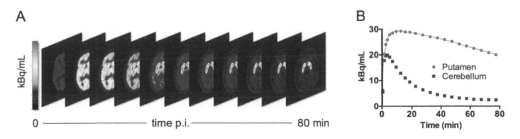

FIGURE 5.2 Dynamic PET scan (A) and time-activity curves with model fit of putamen (B). Colour image available at www.routledge.com/9781138593299.

to the arterial blood and plasma input function respectively, need to be measured during the PET scan. This will be discussed in the next paragraph.

5.3 BLOOD AND PLASMA INPUT FUNCTION

In order to apply a compartment model to describe tracer kinetics, the time course of the radioactivity concentration in arterial plasma and blood needs to be measured together with the PET signal. This is done by (arterial) blood sampling during the dynamic PET scan, either continuously using an on-line sampling system (e.g. [7]), or by rapid manual blood sampling. As such, the arterial whole-blood concentration $C_A(t)$ is measured as a function of time (Figure 5.3A). However, potential tracer uptake by red blood cells reduces the amount of tracer which can interact with the target of interest. Therefore, we need additional discrete blood samples to separate the plasma and cellular blood fraction and determine the activity concentration ratio between plasma and whole-blood. Since this ratio can vary during the course of the scan, several samples need to be taken at different time points after tracer injection (Figure 5.3B). In this way, the whole blood TAC can be multiplied with the appropriate plasma / whole-blood ratios to obtain the plasma TAC, $C_p(t)$. Now, we would be ready if our tracer is stable in plasma and not metabolized during the course of the scan, since we can assume that only intact tracer will be functionally active and interacting with the target of interest. For instance, in brain PET imaging, only intact tracer will be able to pass the blood brain barrier (BBB). Unfortunately, most tracers do undergo peripheral metabolism. If there is peripheral metabolism, the fraction of intact tracer is gradually decreasing as function of time during the PET scan. Therefore, additional arterial blood samples are needed at different time points after tracer injection to determine the fraction of intact tracer in plasma (Figure 5.3C). This is a so-called metabolite analysis. Based on these data, the arterial plasma TAC can be appropriately weighted to determine a metabolite-corrected arterial plasma input function $C_p(t)$ representing the fraction of intact tracer in plasma over time.

While arterial blood sampling is the standard approach to generate the arterial blood and metabolite corrected arterial plasma input function, the procedure requires arterial cannulation and is therefore considered invasive. While the procedure is generally well tolerated by healthy subjects, patients are more reluctant to have this procedure in addition to their diagnostic procedures and therapeutic interventions. Moreover, arterial blood sampling is logistically challenging: Placement and handling of the arterial line requires highly trained and skilled staff and additional resources are needed for the setup and calibration of the measurement device and for the analysis of the blood samples. Therefore, it is not straightforward to schedule this procedure as part of routine clinical practice.

A non-invasive, more cost-effective approach is the use of an image-derived input function (IDIF) where the signal from arterial blood is extracted from the dynamic PET image data to determine the arterial blood input function. However, this is only feasible when a large vascular structure such as the heart or aorta is present within the field of view (FOV). Other blood vessels are relatively small compared to the spatial resolution of PET, resulting in underestimation because of partial-volume effects and making an IDIF approach very challenging. Moreover, the IDIF only estimates the tracer concentration in arterial blood and does not provide information on the metabolization rate of the tracer nor on the time-dependent plasma to whole-blood concentration ratios. Therefore, an IDIF approach needs to be combined with either limited venous sampling to determine the patient-specific tracer metabolization rate and/or plasma to whole-blood activity ratios or with a population-based approach where the average metabolization rate and plasma to whole-blood activity ratios based on arterial blood sampling in a subset of subjects is considered as representative for the whole group.

Some examples of tracers for which a whole-blood curve can be used directly as input curve, or after multiplication with a constant plasma / whole-blood ratio measured using only a few (arterialized) venous samples, are ^{15}O-water,

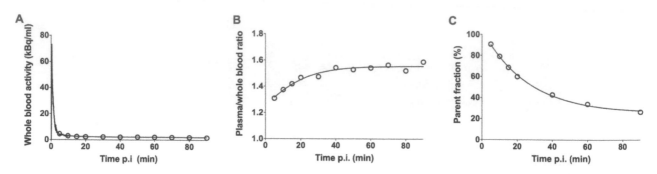

FIGURE 5.3 Typical examples of (A) whole blood time-activity curve, acquired using an on-line sampler during the first 10 min and extrapolated to the full scan duration using discrete blood samples; (B) plasma/whole blood ratio and (C) fraction of intact tracer. The final input function is the product of the solid lines in A, B and C, giving the time-activity curve of intact tracer in plasma.

^{18}F-FDG, and peptides labelled with radiometals such as the somatostatin analogue ^{68}Ga-DOTATOC. Other than that, arterial blood sampling with metabolite analysis is usually necessary to obtain the correct input curve.

5.4 TISSUE TIME-ACTIVITY CURVES

Next to the arterial blood and metabolite-corrected arterial plasma input function, an appropriate tissue TAC is required to quantify tissue tracer kinetics using a compartment model. This tissue TAC should be representative of the underlying tissue of interest. For larger lesions or organs with an almost uniform tracer distribution, extracting a representative TAC is rather straightforward. However, for focal lesions, extraction of an appropriate TAC which represents the kinetic profile of the underlying tumoral tissue is challenging because of the limited PET resolution and, hence, the partial volume effects with surrounding tissues. Extensive research has been done to determine the optimal approach for (semi-)automated and observer-independent lesion segmentation using harmonized PET imaging protocols to improve the reproducibility of PET quantification. In case of brain PET imaging, the standard approach is to spatially normalize the dynamic PET data to a standard space, such as MNI (Montreal Neurological Institute) space, using a (non-)linear transformation. This spatial normalization allows an atlas-based approach where anatomically predefined brain regions in standard space can be projected onto the dynamic PET data using the inverse transformation to extract the corresponding regional TACs (Figure 5.4). If a high-resolution anatomical MR is available, the MR dataset can be used to improve the accuracy of the atlas-based approach. In this case, the dynamic PET data are first aligned with the MR data using a linear transformation, after which the MR data are used to obtain a more accurate spatial normalization and therefore a better automatic delineation of brain regions. This way, the accuracy of the spatial normalizations does not depend on quality or distribution pattern of the dynamic PET data. Moreover, the MR data can be segmented into patient specific distribution maps of grey matter, white matter, and cerebrospinal fluid, which can be used to limit the delineation of brain regions to grey matter or to correct for partial volume effects between different tissue classes.

The most straightforward application of the single-tissue compartment model is in the measurement of perfusion. Blood flow and perfusion are often used interchangeably in PET literature, meaning tissue perfusion, that is, the amount of mL blood that passes through each gram or cm³ tissue per minute.

According to the Fick principle (Figure 5.5), the change in tissue concentration over time is the blood flow multiplied by the difference between arterial and venous concentrations of the tracer:

$$\frac{dC_T(t)}{dt} = FC_A(t) - FC_V(t) \tag{5.4}$$

And, since $C_V(t)$ is related to $C_T(t)$ by the partition coefficient or distribution volume V_T:

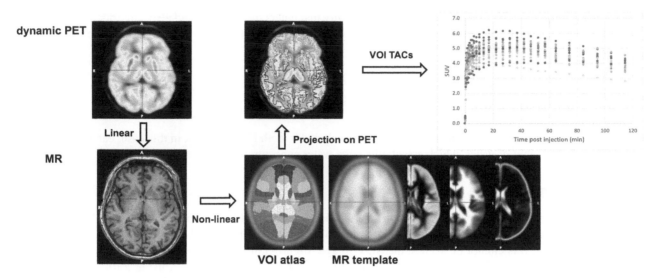

FIGURE 5.4 Time-activity curves of brain PET data using spatial normalization and a VOI atlas. Colour image available at www.routledge.com/9781138593299.

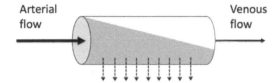

FIGURE 5.5 Schematic description of blood flow through a capillary.

$$\frac{dC_T(t)}{dt} = FC_A(t) - \frac{F}{V_T}C_T(t) \tag{5.5}$$

This equation can be solved:

$$C_T(t) = FC_A(t) \otimes e^{-\frac{F}{V_T}t} \tag{5.6}$$

Clearly, this is the solution of the single-tissue compartment model with K_1 replaced by F and k_2 equalling F/V_T. More generally, the plasma to tissue rate constant K_1 of a PET tracer in a certain tissue is the product of the blood flow and the extraction of the tracer; $K_1 = E \times F$. The extraction of a tracer during each pass through the capillaries in a tissue can be described by

$$E = 100\left(1 - e^{-\frac{PS}{F}}\right)\% \tag{5.7}$$

That is, the extraction is positively correlated to the permeability of the vessel walls for the tracer, expressed by the permeability surface area product PS, whereas it is negatively correlated with the perfusion or blood flow F of the tissue. Only for a tracer with a very high value for PS will extraction be 100 per cent independent of flow, and hence, K_1 will be equal to F. In that case:

$$C_{PET}(t) = (1 - V_A)FC_P(t) \otimes e^{-k_2t} + V_AC_A(t) \tag{5.8}$$

If the tracer is freely diffusible, such as ^{15}O-water, any activity that enters the tissue should also subsequently be cleared from it. In addition, if the tracer does not metabolize, the equation simplifies further by replacing the plasma concentration $C_p(t)$ with the arterial blood concentration $C_A(t)$:

$$C_{PET}(t) = (1 - V_A) F C_A(t) \otimes e^{-\frac{F}{V_T} t} + V_A C_A(t) \tag{5.9}$$

In this case, we only need $C_A(t)$ instead of $C_p(t)$, and F is included in both K_1 and k_2. V_T, in this case, can be interpreted as the partition coefficient of water, which essentially is the water concentration in tissue.

5.5 IRREVERSIBLE TRACER BINDING

Figure 5.6A shows a static image acquired 2 h after administration of the PET tracer ^{68}Ga-ABY025, binding to the HER2 receptor which is overexpressed in HER2-positive breast cancer. Although the patient was known to have a large liver metastasis, this cannot be seen in the SUV image. Figure 5.6B shows an image of the same patient, but now corrected for non-specific signal, that is, tracer in tissue but not bound to HER2, using a dynamic scan and tracer kinetic modelling. This specific uptake images shows that the PET signal in healthy liver tissue nearly completely consists of non-specific, that is non-HER2-related, uptake, and the HER2-positive metastasis can now be seen clearly.

The compartment model for a tracer that is internalized or metabolically trapped in tissue, such as ^{18}F-FDG, was first described by Sokoloff in 1978 [4]. FDG is, just like glucose itself, transported into tissue by the glucose transporter and then converted into 6-FDG-phosphate by the enzyme hexokinase. However, in contrast to glucose-phosphate, 6-FDG-phosphate cannot be further metabolized and is thus metabolically trapped, as shown in Figure 5.7.

It is evident that the fate of ^{18}F-FDG can then be described by the compartment model in Figure 5.7 (and 1B). This model can be described by two differential equations:

$$\frac{dC_F(t)}{dt} = K_1 C_P(t) - k_2 C_F(t) - k_3 C_F(t) \tag{5.10}$$

$$\frac{dC_B(t)}{dt} = k_3 C_F(t) \tag{5.11}$$

Now, k_3 describes the phosphorylation of FDG. The overall trapping rate constant, K_i, which has the same unit mL/g/min as K_1, can be calculated as

$$K_i = \frac{K_1 k_3}{k_2 + k_3} \tag{5.12}$$

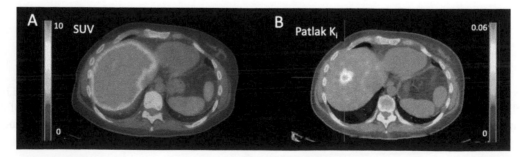

FIGURE 5.6   HER2-positive liver metastasis in a breast cancer patient imaged using ^{68}Ga-ABY025. (A) SUV image at 1 h p.i.; (B) K_i image, showing specific signal only. Image courtesy Dr. Jens Sörensen, Uppsala University. Colour image available at www. routledge.com/9781138593299.

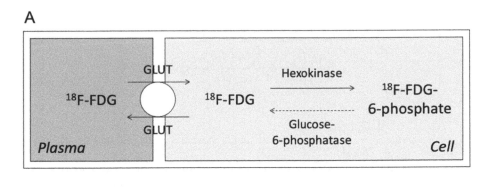

FIGURE 5.7 Schematic depiction of FDG kinetics and corresponding compartment model.

Multiplication of this trapping rate constant, or net influx rate, K_i with the plasma glucose concentration c_{glu}, in μmol/mL, and accounting for differences in metabolism between glucose and FDG using the so-called lumped constant LC, allows us to calculate the metabolic rate of glucose or glucose consumption MR_{glu} in μmol/g/min:

$$MR_{glu} = \frac{c_{glu} K_i}{LC} \tag{15.3}$$

5.5.1 THE PATLAK PLOT

The net influx rate constant K_i can also be calculated using the graphical method first described by Patlak, Gjedde and Blasberg [8, 9]. When steady state is reached in the free compartment, $dC_F(t)/dt=0$. Hence,

$$K_1 C_P(t) = k_2 C_F(t) + k_3 C_F(t) \tag{5.14}$$

$$C_F(t) = \frac{K_1}{k_2 + k_3} C_P(t) \tag{5.15}$$

And,

$$\frac{dC_B(t)}{dt} = k_3 C_F(t) = \frac{K_1 k_3}{k_2 + k_3} C_P(t) = K_i C_P(t) \tag{5.16}$$

Integration of both sides of the equation and adding the free compartment gives

$$C_T(t) = K_i \int_0^t C_P(\tau) d\tau + V_r C_P(t) \tag{5.17}$$

Here, V_r is the so-called apparent distribution volume of the tracer. Dividing both sides of the equation with $C_p(t)$ gives

$$\frac{C_T(t)}{C_P(t)} = K_i \frac{\int_0^t C_P(\tau)d\tau}{C_P(t)} + V_r \tag{5.18}$$

Hence, plotting of $\dfrac{C_T(t)}{C_P(t)}$ versus $\dfrac{\int_0^t C_P(\tau)d\tau}{C_P(t)}$ will, when steady state has been reached, result in a straight line with

a slope of K_i (Figure 5.8). This is referred to as the Patlak (or Patlak-Gjedde) Plot. One major advantage of the Patlak analysis is that the presence of a straight line gives an immediate visual confirmation of the irreversible kinetics of a tracer while the slope allows immediate visual assessment of the tracer uptake rate. Moreover, it is very easy to implement and very fast, such that in can be implemented for tracer kinetic analysis at the voxel level, resulting in the image in Figure 5.6B.

5.6 REVERSIBLE TRACER BINDING

Figure 5.9 shows the image of a healthy volunteer who underwent 80 min dynamic PET scanning with ^{11}C-DASB, a ligand for the serotonin transporter. First, the subject underwent a baseline scan. Then, the subject was given a dose of a selective serotonin reuptake inhibitor (SSRI) binding to the same transporter and competing with the tracer for binding sites, and a second PET scan was done. By measuring the ratio of tracer signal at baseline and tracer signal after the drug was given, an estimate can be made of which percentage of serotonin transporters was occupied by the drug. Figure 5.9A shows PET images at 60–80 min p.i. Based on visual, or even quantitative, analysis of these images alone, one can conclude that the tracer signal has decreased by maybe 50 per cent, probably less, after the drug was given, and hence that at most 50 per cent of the serotonin transporters were occupied by the drug. Figure 5.9B shows the non-displaceable binding potential, BP_{ND}, images of the same scans. BP_{ND} is proportional to the serotonin transporter availability. In contrast to the SUV images, the BP_{ND} images show a 90 per cent reduction in serotonin transporter availability.

To understand the difference between Figure 5.9 A and B, we have to consider the fate of the tracer in the brain. A PET tracer that enters the brain will either be free in tissue, bound specifically to the targeted receptor, transporter, or enzyme, or bound non-specifically to other structures (Figure 5.10A). Hence, we now need three tissue compartments to describe the kinetics of the tracer, involving both a free, a specifically bound, and a non-specifically bound compartment (Figure 5.10B). The measured PET data, however, generally does not provide enough information to be able to fit such a three-tissue compartment model. To reduce the model, the assumption can be made that the free and non-specific compartments interact rapidly, with a much faster interaction than between the free and specific compartments. In that

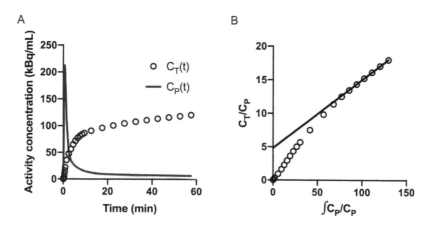

FIGURE 5.8 Plasma and tissue time-activity curves (A) of a tracer with irreversible binding and the corresponding Patlak plot (B), showing a linear relationship for times where the integral of $C_p(t)$ divided by $C_p(t)$ itself is larger than about 80.

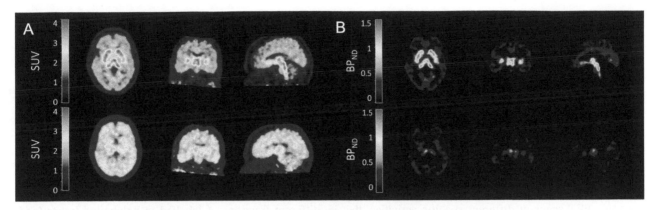

FIGURE 5.9 (A) SUV images (60–80 min p.i.) of the serotonin transporter ligand ^{11}C-DASB, at baseline (top row) and after administration of a selective serotonin reuptake inhibitor (bottom row). (B) Corresponding BP$_{ND}$ images, showing only specific binding to the serotonin transporter. Colour image available at www.routledge.com/9781138593299.

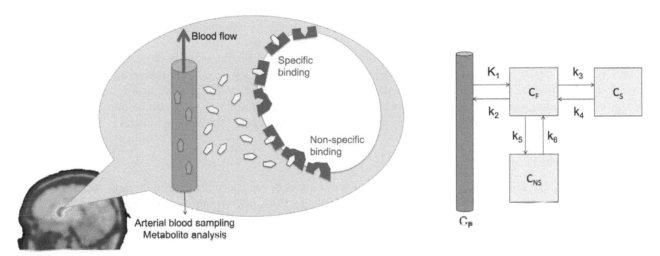

FIGURE 5.10 Distribution of receptor ligands in brain tissue (left) and three-tissue compartment model describing receptor-ligand interaction (right). C$_F$ is free tracer in tissue, C$_s$ is specifically bound tracer, and C$_{NS}$ is non-specifically bound tracer. Colour image available at www.routledge.com/9781138593299.

case, C$_F$ and C$_{NS}$ can be condensed into a single compartment containing both free and non-specifically bound tracer, and the model reduces to that shown in Figure 5.1C.

The reduced, two-tissue compartment model can be described by two differential equations:

$$\frac{dC_{F+NS}(t)}{dt} = K_1 C_P(t) - k_2 C_{F+NS}(t) - k_3 C_{F+NS}(t) + k_4 C_B(t) \tag{5.19}$$

$$\frac{dC_B(t)}{dt} = k_3 C_{F+NS}(t) - k_4 C_B(t) \tag{5.20}$$

The solution of these differential equations results in a function describing the tissue concentration over time C$_T$(t) as a function of K$_1$, k$_2$, k$_3$ and k$_4$. Now, the most interesting macro-parameters are the volume of distribution V$_T$ and the non-displaceable binding potential BP$_{ND}$:

$$V_T = \frac{K_1}{k_2}\left(1 + \frac{k_3}{k_4}\right) \tag{5.21}$$

$$BP_{ND} = \frac{k_3}{k_4} \tag{5.22}$$

V_T is, just like in the single-tissue compartment model, the equilibrium concentration ratio between tissue and plasma. BP_{ND} is the ratio of the influx and clearance rates to the specifically bound compartment, and is directly related to the concentration of available targets B_{avail} and the affinity of the tracer for the target $1/K_D$:

$$BP_{ND} \sim \frac{B_{avail}}{K_D} \tag{5.23}$$

Using two PET scans at different specific activities, that is, different fractions of labelled to unlabelled tracer (and hence different B_{avail}), both B_{avail} and K_D can be estimated. Only a single PET scan is needed to measure BP_{ND} which, although not measuring the absolute concentration of the target, is a measure that is directly proportional to the number of available targets and can be readily compared between subjects and between baseline and interventions. Since the assumption of the tracer principle is valid for most PET scans with a high specific activity, BP_{ND} will closely approximate $\dfrac{B_{max}}{K_D}$ and therefore give information about the receptor density under baseline conditions.

If the PET tracer has a high binding affinity and/or a high density of binding sites is present, tracer kinetics can become very slow because of the very small k_4 value and hence very high BP_{ND} or V_T. For these tracers, V_T or BP_{ND} can only be estimated reliably for dynamic PET data with long scanning times such that the slow tracer clearance rate with the corresponding small k_4 value can still be measured and quantified. If the k_4 value becomes too small, a quantification approach for irreversible tracer binding needs to be considered even if the binding in itself is reversible.

5.6.1 THE LOGAN PLOT

If the rate constant k_4 is much larger than the value for k_2, tracer kinetics can be approximated by single-tissue compartment since tracer clearance will be mainly determined by the clearance from the compartment representing specific binding:

$$\frac{dC_T(t)}{dt} = K_1 C_P(t) - \frac{k_2 k_4}{k_3 + k_4} C_T(t) \tag{5.24}$$

Integration of both sides and rearranging gives the following expression:

$$\frac{\int_0^t C_T(\tau)d\tau}{C_T(t)} = \frac{K_1}{k_2}\left(1 + \frac{k_3}{k_4}\right)\frac{\int_0^t C_P(\tau)d\tau}{C_T(t)} + Int = V_T \frac{\int_0^t C_P(\tau)d\tau}{C_T(t)} + Int \tag{5.25}$$

This equation represents the Logan Plot, which is a linear approach to describe and quantify reversible tracer kinetics (Figure 5.11). It is very similar to the Patlak Plot for irreversible tracer kinetics and is generally valid for quantifying reversible tracer kinetics as it does not make any assumptions on the underlying compartment model. When linearity is achieved, the slope corresponds to the distribution volume V_T. As for the Patlak Plot, the Logan Plot is easy to implement, fast to calculate and therefore very suitable for tracer kinetic analysis at the voxel level, to generate voxel wise V_T maps.

5.7 REFERENCE TISSUE METHODS

Although the reversible two-tissue compartment model provides a useful simplification compared to the full receptor-ligand three-tissue compartment model, it is often still not possible to estimate k_3 and k_4, and hence BP_{ND}, robustly. However, if a so-called *reference region* is available that is devoid of the target, and as such shows no specific binding

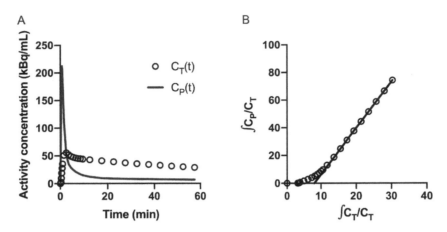

FIGURE 5.11 Plasma and tissue time-activity curves for a tracer with reversible kinetics (A) and the corresponding Logan plot (B), where the slope of the Logan plot is the distribution volume V_T.

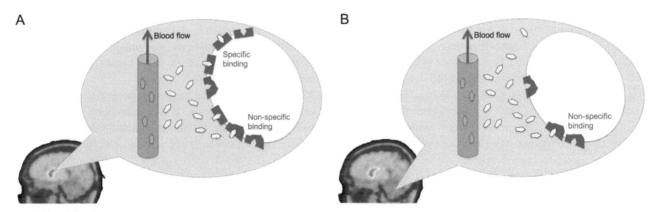

FIGURE 5.12 Distribution of a receptor ligand in brain tissue with (left) and without (right) the specific target. The tissue on the right-hand side can be used as reference tissue. Colour image available at www.routledge.com/9781138593299.

(Figure 5.12), but the same non-displaceable distribution volume K_1/k_2 as the target region, BP_{ND} can be estimated indirectly and is then usually referred to as the distribution volume ratio DVR:

$$DVR = \frac{V_T}{V'_T} = \frac{\dfrac{K_1}{k_2}\left(1 + \dfrac{k_3}{k_4}\right)}{\dfrac{K'_1}{k'_2}} = 1 + \frac{k_3}{k_4} = 1 + BP_{ND} \tag{5.26}$$

This method still requires measurement of V_T in both target and reference regions, for which we need a plasma input function. However, it is possible to rearrange the equations describing the reversible two-tissue compartment model in the target region and the single-tissue compartment model in the reference region in such a way that the plasma concentration $C_p(t)$ disappears from the equations, resulting in the so-called full reference tissue model (FRTM; [10]; Figure 5.13A). Furthermore, if the kinetics in the target region can also be approximated by single-tissue compartment kinetics, this model reduces to the simplified reference tissue model (SRTM; [11]; Figure 5.13B), with the following operational equation:

$$C_T(t) = R_1 C_{REF}(t) + \left[k_2 - \frac{R_1 k_2}{1 + BP_{ND}}\right] C_{REF}(t) \otimes e^{-\frac{k_2}{1+BP_{ND}}t} \tag{5.27}$$

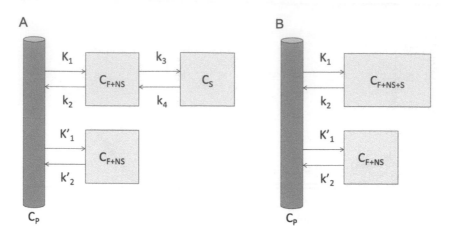

FIGURE 5.13 Full reference tissue model (A) and simplified reference tissue model (B).

Now, the tissue concentration in the target tissue is described as a function of three parameters R_1, k_2 and BP_{ND} and the reference tissue TAC $C_{REF}(t)$, where R_1 equals the ratio of delivery to target and reference region K_1/K'_1. Even if a single-tissue compartment model is not the most suitable model to describe tracer kinetics in the reference and target regions, it has been shown that a simplified reference tissue model is still a valid approach, despite the violation of some of the underlying assumptions [12]. A number of linearizations of the simplified reference tissue model have been published such as the referenced Logan method [13] and multilinear reference tissue methods [14, 15].

It is possible that at some point pseudo-equilibrium is reached for both the reference and target regions. Pseudo-equilibrium basically means that the ratio of tracer concentration in tissue versus plasma is constant. If the assumption of a pseudo-equilibrium for both reference and target tissues are valid, the ratio of the target over reference standardized uptake values (SUVR) can be considered as an approximation of the distribution volume ratio and as such as a valid quantitative endpoint.

5.8   STANDARDIZED UPTAKE VALUE

The standardized uptake value (SUV) is defined as the radioactivity concentration in tissue C_T divided by the injected amount of radioactivity A_{inj} normalized to either body weight (BW), lean body mass, or body surface area:

$$SUV = \frac{C_T(t)}{A_{inj} / BW} \tag{5.28}$$

The Patlak Plot shows that for the linear part of the plot, the tissue activity concentration $C_T(t)$ is proportional to the cumulative tracer concentration in plasma and plasma concentration itself:

$$C_T(t) = K_i \int C_P(t) + V_r C_P(t) \tag{5.29}$$

Dividing both sides of the equation by injected activity per body weight, and neglecting the second term on the right-hand side of the equation, since it is much smaller than the first term, results in

$$\frac{C_T(t)}{A_{inj} / BW} = SUV \approx K_i \frac{\int C_P(t)}{A_{inj} / BW} \tag{5.30}$$

Now, assuming that the plasma integral is proportional to the injected activity per body weight with the same proportionality constant across patients, the following approximation is valid:

$$SUV \sim K_i \tag{5.31}$$

This is a reasonable assumption for tracers that have the whole body as their systemic distribution volume, as has been shown for FDG in non-small cell lung cancer [16]. However, when used for therapy monitoring, systemic treatment effects may affect the plasma integral. For instance, increased leakage of blood vessels due to treatment results in increased uptake in healthy tissues such that normalization of tumour radioactivity concentrations to blood radioactivity concentrations (tumour to blood ratio, TBR, also called standardized uptake ratio, SUR) could provide a simplified measure that correlates better with K_i than SUV does [17, 18].

For tracers with a more specific PET signal, such as receptor ligands like ^{68}Ga-PSMA and ^{68}Ga-DOTATATE, the assumption that the plasma integral is proportional to injected activity per body weight is not necessarily true. Here, the systemic distribution volume for the tracer is rather limited and mainly determined by the tumour volume because of the much higher target expression in tumour tissue than in normal tissue. In a patient with a high tumour load, the tracer will be cleared from the plasma much faster than in a patient with a low tumour load, hence less tracer will be available in plasma, and tumour SUV will be lower in relation to K_i than in a patient with a low tumour volume [19]. For ^{68}Ga-DOTATOC and ^{68}Ga-DOTATATE, it has indeed been shown that TBR rather than SUV is proportional to K_i [17].

5.9 PARAMETRIC IMAGES AND CLINICAL APPLICATIONS

The images in Figures 5B and 8B are so-called parametric images, where tracer kinetic analysis has been done at the voxel level, resulting in color-coded images of the outcome parameter of choice instead of the radioactivity concentration: the net uptake rate K_i in Figure 5.5B and the non-displaceable binding potential BP_{ND} in Figure 5.8B. Although in principle, non-linear regression of the solution of the compartment models at the voxel level could be used to compute parametric images, there are some disadvantages to this. Firstly, NLR is sensitive to noise, resulting in uncertain outcome parameters when applied to inherently noisy single-voxel curves and, hence, noisy parametric images. Secondly, NLR is relatively slow. Even if a single NLR of one voxel can be done in one hundredth of a second, there are of the order of one million voxels in a typical PET volume, so the total computation of the parametric image would take hours on a regular personal computer. Although this may not be a problem for research applications, it makes it unsuitable for routine clinical use where images are expected shortly after the patient leaves the PET scanner. Therefore, faster methods are needed to compute parametric images. Two examples of this have been given above: the Patlak method for irreversible kinetics and the Logan method for reversible kinetics, along with their reference tissue implementations. In addition, a number of variations of the Logan method have been published, mostly focusing on reorganizing the equations to reduce noise-induced biases such as the multilinear reference tissue model [14, 15]. Another frequently used option for computing parametric images is the so-called basis function method [20–22]. Basis function methods involve pre-computing a number of possible tissue response curves by convolving the patient's individual plasma input curve (or reference tissue curve) with a set of plausible tissue impulse response functions, as shown in Figure 5.14. The

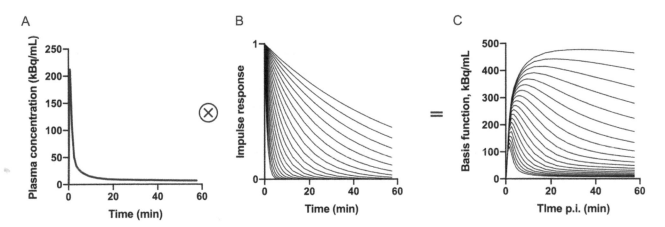

FIGURE 5.14 Basis functions: The radioactivity concentration in tissue can be described as a linear combination of one or more basis functions (C) and a whole blood component. The basis functions are pre-computed as the convolution of the plasma input curve (A) with a set of exponential impulse response functions (B), here with clearance rates ranging between 0.01 and 1 min^{-1}. To describe irreversible kinetics, an irreversible basis function with clearance rate 0, corresponding to the cumulative plasma concentration, can be added.

time-activity curve in each voxel can then be described as a linear combination of any one of these basis functions and a blood volume or reference tissue component. Since a two-tissue compartment model is mathematically equivalent to two parallel single-tissue compartment models, the time-activity curve for a two-compartment model can be described as a linear combination of any two of these basis functions and a blood volume component [6]. This linearization allows for very efficient implementation, enabling calculation of parametric images in seconds for a single-tissue, irreversible two-tissue, or simplified reference tissue model. For example, the images in Figure 5.9B were calculated using a basis function implementation of the simplified reference tissue model [21].

5.10   PET IN DRUG DEVELOPMENT – OCCUPANCY

There are a number of ways in which PET can be used in drug development.

1. First, ^{18}F-FDG, or any tracer that is a suitable marker, can be used for assessment of treatment response. This can be preferable to measurement of anatomical response using CT or MRI, since metabolic response occurs faster than changes in anatomy.
2. The uptake of the drug under investigation can be visualized and quantified by labelling it with a positron-emitting isotope. This is not always straightforward, since developing the labelling method can be a costly and lengthy procedure and may not always be possible.
3. If a specific PET tracer is available for the target of the investigated drug, a more feasible way of assessing drug-target interaction is by measuring changes in tracer signal at baseline and after administration of the investigated drug.

The images in Figure 5.8 are a typical illustration of the use of PET to measure so-called drug occupancy, which equals the drug-induced change in the concentration of available receptors, or the percentage of targets occupied by the drug:

$$Occ = \left(\frac{BP_{ND} - BP'_{ND}}{BP_{ND}} \right) \times 100\% \tag{5.32}$$

Here, BP_{ND} is the binding potential at baseline and BP'_{ND} is the binding potential after administration of the drug. A classic example of the application of this method in drug development are two studies wherein the optimal concentration and optimal dosing regimen of the neuroleptic drug ziprasidone, targeting D2 receptors, were evaluated using a PET study with the specific D2 ligand [^{11}C]raclopride [23, 24]. Seven healthy control subjects were given different doses of the drug, and one subject placebo, prior to a dynamic PET scan with [^{11}C]raclopride. BP_{ND} at each drug dose can then be calculated using SRTM and receptor occupancy at each of the doses can be calculated by relating BP_{ND} at that dose to BP_{ND} in the placebo subject. Then, once the optimal dose is known, the time course of the receptor occupancy can be assessed. [^{11}C]raclopride in a number of subjects at varying times after drug administration, and the dosage regimen required to maintain a certain level of occupancy was established. A study like this can be done with about 20 subjects, compared to hundreds of subjects that typically need to be included for conventional dose-escalation protocols.

A challenge arises for tracers that have no suitable reference region lacking specific binding, and for which BP_{ND} can also not be robustly determined using a two-tissue compartment model. In that case, the specific and non-specific contributions to the tissue signal cannot be separated, and only the total distribution volume V_T can be measured. In this case, the Lassen Plot can be used to estimate occupancy using two PET scans at baseline and after drug administration [25]:

$$V_T - V'_T = Occ \times V_T + V_{ND} \tag{5.33}$$

Here, V_T is the volume of distribution at baseline (tracer alone), V'_T the volume of distribution after drug administration, and V_{ND} is the non-displaceable volume of distribution. If V_{ND} is assumed to be the same for all regions across the grey matter, which is a reasonable assumption, plotting V_T-V'_T versus V_T for a number of regions should result in a straight

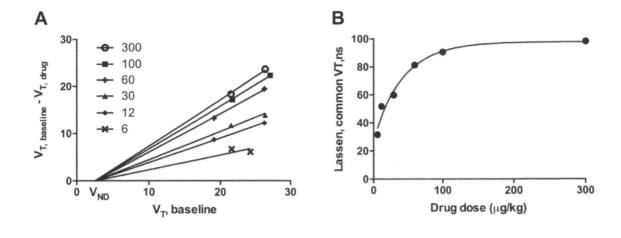

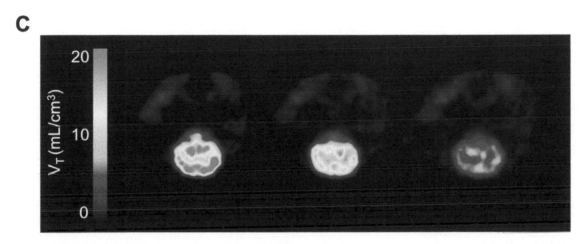

FIGURE 5.15 (A) Lassen plots (V_T. V'_T versus V_T) for six different doses of an SV2A binding drug in µg/kg as measured with the SV2A ligand [^{11}C]UCB-A in a pig study. The solid lines are multi-linear regressions with a common x-axis intercept equal to V_{ND}, assuming identical V_{ND} across scans. (B) Occupancy versus drug dose based on Lassen plots with common V_{ND}. (C) Corresponding [^{11}C]UCB-A V_T images at baseline and at drug doses of 30 and 100 ug/kg, resulting in 52 and 81 per cent occupancy (left to right). Reprinted with permission from Estrada et al [26]. Colour image available at www.routledge.com/9781138593299.

line, the slope of which equals Occ, and the intercept equals V_{ND}. An example of this, using only two regions, is given in Figure 5.15.

5.11 SUMMARY

The aim of this chapter was to provide the reader with insight into the different steps necessary to be able to use PET as a tool for measurement of (patho)physiology (Figure 5.16), along with examples of a number of applications, but also to describe how different outcome measures are related and can be simplified. In addition to being a valuable clinical diagnostic imaging modality, the added value of PET lies very much in its inherent capabilities as a tool for *measurement* of biological processes. This can be applied to basic research in the understanding of these processes, in the understanding of disease, or in drug development research. However, simplification and automation of the quantitative methods described in this chapter also allows for use of quantitative information in clinical practice, exceeding simple uptake measures such as SUV. Examples for this are given in chapter 15 in Volume III by Trägårdh et al. on cardiac perfusion imaging, where true quantitative PET has found one of its first routine clinical applications.

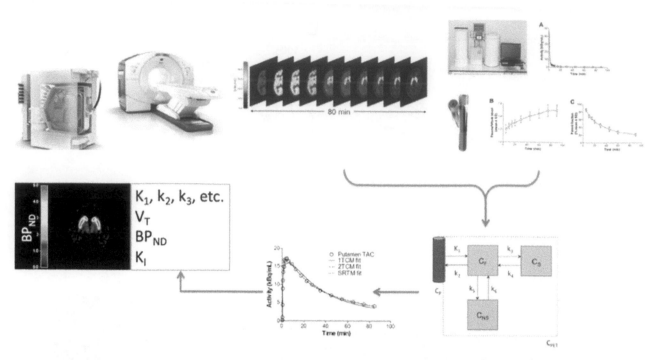

FIGURE 5.16 Summary of steps in a quantitative PET study. Colour image available at www.routledge.com/9781138593299.

REFERENCES

[1] L. A. Hahn, G. C. Hevesy, and E. C. Lundsgaard, "The circulation of phosphorus in the body revealed by application of radioactive phosphorus as indicator," *Biochem J,* vol. 31, no. 10, pp. 1705–9, 1937, doi: 10.1042/bj0311705.

[2] G. Hevesy, "The Absorption and Translocation of Lead by Plants: A Contribution to the Application of the Method of Radioactive Indicators in the Investigation of the Change of Substance in Plants," *Biochem J,* vol. 17, no. 4–5, pp. 439–45, 1923, doi: 10.1042/bj0170439.

[3] S. S. Kety, "The theory and applications of the exchange of inert gas at the lungs and tissues," *Pharmacological reviews,* vol. 3.1, pp. 1–41, 1951.

[4] L. Sokoloff *et al.,* "The [14C]deoxyglucose method for the measurement of local cerebral glucose utilization: theory, procedure, and normal values in the conscious and anesthetized albino rat," *J.Neurochem.,* vol. 28, no. 5, pp. 897–916, 1977.

[5] M. A. Mintun, M. E. Raichle, M. R. Kilbourn, G. F. Wooten, and M. J. Welch, "A quantitative model for the in vivo assessment of drug binding sites with positron emission tomography," *Ann Neurol,* vol. 15, no. 3, pp. 217–27, 1984, doi: 10.1002/ana.410150302.

[6] R. N. Gunn, S. R. Gunn, and V. J. Cunningham, "Positron emission tomography compartmental models," *J Cereb Blood Flow Metab,* vol. 21, no. 6, pp. 635–52, 2001.

[7] R. Boellaard, A. Van Lingen, S. C. Van Balen, B. G. Hoving, and A. A. Lammertsma, "Characteristics of a new fully programmable blood sampling device for monitoring blood radioactivity during PET," *Eur J Nucl Med,* vol. 28, no. 1, pp. 81–89, 2001.

[8] C. S. Patlak, R. G. Blasberg, and J. D. Fenstermacher, "Graphical evaluation of blood-to-brain transfer constants from multiple-time uptake data," *J.Cereb.Blood Flow Metab,* vol. 3, no. 1, pp. 1–7, 1983.

[9] A. Gjedde, "Calculation of cerebral glucose phosphorylation from brain uptake of glucose analogs in vivo: A re-examination," *Brain Res,* vol. 257, no. 2, pp. 237–74, 1982, doi: 10.1016/0165-0173(82)90018-2.

[10] A. A. Lammertsma *et al.,* "Comparison of methods for analysis of clinical [C-11]raclopride studies," *Journal of Cerebral Blood Flow and Metabolism,* vol. 16, no. 1, pp. 42–52, 1996.

[11] A. A. Lammertsma and S. P. Hume, "Simplified reference tissue model for PET receptor studies," *Neuroimage,* vol. 4, no. 3 Pt 1, pp. 153–58, 1996.

[12] C. A. Salinas, G. E. Searle, and R. N. Gunn, "The simplified reference tissue model: model assumption violations and their impact on binding potential," *J Cereb Blood Flow Metab,* vol. 35, no. 2, pp. 304–11, 2015, doi: 10.1038/jcbfm.2014.202.

[13] J. Logan, J. S. Fowler, N. D. Volkow, G. J. Wang, Y. S. Ding, and D. L. Alexoff, "Distribution volume ratios without blood sampling from graphical analysis of PET data," *J Cereb.Blood Flow Metab,* vol. 16, no. 5, pp. 834–40, 1996.

[14] M. Ichise *et al.*, "Linearized reference tissue parametric imaging methods: application to [11C]DASB positron emission tomography studies of the serotonin transporter in human brain," *J Cereb Blood Flow Metab,* vol. 23, no. 9, pp. 1096–112, 2003, doi: 10.1097/01.WCB.0000085441.37552.CA.

[15] M. Ichise, H. Toyama, R. B. Innis, and R. E. Carson, "Strategies to improve neuroreceptor parameter estimation by linear regression analysis," *J Cereb Blood Flow Metab,* vol. 22, no. 10, pp. 1271–81, 2002, doi: 10.1097/00004647-200210000-00015.

[16] C. J. Hoekstra *et al.*, "Methods to monitor response to chemotherapy in non-small cell lung cancer with 18F-FDG PET," *J Nucl Med,* vol. 43, no. 10, pp. 1304–09, 2002.

[17] E. Ilan, I. Velikyan, M. Sandstrom, A. Sundin, and M. Lubberink, "Tumor-to-Blood Ratio for Assessment of Somatostatin Receptor Density in Neuroendocrine Tumors Using (68)Ga-DOTATOC and (68)Ga-DOTATATE," *J Nucl Med,* vol. 61, no. 2, pp. 217–21, 2020, doi: 10.2967/jnumed.119.228072.

[18] J. van den Hoff *et al.*, "The PET-derived tumor-to-blood standard uptake ratio (SUR) is superior to tumor SUV as a surrogate parameter of the metabolic rate of FDG," *EJNMMI research,* vol. 3, no. 1, p. 77, 2013, doi: 10.1186/2191-219X-3-77.

[19] I. Velikyan *et al.*, "Quantitative and qualitative intrapatient comparison of 68Ga-DOTATOC and 68Ga-DOTATATE: Net uptake rate for accurate quantification," *J Nucl Med,* Research Support, Non-U.S. Gov't vol. 55, no. 2, pp. 204–10, 2014, doi: 10.2967/jnumed.113.126177.

[20] R. Boellaard, P. Knaapen, A. Rijbroek, G. J. Luurtsema, and A. A. Lammertsma, "Evaluation of basis function and linear least squares methods for generating parametric blood flow images using 15O-water and Positron Emission Tomography," *Mol Imaging Biol,* vol. 7, no. 4, pp. 273–85, 2005.

[21] R. N. Gunn, A. A. Lammertsma, S. P. Hume, and V. J. Cunningham, "Parametric imaging of ligand-receptor binding in PET using a simplified reference region model," *Neuroimage,* vol. 6, no. 4, pp. 279–87, 1997.

[22] H. Watabe *et al.*, "Parametric imaging of myocardial blood flow with 15O-water and PET using the basis function method," *J Nucl Med,* vol. 46, no. 7, pp. 1219–24, 2005.

[23] C. J. Bench *et al.*, "Dose dependent occupancy of central dopamine D2 receptors by the novel neuroleptic CP-88,059-01: A study using positron emission tomography and 11C-raclopride," *Psychopharmacology (Berl),* vol. 112, no. 2–3, pp. 308–14, 1993.

[24] C. J. Bench *et al.*, "The time course of binding to striatal dopamine D2 receptors by the neuroleptic ziprasidone (CP-88,059-01) determined by positron emission tomography," *Psychopharmacology (Berl),* vol. 124, no. 1–2, pp. 141–47, 1996.

[25] N. A. Lassen *et al.*, "Benzodiazepine receptor quantification in vivo in humans using [11C]flumazenil and PET: Application of the steady-state principle," *J Cereb.Blood Flow Metab,* vol. 15, no. 1, pp. 152–65, 1995.

[26] S. Estrada *et al.*, "[(11)C]UCB-A, a novel PET tracer for synaptic vesicle protein 2A," *Nucl Med Biol,* vol. 43, no. 6, pp. 325–32, 2016, doi: 10.1016/j.nucmedbio.2016.03.004.

6 Principles of Radiological Protection in Healthcare

Sören Mattsson

CONTENTS

DOI: 10.1201/9780429489549-6

6.1   INTRODUCTION

The use of ionizing radiation and radioactive substances for diagnostic, interventional, and therapeutic procedures in healthcare provides benefits to millions of people each year. The use of X-rays and radiopharmaceuticals for imaging (especially in CT and hybrid imaging like PET/CT and SPECT/CT) has increased much over the past thirty years [1] and has revolutionized medicine. Therapies in the form of external beam radiation therapy, brachytherapy, and therapy with radiopharmaceuticals (now often named molecular radiotherapy) are increasingly planned and given to delivering the required radiation absorbed dose to the treatment volumes and at the same time reducing the absorbed dose to healthy tissues. All this has also made the use of ionizing radiation in medicine the single largest artificial source of ionizing radiation for the population in many countries. Since ionizing radiation also has harmful effects, a radiation protection approach is needed. The International Commission on Radiological Protection (ICRP) has formulated the primary aim of radiation protection. It is "to contribute to an appropriate level of protection for people and the environment against the detrimental effects of radiation exposure without unduly limiting the desirable human actions that may be associated with such exposure" [2]. ICRP is developing recommendations and guidance based on the most recent advances in our knowledge of radiation risks to humans and to the environment, and in application and control of radiation. ICRP is a non-profit organization and acts independently of governments and organizations, including industry and other users of radiation. Although ICRP just provides recommendations, governments and international organizations throughout the world rely on its estimates and follow its recommendations. ICRP bases much of its work on the results reported by the United Nations Scientific Committee on the Effects of Atomic Radiation (UNSCEAR), which was established by the General Assembly of the United Nations in 1955. Its mandate is to assess and report levels and effects of exposure to ionizing radiation (www.unscear.org).

The understanding of the effects of exposure to radiation is based on radiation epidemiology and radiation biology. Radiation epidemiology relies on statistical analyses of observed effects on large populations that have been exposed to radiation. For effects of radiation exposure on humans, the gold standard today is the work being done by the Radiation Effects Research Foundation (www.rerf.or.jp/en/) with survivors of the nuclear weapons detonated over the Japanese cities of Hiroshima and Nagasaki in 1945. This is supplemented by studies of other population groups, such as workers in mines and nuclear facilities, patients, and people exposed to radon in homes, and others, as summarized and reviewed by ICRP and UNSCEAR [2, 3], the United States National Research Council (NRC), and other national organizations. The NRC committee on the biological effects of ionizing radiation (BEIR) develops risk estimates for cancer and other health effects from exposure to low-level ionizing radiation. The BEIR VII report [4] is the latest in a series on the biological effects of ionizing radiation. The BEIR committee's risk models for exposure to low-level ionizing radiation are based on a sex and age distribution similar to that of the entire U.S. population and refer to the risk that an individual would face over his or her lifespan.

Basic risk data are also gained from research in radiation biology investigating how radiation exposure affects people, animals, and plants at the individual, tissue, cellular, and even subcellular level. This work is often done in laboratories using cell cultures or mice.

This chapter deals with principles for radiological protection and safety of patients, staff and the general public. It will also discuss the situation for persons who assist and support patients as well as for volunteers in biomedical research. A special section is devoted to pregnant and breast-feeding women among patients and staff members. How the principles for the radiation protection of the environment influence healthcare and the necessity to protect strong radiation sources will also be briefly discussed as will the importance of radiological protection and medical service in connection with radiological and nuclear emergencies.

6.2   EFFECTS OF EXPOSURE TO IONIZING RADIATION

The biological effects of radiation can be grouped as follows:

1. Tissue reactions (deterministic effects) and
2. an increased likelihood for cancer during the rest of life and hereditary effects (both are stochastic effects).

Tissue reactions result from cell killing, cell loss, or inflammation and occur if the absorbed dose to tissue is above a certain threshold [5]. The goal of radiotherapy is to kill the cells in the tumour volume, but tissue reactions can also be reached in normal tissues during radiotherapy. Also, in complex fluoroscopically controlled intervention procedures, this may happen. Tissue reactions in normal tissues have to be prevented, avoided or, if clinically unavoidable, handled carefully.

An increased total likelihood of cancer over the baseline incidence of cancer (in a number of different organs and tissues) may occur in a population exposed to ionizing radiation. Some groups show higher than average sensitivity to cancer induction, for example, embryo-foetuses, infants, adolescents, and young women (breast cancer).

The linear no threshold (LNT) hypothesis has been used in radiation protection for over forty years [6]. A cancer risk model conforms to the LNT hypothesis if the excess risk of cancer at low doses or dose rates increases approximately proportionally to the absorbed dose, with no threshold. It has been shown that also risk models with a linear-quadratic dose response can satisfy the LNT hypothesis for low doses [6, 7]. The LNT model relies heavily on human epidemiology, with support from radiobiology and the LNT model (with the steepness of the dose-response slope perhaps reduced by a dose and dose-rate effectiveness factor (DDREF) should continue to be utilized for radiation protection purposes [6]. Also, the most recent epidemiologic studies with dose response functions that are essentially linear or LQ argue for some risk at low doses [8]. The scientific underpinnings of the LNT model include the early mentioned reports: UNSCEAR [9], ICRP Publication 99 [10], and the US National Academies of Sciences, National Research Council BEIR VII Report [4]. These authoritative scientific bodies have repeatedly endorsed the use of LNT models for estimating and regulating risks from ionizing radiation and concluded that despite uncertainties at low dose and dose rates, the LNT model remains the most practical and implementable model for radiation protection.

6.3　ABSORBED DOSE ESTIMATION

Accurate radiation dosimetry is a requirement of radiation oncology, diagnostic radiology, and nuclear medicine. It is necessary for therapeutic and diagnostic optimization, patient risk estimations, and retrospective epidemiological studies of the biological effects resulting from low absorbed doses of ionizing radiation.

A detailed description of methods for absorbed dose estimations for organs and tissues as well as of the effective dose for patients in diagnostic nuclear medicine are given in Chapter 3 (Diagnostic Dosimetry). Dose estimates for various investigations and age groups have been published by ICRP [11]. There are various software codes available to calculate organ absorbed doses and effective doses to patients in diagnostic nuclear medicine. A software code named "IDAC-Dose2.2" [12] was developed specifically for ICRP, and the code was benchmarked against the software "DCAL" by Eckerman and colleagues [12, 13]. Both DCAL and IDAC-Dose are codes which use the radionuclide data of ICRP Publication 107 [14], and the Specific Absorbed Fraction data of Publication 133 [15] and strictly follow the ICRP computational framework for internal dose assessment of the reference person to estimate the effective dose [2].

The Medical Internal Radiation Dose (MIRD) Committee of the United States Society of Nuclear Medicine and Molecular Imaging (SNMMI) develops standard methods, models, assumptions, and mathematical schema for assessing internal radiation doses from administered radiopharmaceuticals. The advantage of the MIRD method is that it systematically reduces complex dosimetry analyses to relatively simple methods, including software tools for experimental and clinical use. The Radiation Dose Assessment Resource (RADAR) [16] seeks to bring together the various resources that exist in the areas of internal and external dose assessment and integrate them into a single system. Its software code OLINDA-EXM version 2.0 calculates the effective dose using their own absorbed fractions, based on the anatomical and physiological data given in ICRP Publication 89 [17].

6.4　PRINCIPLES OF RADIOLOGICAL PROTECTION

Scientific facts in combination with ethical values are ingredients necessary for making recommendations on how to behave in light of our often-limited scientific knowledge. The recommendations also rely on experience to help make them practical.

Radiological protection is based on society's fundamental values in ethics [18–20].

The ethical questions in medicine are often addressed by referring to four basic principles [17, 21, 22]:

- Respect for autonomy (of the individual)
- Non-maleficence (do not harm – "an appropriate level of protection")
- Beneficence (do good – "without unduly limiting … desirable human actions"), and
- Justice (be fair).

There are also additional values which may be implied in the above principles but deserve to be mentioned, namely,

- Prudence: (keep in mind possible long-term risks of actions) and
- Honesty: (truthful sharing of knowledge with concerned groups and individuals).

The concept of prudence is generally understood to be at the heart of the Precautionary Principle, which is highly valued in dealing with scientific problems where action is required in the absence of definitive data. Honesty, in the sense used here is often thought as "working in an open and transparent manner".

The core ethical values support the aims of the system of radiological protection defined by the International Radiological Protection Commission [2] and its *three fundamental principles: justification, optimization,* and *individual dose limitation.* Three procedural values are highlighted to aid the practical implementation of radiological protection: accountability, transparency, and inclusiveness (stakeholder participation). These principles include exposures that arise from both medical and non-medical applications.

The principle of *justification*, states that any decision that alters the exposure situation should do more good than harm. This means that by introducing a new radiation source in planned exposure situations, or by reducing exposures in existing and emergency exposure situations, one should achieve sufficient benefit to offset any costs or negative consequences. The benefits are deemed to apply to specific individuals, society as a whole, and also to the environment.

The principle of *optimization*, stipulates that all exposures should be kept as low as reasonably achievable, taking into account economic and societal factors. It is a source-related process, aimed at achieving the best level of protection under the prevailing circumstances through an ongoing, iterative process. This principle is the cornerstone of the system of protection. Furthermore, in order to avoid inequitable distributions of individual exposures, the ICRP recommends restricting doses to individuals and nonhuman biota from a particular source.

The principle of *limitation*, states that individual exposures should not exceed the dose limits recommended by the ICRP. It applies to planned exposure situations, other than medical exposure of patients, or exposure of non-human biota.

These three fundamental principles of protection are central to the system of radiological protection, which applies to different types of exposure situations (planned, emergency, and existing) and to categories of exposure (occupational, public, medical, and environmental).

For human health, the system aims to "manage and control exposures to ionizing radiation so that deterministic effects are prevented, and the risks of stochastic effects are reduced to the extent reasonably achievable" [2].

6.5 EXPOSURE CATEGORIES

The ICRP [2] distinguishes between three categories of exposures: occupational, public, and medical exposures.

6.5.1 MEDICAL EXPOSURE

Medical exposure includes radiation exposure of patients and occurs in diagnostic, interventional, and therapeutic procedures. There are several features of radiological methods in medicine that require an approach that differs from the radiological protection in other planned exposure situations. In healthcare, the exposure is deliberate and directly beneficial to the irradiated patient. The principles of radiation protection in medical exposure are discussed in detail in ICRP Publication 105 [23]. Another type of medical exposure is the exposure of volunteers in biomedical research. Such an exposure has no direct benefit for the exposed person. The exposure of carers and helpers (as family members and close friends) is also classified as a medical exposure. Figure 6.1 shows some of the ICRP publications related to radiological protection in medicine from the period 2016–2020.

6.5.2 OCCUPATIONAL EXPOSURE

Occupational exposure is defined as all radiation exposure to workers that occurs during their work. The employer has the main responsibility for the protection of the employee.

6.5.3 EXPOSURE OF THE PUBLIC

This category covers all exposures except occupational exposures and medical exposures. Such exposure can be caused by various sources of radiation. The contribution from natural radiation sources is by far the largest, but there are also a

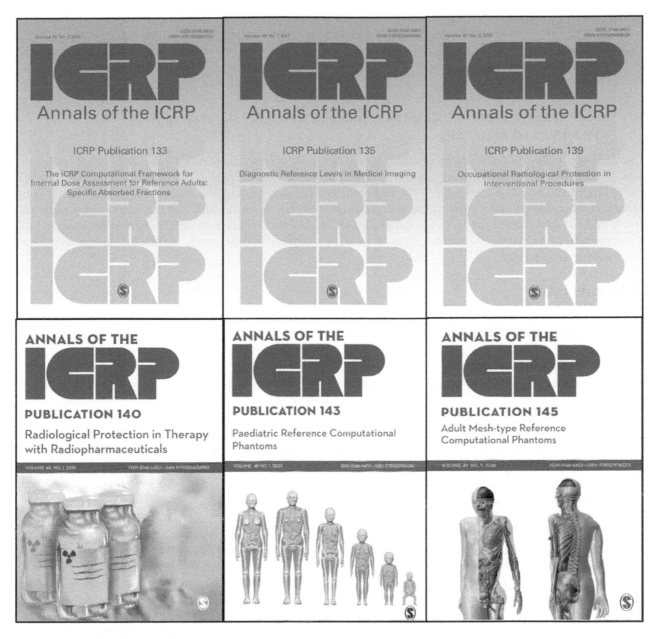

FIGURE 6.1 Some ICRP publications related to radiological protection in medicine (2016–2020).

number of artificial sources for which the exposure can be controlled. In view of the protection of embryos and foetuses, exposure of pregnant workers is considered and regulated as public exposure [2]. This is also the case for young children and infants as well as visitors not engaged in direct care or comforting a patient.

6.5.4 SPECIAL SITUATIONS FOR RADIOLOGICAL PROTECTION OF PATIENTS IN HEALTHCARE

Medical use of radiation for patients is voluntary and combined with an expectation of a result of direct relevance to the individual patient's health. The voluntary decision is made with varying degrees of informed consent, which should cover the expected benefit and also the potential risks. The amount of information provided to obtain informed consent varies depending on the level of exposure (e.g., different levels in diagnostic, interventional, or therapeutic procedures) and the patient's medical condition. An exception to the concept of voluntary exposure that leads to a direct individual medical benefit is the use of radiation in biomedical research. Here, the voluntary exposure is something that is an advantage for the society rather than for the exposed individual. Therefore, informed consent is always needed. Screening is performed to identify a disease process that has not been clinically proven. Any application of ionizing radiation for screening asymptomatic individuals in specific populations must be evaluated and motivated for their clinical benefit and associated risks. Patients undergoing screening should be fully informed of the potential benefits and risks, including radiation risks.

6.6 APPLICATION OF THE PRINCIPLES FOR RADIOLOGICAL PROTECTION TO PATIENTS IN HEALTHCARE

In the case of patients, the basic radiation protection principles apply to justification and optimization. It is not appropriate to apply dose limits, since there are often chronic, severe or even life-threatening medical conditions that are more critical than the radiation exposure. The emphasis then lies on justifying the medical procedures and on optimizing radiological protection. In diagnostic and intervention procedures, justification for procedures (for a particular purpose and for an individual patient) and management of the patient radiation dose in proportion to the medical task are mechanisms to avoid unnecessary investigations or unnecessary radiation exposure. In radiation therapy, avoidance of accidents is a major issue.

6.6.1 Justification

Three levels of justification (generally for the method, for the particular examination/ treatment, for the individual patient) are considered in medical exposures.

6.6.1.1 Generally for the Method

At the first and most general level, appropriate use of radiation in healthcare is more beneficial than harmful for patients and society.

6.6.1.2 For a Specific Examination/Treatment with a Specified Target

The second level of justification defines and motivates a specified procedure with a specified target. The purpose is to assess whether the radiological procedure will improve the diagnosis or treatment or provide the necessary information about the exposed individuals. Such assessments need to be reviewed from time to time – for example, is a chest X-ray for diagnostic purposes for patients showing relevant symptoms justified.

6.6.1.3 For an Individual Patient

At the third level, the application of the procedure to an individual patient should be justified. Therefore, all individual medical exposures should be justified in advance, taking into account the specific objectives of the exposure and the person's characteristics. The procedure should be judged to be more beneficial than harmful to the patient. This includes checking that the required information is not already available and that the proposed procedure is the most appropriate.

There are numerous reports indicating that a substantial fraction of diagnostic imaging examinations is unjustified. This means that an unnecessary radiation burden is placed on the population and where radiation protection of patients can be more efficient [24]. Medical practitioners will require quantitative guidance as to the risk–benefits arising from modern X-ray imaging methods if they are to make rational judgements as to the applicability of modern high-dose techniques to particular diagnostic and therapeutic tasks. At present such guidance is variable due to the lack of a rational framework for assessing the clinical impact of medical imaging techniques [25].

6.6.2 Optimization

Optimization of radiological protection for patients in medicine is usually applied at two levels: (1) design, appropriate selection and construction of equipment and installations; and (2) the daily working methods. The basic purpose of this optimization of protection is to adjust the protective measures for a radiation source in such a way that the net benefit is maximized. Optimization of protection in medical exposures for diagnostic nuclear medicine procedures does not necessarily mean reducing administered activities to the patient. Optimization of radiological protection means that the doses are *as low as reasonably achievable* (ALARA), taking into account economic and societal factors, and are best described as managing the radiation dose to the patient in proportion to the medical purpose. We should give attention to both what "as low as" and "reasonable" means in ALARA. Optimization does not always mean minimization of radiation absorbed doses for a fixed image quality. Using new imaging systems with higher sensitivity may give improved image quality and therefore improved diagnostic possibilities. Therefore, the optimal conditions could be reached for a better image quality, hopefully, but not necessarily, also for a lower absorbed dose. For therapeutic application, the goal is to give such a high dose that the tumour is eradicated. Sometimes the dose to the tumour tissue has to be reduced not to exceed the tolerance doses for critical organs / tissues.

An optimization of the absorbed dose to healthy tissues should also be performed. For nuclear medicine this can, for example, be done by reducing the total amount of unnecessary non-clinically relevant decays in the body through increased voiding or hydration. In X-ray imaging it can be done by shielding of organs.

Thus, the absorbed dose to the patient should be managed to ensure that it corresponds to the medical purpose (the required radiation dose – neither more nor less) to obtain the desired image or deliver an effective treatment.

6.6.3 Dose Limiting

As earlier mentioned, the principle of dose limitation does not apply to medical exposures of patients. However, some management of patient exposure is needed. The use of diagnostic reference levels (discussed below) is one way to help towards optimization of diagnostic procedures.

For therapeutic procedures, however, as previously stated, consideration of tolerance radiation doses for critical organs may limit the radiation absorbed dose to the tumour tissue in both external radiation therapy and in radiopharmaceutical therapy.

6.7 MANAGEMENT OF PATIENT EXPOSURE FROM DIAGNOSTIC PROCEDURES – DIAGNOSTIC REFERENCE LEVELS, DRLS

Diagnostic reference levels, DRLs, are used to evaluate whether the amount of radiation is unusually high or low for a particular diagnostic procedure or in line with those of peers [18]. The reasons for significant differences should be investigated. A DRL indicates a form of investigation level for medical exposure. DRL is a help to a professional assessment and is not a dividing line between "good" and "bad" medicine. The numerical values for DRL are advisory; however, the concept may be a legal requirement. DRLs should be set by regional/national/local bodies. The values should be reviewed at regular intervals, which is a trade-off between the necessary stability and consideration for the long-term changes in the observed dose distributions. A DRL can be used to improve a regional, national, or local distribution of observed results for a medical activity by reducing the frequency of too-high or too-low values. DRLs also bring an important harmonization of diagnostic procedures between different hospitals. DRLs should be easily measured, for example, using: entrance skin dose (ESD), dose-area product (DAP), dose length product (DLP), or administered activity (A). DRL is normally set at the 75th percentile dose, which is that dose for a group of patient doses below which 75 per cent of observations (patient doses) fall. DRLs apply to groups, not to single patients. It is inappropriate to use the numerical values for DRL as regulatory limits or for commercial purposes.

6.8 EXPOSURE RESULTING FROM RADIATION THERAPY

The use of ionizing radiation for the treatment of cancer is constantly increasing, giving rise to several new issues and concerns. One of the most important radiation protection aspects is the associated radiation dose given to healthy tissues. This undesirable dose contribution is a result of both radiotherapy and diagnostic imaging. The absorbed dose to healthy tissues from external radiation therapy derives mainly from the primary therapy beam. However, the patient also receives non-negligible organ doses derived from secondary radiation produced in the treatment machine and within the patient's body. This secondary radiation, in particular photons and neutrons, can travel long distances and consequently give radiation doses to organs that are far from the primary treatment volume. The dose contribution to healthy organs from diagnostic procedures is growing due to the increase of repeated imaging performed in radiotherapy. Patients undergoing both external radiotherapy and treatment with radiopharmaceuticals may also receive a high absorbed dose to healthy tissues.

6.9 EMBRYO/FOETUS OR INFANT DURING EXPOSURE OF PATIENTS, WHO ARE PREGNANT OR BREAST-FEEDING

Before a woman of childbearing age (15–45 years) is examined with X-rays or radiopharmaceuticals or treated with various forms of radiotherapy, it is important to find out whether she is pregnant or not, and if she is breastfeeding or caring for an infant [26]. Some procedures in nuclear medicine (e.g. use of radioactive iodine) can impose increased risks to the embryo/foetus [26, 27].

If pregnancy or breastfeeding has been confirmed, it is important to examine if the nuclear medicine procedure can be postponed or if there are alternatives involving non-ionizing radiation. For diagnostic nuclear medicine investigations, pregnancy is not an absolute contraindication and may in many situations provide essential diagnostic information: for example, confirmation or exclusion of pulmonary embolism. Dose estimates are available for four stages of pregnancy (early pregnancy, 3 months', 6 months' and 9 months' gestation) and for a large number of radiopharmaceuticals [28]. Nevertheless, there are considerable uncertainties about how much activity may cross the placenta barrier and about the biokinetics in the foetus.

A pregnant woman should not undergo therapeutic nuclear medicine procedures unless there are implications to save her life. If the procedure is justified, the possible foetal radiation dose should be calculated, the risk for malformations and childhood cancer should be estimated, and the information shared with the patient.

Many radiopharmaceuticals are excreted through the breast milk of nursing mothers [29]. For radiopharmaceuticals used for diagnostic procedures, breast feeding interruption schedules are recommended keeping the effective dose to the infant under 1 mSv. Before start of therapy with radiopharmaceuticals, breast feeding has to be stopped. Higher doses, such as those from therapeutic procedures, can result in significant foetal harm and risk for the nursing infant. More detailed information is given in ICRP Publication 84 [26].

6.10 PRINCIPLES FOR RADIOLOGICAL PROTECTION OF HEALTHY VOLUNTEERS IN BIOMEDICAL RESEARCH

Research involving humans form a valuable, often unavoidable, step in the development of new knowledge in medicine and biology and for the development of new pharmaceuticals.

Volunteers are of two groups:

1. Patients, who have a diagnosis and are suffering from a disease;
2. Healthy persons who are not suffering from any disease.

The participation of volunteers in biomedical research and its justification is discussed in ICRP Publication 62 [30] – a discussion based on the Declaration of Helsinki (reproduced in ICRP Publication 62, 1992), and continuously augmented www.wma.net/policies-post/wma-declaration-of-helsinki-ethical-principles-for-medical-research-involving-human-subjects/). The potential harm for the volunteer should be weighed against the potential societal benefit of the investigation, which has to substantially exceed the risk for the volunteers. No one should be subjected to medical or scientific investigations without giving free and informed consent. This means that the risks and likely benefits of the proposed research should be explained in advance. The subject has the right to accept the risk voluntarily and has an equal right to refuse.

By free and informed consent is meant genuine consent, freely given, with a proper understanding of the nature and consequence of what is proposed, obtained from adults who are of sound mind. Therefore, such investigations should not be carried out on children or those who are mentally ill or defective, as they cannot give free and informed consent in this sense. In exceptional circumstances, as when proposed investigations are likely to benefit children or mental defectives and the risks are sufficiently small, those responsible for such individuals might be able to agree to their participation.

Pregnant women should not be asked to take part in research projects involving irradiation of the foetus unless the pregnancy itself is central to the research, and then only if other techniques involving less risk cannot be used. If the subject is in a dependent position vis-à-vis the investigators, for example as an employee, a student or even a patient, or can expect some non-health benefit such as promotion, special privileges or payment, a difficult situation arises. It is particularly important that consent under such circumstances can be given freely. Even though a subject may have given consent to the investigation at the start, this consent can be withdrawn at any time by the subject. If the subject withdraws consent, the investigator must at once terminate the subject's involvement in the study.

All research involving human subjects must be carefully planned to gain the maximum medical or scientific knowledge with the minimum risk and inconvenience to the subject. To ensure an impartial and independent view of the need for the investigation and the balance between the likely benefits and the risks, proposals should be vetted by an "Ethics Committee" composed of persons not engaged in the research project.

TABLE 6.1
Dose Limitations for Volunteers Under Different Conditions [31]

Benefit for the society	"Acceptable" effective dose
Minor	<0.1 mSv
Intermediate	0.1–1 mSv
Moderate	1–10 mSv
Substantial	> 10 mSv

The ICRP [30] also recommends dose constraints for volunteers under different conditions as summarized in Table 6.1 below.

6.11 PRINCIPLES FOR RADIOLOGICAL PROTECTION OF PERSONNEL, CARERS AND HELPERS, INFANTS, SMALL CHILDREN AND VISITORS, AND MEMBERS OF THE PUBLIC

6.11.1 PERSONNEL

Exposure of workers may arise from unsealed sources, either through external irradiation of the body or through entry of radioactive substances into the body. The principles for the protection of workers from ionizing radiation, including those in medicine, are discussed in Publication 75 [32] and in Publication 103 [2]. Generally, the annual effective dose to staff working full time in nuclear medicine with optimized protection should be below 5 mSv.

6.11.2 CARERS AND HELPERS (AS FAMILY MEMBERS AND CLOSE FRIENDS)

While exposures in healthcare are predominantly delivered to individuals (patients), other individuals caring for and comforting patients are also exposed to radiation. These individuals include parents and others, normally family or close friends, who may come close to patients following administration of radiopharmaceuticals. These exposures are considered medical exposures [2]. Publication 94 [33] recommends that for individuals directly involved in comforting and caring (other than young children and infants) a dose constraint of 5 mSv per episode (e.g. for the duration of a given release from hospital after therapy) is reasonable [2, 33]. The restriction needs to be used flexibly. Higher doses may for example be suitable for parents of very ill children.

6.11.3 INFANTS, SMALL CHILDREN AND VISITORS, AND MEMBERS OF THE PUBLIC

ICRP Publication 94 [33] recommends that young children and infants as well as visitors not engaged in direct care or comforting should be treated as members of the public and be subject to the public dose limit of 1 mSv/year.

Dose criteria serve as boundaries within which the optimization process takes place and serve to eliminate unnecessary or unauthorized exposure. The three types of dose criteria are the following:

- **reference levels** – in emergency or existing controllable exposure situations, this represents the level of dose or risk, above which exposures are considered inappropriate, and below which optimization of protection should be implemented; the chosen value for a reference level will depend upon the circumstances of the exposure under consideration for the public and non-human biota.
- **dose constraints** - a prospective and source-related restriction on the individual dose from a source, which provides a basic level of protection for the most highly exposed individuals from a source and serves as an upper bound on the dose in optimization of protection for that source.
- **dose limits** - the value of the effective dose or the equivalent dose from planned exposure situations that shall not be exceeded.

6.12 PRINCIPLES FOR RADIOLOGICAL PROTECTION OF THE ENVIRONMENT

According to ICRP [34], the aims of environmental protection are to prevent or reduce the frequency of deleterious radiation effects on flora and fauna to a level where they would have a negligible impact on the maintenance of biological diversity, the conservation of species, and the health and status of natural habitats, communities, and ecosystems.

In nuclear medicine a waste management plan should consider all forms of waste – sealed sources and unsealed sources in solid, liquid, or airborne form. The plan should also take into account mixed waste hazards, for example, if the waste is also flammable, toxic, or infectious. The effective management of low-level and intermediate-level waste depends on knowledge of the waste characteristics and the contained activity. Non-radioactive waste and very low-level waste (that is, below the exemption levels set by the regulatory authority) should be kept separate from waste that needs to be disposed of as radioactive waste. This waste should be monitored to confirm its status before being removed from a controlled area. It is useful to segregate radioactive waste on the basis of half-life in order to facilitate appropriate storage and disposal. For example, waste can be segregated into short-lived and long-lived radionuclide bins. The bins should be well shielded, and the content disposed of when the activity drops to a sufficiently low level (for example after 10 half-lives). As a general rule, the majority of liquid radioactive waste from nuclear medicine departments may be disposed of in the sewage system while most solid waste can be allowed to decay to levels when it may be disposed of as non-radioactive waste. If possible, sealed sources should be returned to the supplier when no longer required.

6.13 PRINCIPLES FOR THE PROTECTION OF STRONG MEDICAL RADIATION SOURCES

The security of sealed radioactive sources has to be in focus due to the increased risk for such sources to be used in terrorism. For security purposes, nuclear medicine facilities should be located in areas where access by members of the public to the rooms where sources, including radionuclide generators, and radiopharmaceutical dispensing equipment, are used and stored can be restricted. Furthermore, the proximity of source storage facilities to personnel that may need to respond in the event of a security breach should also be considered. As a general rule, the design of the nuclear medicine facility should make provision for safety systems or devices associated with the equipment and rooms. This includes electrical wiring relating to emergency off switches, as well as safety interlocks and warning signs and signals.

Hospitals and departments must have special routines and systems for disposal of all radioactive material, including contaminated cloths, paper, and other items that patients and / or staff contaminate. The manufacturer, dealer, owner, and user are obliged to ensure that radiation sources and equipment are in a state that the risk for accidents and abnormal events and undesired radiation exposure of users, patients, and other persons is as low as practically achievable. Ionizing radiation sources shall be marked with standard symbol for ionizing radiation. For radioactive sources, information concerning radionuclide, activity on a specified date, serial number, or other data suitable to uniquely identify the radiation sources, shall appear on the marking. For each individual apparatus, a technical measurement protocol shall be available, showing results from completion, acceptance testing, and periodic checks on the equipment, as well as maintenance and service reports.

Using a risk-management methodology based on the International Atomic Energy Agency's [35] categorization, radioactive sources fall into five categories with security outcomes commensurate with the risk they pose. While the Code of Practice sets clear objectives for improving the security of radioactive sources, its effective implementation relies on the development and maintenance of an effective security culture. Such a culture consists of characteristics and attitudes in organizations, and of individuals, that ensure security issues receive the attention warranted by their significance. It is vital that this culture be instilled as early as possible.

6.14 PRINCIPLES FOR SCREENING INVESTIGATIONS

Screening is significantly different from clinical healthcare, because apparently healthy individuals are offered a test. An effective screening intervention detects either pathology demonstrating risk factors for developing a disease, or the disease itself at an early stage, where treatment can improve clinical outcome. Concerning screening, two scenarios have tended to be considered together but in fact should be clearly distinguished:

6.14.1 SCREENING AS PART OF A PROGRAM

Screening programs systematically invite all members of a certain population to take a screening test. Examples of this are the breast screening programs in Europe where all women, for example, between 50 and 74 years of age, routinely receive invitations to have an X-ray mammography.

6.14.1.1 Screening Programs

Screening programs

1. have to be evidence based, and
2. have to meet stringent quality requirements, taking into account the need to include all parts of the program (i.e. invitation, X-ray devices, performance and reading of X-ray procedure, diagnostic workup, training and education, documentation, evaluation, etc.),
3. have to be approved by competent national health authorities.

The International Atomic Energy Agency (IAEA) [36], claims that "[J]ustification for radiological procedures to be performed as part of a health screening program of asymptomatic populations shall be carried out by the health authority in conjunction with appropriate professional bodies".

Where possible, the risk to the individual associated with any examination performed as part of a screening program should be low. However, even for well-established screening programs, such as breast cancer screening, the balance between benefits and undesired adverse health effects – such as radiation-induced cancer or false positive results and over diagnosis – is narrow. In addition, it has to be considered that due to the typically low prevalence of serious diseases in an asymptomatic population, the vast majority of individuals undergoing even a well-established screening program are not affected by the disease. These individuals do not derive a direct health effect but can only be harmed.

6.14.2 Opportunistic "Screening" or Individual Health Assessment

This scenario, often occurring as a result of patient desire, is usually denoted as "opportunistic screening" or "individual health assessment". A range of difficulties exist with examinations for individual health assessment. By definition, they apply to individuals and not large populations, and there is typically a lack of evidence to support their use. In addition, lack of follow-up from inclusion of individuals and lack of embedding these examinations within a clinical care pathway do not increase this evidence base. Failure to include these medical exposures within the healthcare pathway seriously reduces their potential benefit and may be considered by some to undermine their justification. The isolation of these services may hinder quality assurance. Information about the tests, their efficacy, and the need and conduct of follow-up tests can be poor. In summary, there is potential for a large number of individuals receiving more harm than good, particularly if the individual examination used carries a higher risk, and the false positive rate from the examination is high. With the evolving new technology of multi-slice spiral CT, predominantly CT procedures are discussed in the context of individual health assessment:

1. lung CT for early detection of lung cancer, in particular in smokers;
2. virtual CT colonoscopy – also denoted as CT colonography – for early detection of intestinal polyps (which might be pre-cancerous lesions) and colorectal cancer;
3. CT quantification of coronary artery calcification (which is considered as a sensitive marker of arteriosclerosis);
4. whole-body CT, particularly for early detection of cancer; and
5. cancer screening in asymptomatic subjects using PET/CT or PET/MR.

Due to the typically low prevalence of serious diseases in an asymptomatic population, it is questionable whether radiological procedures as part of an individual health assessment may be assigned to the healthcare scenario or whether it shall be assigned to a separate scenario somewhere between healthcare and screening programs.

6.15 PRINCIPLES FOR THE RADIOLOGICAL PROTECTION IN CONNECTION WITH RADIOLOGICAL AND NUCLEAR EMERGENCY SITUATIONS

The fundamentals of radiation protection allow all ionizing radiation exposures to be classified into three types of exposure situations: planned, existing, and emergency situations. Planned exposure situations are controlled and regulated but must consider arrangements for preparedness and response to an incident.

A nuclear or radiological emergency situation is defined as a non-routine situation of radiation exposure that arises as a result of an accident, a malicious act, or other unexpected event, and requires prompt action in order to avoid or reduce adverse consequences.

The healthcare community should be prepared to deal with contaminated and exposed patients and also with rescue personnel and members of the society. For that, there is a need for training. Existing exposure situations are exposure situations that already exist when a decision on control has to be taken, including prolonged exposure situations after emergencies. For the purpose of protection, reference levels for emergency exposure situations should be set in the range of 20–100 mSv effective dose (acute or per year). The reference level represents the level of residual dose or risk above which exposures are considered inappropriate. The ICRP considers that a dose rising towards 100 mSv will almost always justify protective measures.

When urgent protective actions must be taken promptly, it may be acceptable for emergency workers to receive, on the basis of informed consent, doses that exceed occupational dose limits. Accepted maximum values for personal dose equivalent are 100 mSv for actions to avert a large collective dose and 500 mSv for life-saving actions and actions to prevent severe deterministic effects or the development of catastrophic conditions [31, 37]. Protection against all exposures, above or below the reference level, should be optimized [31].

6.16 FUTURE ACTIONS TO IMPROVE RADIOLOGICAL PROTECTION IN MEDICINE

In 2012, the International Atomic Energy Agency (IAEA) and the World Health Organization (WHO) held a conference on radiation protection in medicine. An important outcome of the conference was the "Bonn Call-for-Action", highlighting ten main actions to improve radiation protection in medicine over the next decade (www.iaea.org/sites/default/files/17/12/bonn-call-for-action.pdf). These are (not listed in order of importance):

1. Enhance the implementation of the principle of justification.
2. Enhance the implementation of the principle of optimization of protection and safety.
3. Strengthen manufacturers' role in contributing to the overall safety regime.
4. Strengthen radiation protection education and training of health professionals.
5. Shape and promote a strategic research agenda for radiation protection in medicine.
6. Increase availability of improved global information on medical exposures and occupational exposures in medicine.
7. Improve prevention of medical radiation incidents and accidents.
8. Strengthen radiation safety culture in healthcare.
9. Foster an improved radiation benefit–risk dialogue.
10. Strengthen the implementation of safety requirements globally.

IAEA's Radiation Protection of Patients website is a leading source of information on the topic and presents a new online toolkit to support implementation of the Bonn Call for Action https://gnssn.iaea.org/main/bonn-toolkit/SitePages/Home.aspx. The toolkit enables the sharing of information and knowledge about the safe use of radiation, providing for better protection of patients and workers.

6.17 EDUCATION AND TRAINING

Referring physicians, radiological medical practitioners, medical physicists, technicians, and nurses must be aware of the radiation risks as well as the benefits of medical exposure and understand and implement the principles of radiation protection for patients. In particular, the concepts of justification and ALARA (doses as low as reasonably achievable) applied to medical exposures should be assessed in terms of their relevance in a rapidly changing technology-led healthcare system. Radiation protection is an integral part of patient safety in medical practice and must be evidence-based and receptive to the scientific process. In particular, physicians will require quantitative guidance on the risk/benefits of modern X-ray techniques if they are to make rational assessments of the applicability of modern high-dose techniques for particular diagnostic and therapeutic tasks. Currently, such guidance is variable due to the lack of a rational framework for assessing clinical effects of medical imaging.

6.18 SUMMARY

There is international consensus about the goal and principles for protection against ionizing radiation. Essentially all international intergovernmental organizations (IAEA, WHO, etc.) as well as individual countries incorporate ICRP concepts in their radiation protection regulations and operations. For human health, the system aims to manage and control exposures to ionizing radiation so that deterministic effects are prevented, and the risks of stochastic effects are reduced to the extent reasonably achievable. The principles are based on a combination of scientific facts from radiation epidemiology and radiation biology, ethical values of the society and practical experiences. Radiological protection is based on three fundamental principles: justification, optimization, and dose limitation. These principles apply to different types of exposure situations (planned, emergency, and existing) and categories of exposure (occupational, public, medical, and environmental). The principle of dose limitation applies to planned exposure situations other than medical exposure of patients, or exposure of non-human biota. For patients, the use of diagnostic reference levels is one way to help towards optimization of diagnostic procedures.

REFERENCES

[1] UNSCEAR, *United Nations Scientific Committee on the Effects of Atomic Radiation. UNSCEAR 2010 Report, Includes Scientific Report: Summary of low-dose radiation effects on health*, United Nations, New York, 2010.

[2] ICRP, 2007. *The 2007 Recommendations of the International Commission on Radiological Protection*, ICRP Publication 103, Ann. ICRP (2–4).

[3] UNSCEAR, *United Nations Scientific Committee on the Effects of Atomic Radiation. UNSCEAR 2008 Report Vol. I. Sources and Effects of Ionizing Radiation. Annexes A and B*. United Nations, New York, 2008.

[4] BEIR, "BEIR VII – Health Risks from Exposure to Low Levels of Ionizing Radiation," The National Academies Press, Washington, DC, 2006. www.nap.edu/catalog/11340/health-risks-from-exposure-to-low-levels-of-ionizing-radiation.

[5] ICRP, 2012. *ICRP statement on tissue reactions / Early and late effects of radiation in normal tissues and organs – Threshold doses for tissue reactions in a radiation protection context*, ICRP Publication 118, Ann. ICRP 41 (1/2).

[6] J. D. Boice, Jr., "The linear nonthreshold (LNT) model as used in radiation protection: An NCRP update," *Int J Radiat Biol*, vol. 93, no. 10, pp. 1079–92, 2017, doi: 10.1080/09553002.2017.1328750.

[7] D. Pawel and M. Boyd, "Studies of radiation health effects inform EPA actions," *J Radiol Prot*, vol. 39, no. 4, pp. 40–57, 2019, doi: 10.1088/1361-6498/ab2197.

[8] NCRP, "Implications of recent epidemiologic studies for the linear-nonthreshold model and radiation protection," NCRP Commentary No 27, Bethesda, MD, 2018.

[9] UNSCEAR, *Sources and effects of ionizing radiation UNSCEAR 2000 report to the General Assembly, with scientific annexes Volume I: Sources*. UN, United Nations (UN), 92-1-142238-8, 2000, http://inis.iaea.org/search/search.aspx?orig_q=RN:32002971.

[10] ICRP, 2005. *Low-dose Extrapolation of Radiation-related Cancer Risk*, ICRP Publication 99, Ann. ICRP 35 (4).

[11] ICRP, 2015. *Radiation Dose to Patients from Radiopharmaceuticals: A Compendium of Current Information Related to Frequently Used Substances*. ICRP Publication 128, Ann. ICRP 44 (2S).

[12] M. Andersson, L. Johansson, K. Eckerman, and S. Mattsson, "IDAC-Dose 2.1, an internal dosimetry program for diagnostic nuclear medicine based on the ICRP adult reference voxel phantoms," *EJNMMI Res*, vol. 7, no. 1, p. 88, 2017, doi: 10.1186/s13550-017-0339-3.

[13] K. F. Eckerman *et al.*, "User's Guide to the DCAL System," in ORNL/TM-2001/190. 2006.

[14] ICRP, 2008. *Nuclear Decay Data for Dosimetric Calculations*. ICRP Publication 107, Ann. ICRP 38 (3).

[15] ICRP, 2016. *The ICRP Computational Framework for Internal Dose Assessment for Reference Adults: Specific Absorbed Fractions*. ICRP Publication 133, Ann. ICRP 45 (2).

[16] M. Stabin and A. Farmer, "OLINDA/EXM 2.0: The new generation dosimetry modeling code," *J Nucl Med*, vol. 53, no. supplement 1, p. 585, 2012.

[17] ICRP, 2002. *Basic Anatomical and Physiological Data for Use in Radiological Protection: Reference Values*. ICRP Publication 89, Ann. ICRP 32 (3–4).

[18] ICRP, 2017. *Diagnostic Reference Levels in Medical Imaging*. ICRP Publication 135, Ann. ICRP 46 (1).

[19] A. Brandl and M. Tschurlovits, "Professional ethics in radiological protection," *J Radiol Prot*, vol. 38, no. 4, pp. 1524–34, 2018, doi: 10.1088/1361-6498/aadd23.

[20] J. Malone and F. Zölzer, "Pragmatic ethical basis for radiation protection in diagnostic radiology." *Br J Radiol*, vol. 89, no. 1059, p. 20150713, 2016, doi: 10.1259/bjr.20150713.

[21] T. L. Beauchamp and J. F. Childress, *Principles of Biomedical Ethics*. New York: Oxford University Press, 2012.

[22] J. Malone, F. Zölzer, G. Meskens, and C. Skourou, *Ethics for Radiation Protection in Medicine*. 2018.

[23] ICRP, 2007. *"Radiological Protection in Medicine,"* ICRP Publication 105, Ann. ICRP 37 (6).

[24] O. Holmberg, J. Malone, M. Rehani, D. McLean, and R. Czarwinski, "Current issues and actions in radiation protection of patients," *Eur J Radiol*, vol. 76, no. 1, pp. 15–19, 2010, doi: 10.1016/j.ejrad.2010.06.033.

[25] B. M. Moores and D. Regulla, "A review of the scientific basis for radiation protection of the patient," *Radiat Prot Dosimetry*, vol. 147, no. 1–2, pp. 22–29, 2011, doi: 10.1093/rpd/ncr262.

[26] ICRP, 2000. *Pregnancy and medical radiation*. ICRP Publication 84, Ann. ICRP 30 (1).

[27] S. Mattsson, S. Leide-Svegborn, and M. Andersson, "X-ray and molecular imaging during pregnancy and breastfeeding – when should we be worried?" *Radiat Prot Dosimetry,* 2021, ncab041. https://doi.org/10.1093/rpd/ncab041

[28] M. G. Stabin, "Radiation dose and risks to fetus from nuclear medicine procedures," *Phys Med,* vol. 43, pp. 190–98, 2017, doi: 10.1016/j.ejmp.2017.04.001.

[29] S. Leide-Svegborn, L. Ahlgren, L. Johansson, and S. Mattsson, "Excretion of radionuclides in human breast milk after nuclear medicine examinations. Biokinetic and dosimetric data and recommendations on breastfeeding interruption." *Eur J Nucl Med Mol Imaging,* vol. 43, no. 5, pp. 808–21, 2016, doi: 10.1007/s00259-015-3286-0.

[30] ICRP, 1992. *Radiological protection in biomedical research.* ICRP Publication 62, Ann. ICRP 22 (3).

[31] ICRP, 2009. *Application of the Commission's recommendations for the protection of people in emergency exposure situations.* ICRP Publication 109, Ann. ICRP 39 (1).

[32] ICRP, 1997. *General Principles for the Radiation Protection of Workers.* ICRP Publication 75, Ann. ICRP 27 (1).

[33] ICRP, 2004. *Release of Patients after Therapy with Unsealed Radionuclides.* ICRP Publication 94, Ann. ICRP 34 (2).

[34] ICRP, 2014. *Protection of the environment under different exposure situations.* ICRP Publication 124, Ann. ICRP 43 (1).

[35] IAEA, "Categorization of radioactive sources. General safety guides No RS-G-1.9," IAEA, Vienna, 9789201111043, 2005. https://books.google.se/books?id=U05RAAAAMAAJ.

[36] IAEA, *Radiation protection and safety in medical uses of ionizing radiation. Specific safety guides No. SSG-46.* IAEA, Vienna, 2018. https://books.google.se/books?id=U05RAAAAMAAJ.

[37] IAEA, *Criteria for use in preparedness and response for a nuclear or radiological emergency. IAEA Safety Standards Series No. GSG-2,* IAEA, Vienna, 2011. https://books.google.se/books?id=U05RAAAAMAAJ

7 Controversies in Nuclear Medicine Dosimetry

Michael G. Stabin

CONTENTS

7.1 THE NEED FOR DOSE CALCULATIONS IN THERAPY WITH RADIOPHARMACEUTICALS

Radiation dose calculations are required for the approval of any new radiopharmaceutical agent, diagnostic or therapeutic. In the United States, the US Food and Drug Administration (FDA) requires dose calculations, first by extrapolation in animal studies, then in multiple human patients in Phase I, II, and III clinical trials [1]. Once a radiopharmaceutical is approved, the best dosimetry is included in the 'package insert' (an information document included with the pharmaceutical packaging that gives much information about the drug and its approved uses). For diagnostic pharmaceuticals, this information is rarely used, except in the case of a pharmaceutical misadministration (as state laws require reporting of misadministrations if an organ or effective dose is different than expected by a certain amount), or in the case of accidental administration to a pregnant or potentially pregnant patient. Individualized dose calculations are also not calculated for individual patients in radiopharmaceutical therapy. There has been significant discussion about whether such dose calculations should be performed, as ALL patients receiving external beam therapy receive an individualized dosimetry analysis.

Siegel and colleagues [2] noted the following:

> If one were to approach the oncologist or medical physicist in an external beam therapy program and suggest that all patients with a certain type of cancer should receive the exact same protocol (beam type, energy, beam exposure time, geometry, etc.), the idea would certainly be rejected as not being in the best interests of the patient. Instead, a patient-specific treatment plan would be implemented in which treatment times are varied to deliver the same radiation dose to all patients. Patient-specific calculations of doses delivered to tumors and normal tissues have been routine in external beam radiotherapy and brachytherapy for decades. The routine use of a fixed GBq/kg, GBq/m^2, or simply GBq, administration of radionuclides for therapy is equivalent to treating all patients in external beam radiotherapy with the same protocol. Varying the treatment time to result in equal absorbed dose for external beam radiotherapy is equivalent to accounting for the known variation in patients' uptake and retention half-time of activity of radionuclides to achieve equal tumor absorbed dose for internal-emitter radiotherapy. It has been suggested that fixed activity-administration protocol designs provide little useful information about the variability among patients relative to the normal organ dose than can be tolerated without dose-limiting toxicity compared to radiation dose-driven protocols.

DOI: 10.1201/9780429489549-7

Brans and colleagues [3] wrote an article cleverly titled 'Clinical radionuclide therapy dosimetry: the quest for the "Holy Gray"', in which they argued that 'dosimetry may be considered an inherent part of therapy to establish the maximum tolerated dose and dose-response relationship'. They suggested that individual patient dosimetry has the following goals:

- To establish individual minimum effective and maximum tolerated absorbed doses;
- To establish a dose–response relation to predict tumour response and normal organ toxicity on the basis of pretherapy dosimetry;
- To objectively compare the dose–response results of different radionuclide therapies, either between different patients or between different radiopharmaceuticals, as well as to perform comparisons with the results routinely obtained with external radiotherapy;
- To increase the knowledge of clinical radionuclide radiobiology, in part with the aim of developing new approaches and regimens.

They discussed the successes of dosimetry with a number of different therapy agents and concluded that 'recent developments in molecular medicine, PET/CT and SPECT/CT cameras and radiobiology offer major scientific and clinical opportunities in radionuclide therapy dosimetry. However, only prospective, randomised trials with adequate methodology can provide the evidence that applied clinical dosimetry results in better patient outcome than is achieved with fixed activity dosing methods.'

In the same year, Stabin wrote an article entitled 'The Case for Patient-Specific Dosimetry in Radionuclide Therapy' [4]. He noted that patient-individualized dose calculations are mostly not done in radiopharmaceutical therapy; instead, patients generally receive a 'fixed dosing' approach, in which all patients receive the same fixed amount of the pharmaceutical, perhaps only adjusted for patient body size. Stabin addressed a number of arguments that are generally offered for not performing patient-individualized dose calculations, including

- Performing such calculations is difficult and expensive, requiring too much effort.
- There are no standardized methods for performing individualized dose calculations, and methods vary significantly among different institutions.
- Dose calculations calculated to date have had poor success in predicting tissue response.
- With the level of difficulty involved, there must be some objective evidence that the use of radiation dose calculations provides positive benefit that justifies the extra effort and cost.

All arguments were answered, with citation of literature data. It is interesting to note that Dr. Brans is a nuclear medicine physician who has written and spoken many times in favour of performing dose calculations for nuclear medicine therapy patients. However, resistance to performing such dose calculations remains strong among physicians in the United States, with very few exceptions. In Europe, pressure from European Union regulations and some successes in clinical trials and clinical practice have influenced some to consider the practice.

7.2 THE LINEAR, NO-THRESHOLD (LNT) MODEL OF RADIATION CARCINOGENESIS

It would be impossible in this limited space to give a comprehensive review of the radiobiological literature on low-dose radiation effects. The issue of LNT continues to be contentious. Some are ardent believers and not likely to be swayed to change their opinion based on literature evidence. Others contend equally ardently that the theory is wrong, and that there may even be *beneficial* effects of low-dose radiation exposure (the concept of radiation hormesis). Debates in the literature continue, and many scientific meetings hold public verbal discussions at times. Edward Calabrese, in a number of publications (e.g. [5]) argues that Hermann Muller's proclamation that any dose of radiation, no matter how small, may be dangerous, was belied by his own internal writings. Nonetheless, his proclamation in his 1946 Nobel Prize acceptance speech ushered in the era of LNT, with the mantra, 'there is no safe dose of radiation', driving public policy and the practice of radiation protection until today. Evidence has mounted to contradict the theory, as will be very briefly discussed here, but regulators, radiation-safety professionals and others are hesitant to change policies, in the interest of 'prudence'. The mantra is firmly imprinted on the mind of the general public, to the point that many are afraid of the smallest doses of radiation, avoid necessary medical scans, and feel ostracized by family members and friends if they become even slightly contaminated with radioactive materials. This also has implications on the practice of releasing nuclear medicine therapy patients, as will be discussed below. The main points of the LNT theory and counter arguments will be very briefly discussed here.

The fundamental suppositions of the LNT ('point mutation') theory are the following:

1. One radiation hit can cause a DNA mutation that can cause a cancer that can cause death. But,
    a. 10^6 DNA mutations/cell/day are produced by about x 10^9 free radicals/cell/day derived from the metabolism of oxygen.
    b. 10^7 mutations/cell/day are produced by low linear energy transfer (LET) background radiation (x- and γ-rays, $\beta-$ particles) amounting to 0.1 cGy (rad) per year. These mutations are also caused by free radicals.
2. All radiation doses are additive, and the dose rate does not matter, so a dose received instantaneously causes the same damage as the same dose received very slowly over a long period of time. But,
    a. incontrovertible research has shown that doses received gradually are far less hazardous and carcinogenic than the same radiation dose received instantaneously. This is because only permanent damage would accumulate, but repair or removal of damaged cells prevents such accumulation when the dose rate is low enough for such protective mechanisms to keep up with the rate of damage.

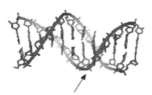   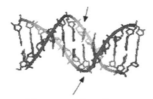

Single strand breaks occur 10,000 times per day per cell. 100 mSv/y radiation add 12 per day per cell. So EPA's 12 mrem causes an increase to 10,000.01 per day per cell

Double strand breaks occur 10 times per day – 1 per week per cell. 100 mSv/y radiation adds 1 per years

FIGURE 7.1 DNA strand breaks occur frequently where ionized oxygen molecules from metabolism are the principal causes. Colour image available at www.routledge.com/9781138593299.

DNA REPAIR MECHANISM

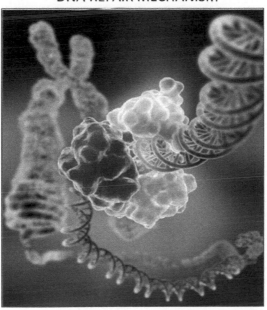

FIGURE 7.2 Special enzyme DNA ligase encircles the double helix to repair a broken strand of DNA. Colour image available at www.routledge.com/9781138593299.

b. The International Commission on Radiological Protection (ICRP), an absolutely committed LNT advocacy organization, introduced a 'dose and dose rate effectiveness factor' of 2 to recognize the decreased effect of low dose rate. While this factor is not nearly enough, the admission of decreased low dose-rate effect is basically an admission that LNT is not true. The use of such a made-up factor is merely an attempt to preserve, within two different dose-rate ranges, the very linear feature that it negates and denies.

No processes exist at low dose that do not exist at high dose. Therefore, there is no such thing as radiation repair. But:

a. Over 3,000 papers have shown repair mechanisms for DNA (Figures 7.1 and 7.2).
b. Over 150 genes have been identified that make compounds involved in DNA repair (Figure 7.1).
c. There are three general classes of repair;
   1. antioxidant prevention,
   2. enzymatic repair of DNA damage, and
   3. *removal* of DNA alterations by apoptosis, differentiation, and the immune system.
d. These repair systems sequentially reduce DNA damage from about 10^6 alterations/cell/day to about 1 fixed damage (mutation)/cell/day. These mutations in stem cells accumulate for a lifetime, with progression of DNA damage that is associated with aging and cancer.
e. Even the Atomic Bomb Survivor Cancer Mortality Data, used by LNT-advocates, show that effects are nonlinear at low doses, and may even suggest a *beneficial* influence [6] (Figure 7.3).

Thus, the idea that every single radiation interaction in the body can produce a lethal cancer is arguably in conflict with much published data. Resistance to changes in regulations and practice has a number of consequences that LNT proponents understand:

– Thousands of regulators would lose their jobs if low doses were admitted to be harmless or beneficial.
– Many lawyers would no longer make a living from radiation-damage lawsuits.
– Many scientists would lose their grants, graduate programs, and government-related impressive consultant positions involved in the pursuit of links between trivial radiation doses and cancers.
– Many politicians would no longer be able to use radiation hysteria to gain votes.

On the other hand, multitude important *benefits* could be realized:

– Financial resources could be diverted from chasing phantom radiation effects from trivial radiation doses to activities that actually save human lives.

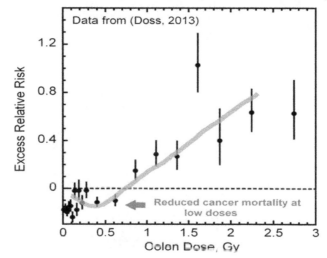

FIGURE 7.3 The shape of dose-response curve, with the correction for the negative bias in the baseline cancer rate, is consistent with the concept of radiation hormesis. The references for the research by Ozasa and Doss are listed as [7] and [6], respectively.

- Radiation Safety Officers (RSOs) could have to stop collecting useless paperwork for inspectors to inspect and instead focus their time on real radiation hazards
- The public could be relieved of the stress caused by low-dose radiophobia. They could stop worrying about getting badly needed medical procedures involving radiation, among other issues. A tragic case was that of Bryan Salinas, who fell from a window and sustained a head trauma. Physician decided against a necessary CT, which could have detected the state of the trauma, due to radiophobia. Unfortunately, Bryan was sent home, and died several hours later. For more information about this incident see the following webpage [8].
- Zanzonico [9] calculated the number of excess deaths that would result if medical procedures involving ionizing radiation were abandoned, and inferior methods, with clearly documented rates of morbidity and mortality replaced them.

7.3 CALCULATIONS FOR THE RELEASE OF RADIOPHARMACEUTICAL THERAPY PATIENTS

The US Nuclear Regulatory Commission (NRC) regulations for the release of patients administered radioactive material, pursuant to x 10 CFR 35.75, authorize patient release according to a dose-based limit – that is, the dose to other individuals exposed to the patient (U.S. NRC 1997). The dose-based limit, which replaced the activity or dose-rate-based release limit, <1,110 MBq (30 mCi) or <0.05 mSv h^{-1} (5 mrem h^{-1}). Siegel and colleagues [10] gave a thorough scientific analysis of the scientific weaknesses of the NRC's NUREG-1556, Appendix U guidance on patient-release values for individual radionuclides. Many radiation safety professionals in the United States believe that this NUREG *must* be followed in the release of patients who have received radiopharmaceuticals, both diagnostic and therapeutic, but a NUREG is *not a regulatory document*, it is a scientific guidance document meant to help licensees comply with the x 10CFR 35 dose limit, <u>which is a regulation</u>.

Siegel and colleagues showed that the external dose component calculated in the NUREG was deficient, as it did not account for the following:

- The biological clearance of radioiodine from the body, relying solely on the physical half-life for clearance.
- Includes nonrealistic 'non-void' model assumptions.
- Treated the patient as an unshielded point source, with no patient self-attenuation of the photons, which Siegel and colleagues measured to be about 30 per cent [11].

They also showed that the internal dose component, assumed to be received by members of the patients' families from ^{131}I contamination of the household by patient body fluids, was overly conservative, and that 'no such "highly exposed" individual [as cited in the NUREG] has ever been found, and no documentation substantiates that [the NUREG's] "factor of x 10" conservative approach is advisable, necessary, or accurate'.

Willegaignon and colleagues [12] used thermoluminescent dosimeters to measure actual doses in the households of x 100 released ^{131}I NaI therapy patients and found that caregivers' doses were mostly below 1 mSv, and that surface contamination levels were much lower that model predictions from the NUREG, and generally not of concern.

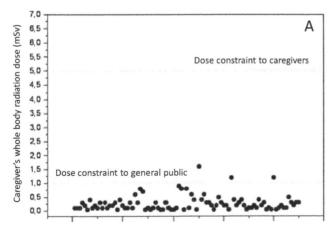
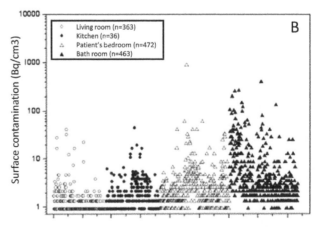

FIGURE 7.4 Findings of Willegaignon et al. regarding release of radioiodine patients.

Ignoring the science, released radiopharmaceutical patients are held for inappropriate times, and released with restrictions on sleeping with their spouses, having contact with their family members, and even having contact with their pets for irrationally long periods of time. This radiophobia, inextricably linked to the LNT hypothesis discussed above, is creating hardships on patients and their families, including embarrassment and ostracism from friends and neighbours, and should be replaced with a science-based approach that recognizes the real hazards (or lack thereof).

7.4 THE PHANTOM MENACE

As noted in Chapter 9, in the 1980s and 1990s there was only one set of anthropomorphic models used for dosimetry, the Cristy/Eckerman adult and pediatric series [13] and the Stabin and colleagues pregnancy series [14]. In the early 2000s a proliferation of phantom series was generated by various authors, mostly based on more realistic, image-based models. The availability of high-quality CT images of persons (and animals!) and increases in computing speeds facilitated Monte Carlo calculations of organ- and body-absorbed fractions by various researchers. The models of the Radiation Dose Assessment Resource (RADAR) Committee of the Society of Nuclear Medicine and Molecular Imaging [15], including 12 adult and pediatric phantoms (male and female adults, 15-yr-olds, 10-yr-olds, 5-yr-olds, 1-yr-olds and newborns), scaled to represent the standard masses in International Commission on Radiological Protection (ICRP) Publication 89 [16], and three models of the pregnant woman, are incorporated in the OLINDA/EXM nuclear medicine dosimetry software [17], and have been used to generate two radiopharmaceutical compendia [18, 19]. RADAR has also generated absorbed fractions for several animal models [20] (3 mice, 5 rats, and 2 beagle dogs) and implemented them in the OLINDA/EXM software.

As noted in Chapter 9, the GSF (Research Center for Environment and Health) in Germany developed a number of phantoms based on CT images of living subjects. Their two adult models have been adopted by the (ICRP) for use in standard dose calculations for radiation workers [21]. Another series of phantoms, developed at the University of Florida, is also pending for adoption by the ICRP [22]. These phantoms will be used to develop dose estimates for ICRP publications, principally for use in occupational radiation dose calculations.

So now there are two phantom series, one for use in nuclear medicine and the other for use with radiation worker and general public dose calculations from occupational uses of radiation. RADAR attempted to work with the ICRP to develop a single set of adult, pediatric, and pregnant female phantoms, in a shared effort, but was not permitted even to make a presentation to the ICRP regarding its efforts. As noted in Chapter 9, many other good phantoms, representing individuals from different countries and other cases, have been developed as well. Which phantoms to use for which applications is now a matter of discussion, whereas in the 1980s and 1990s only the Cristy/Eckerman and Stabin and colleagues phantoms were available. The phantoms are generally all of good quality; use of one or another will not substantially provide 'better' dose calculations. Interestingly, Stabin noted that even the change from the 'stylized' Cristy/Eckerman phantoms to the newer, realistic RADAR anthropomorphic phantoms, has a minimal effect on effective doses for radiopharmaceuticals, which is encouraging (see Table 3.3 in Chapter 9).

REFERENCES

[1] *Guidance for Industry Developing Medical Imaging Drug and Biological Products Part 3: Design, Analysis, and Interpretation of Clinical Studies.* US Food and Drug Administration, 2004.

[2] J. A. Siegel, M. G. Stabin, and A. B. Brill, "The importance of patient-specific radiation dose calculations for the administration of radionuclides in therapy," *Cell Mol Biol (Noisy-le-grand),* vol. 48, no. 5, pp. 451–59, 2002.

[3] B. Brans *et al.*, "Clinical radionuclide therapy dosimetry: The quest for the "Holy Gray"," *Eur J Nucl Med Mol Imaging,* vol. 34, no. 5, pp. 772–86, 2007, doi: 10.1007/s00259-006-0338-5.

[4] Stabin MG. The Case for Patient-Specific Dosimetry in Radionuclide Therapy. *Cancer Biotherapy & Radiopharmaceuticals,* vol. 23 no. 3, pp. 273–284, 2008.

[5] E. J. Calabrese, "From Muller to mechanism: How LNT became the default model for cancer risk assessment," *Environ Pollut,* vol. 241, pp. 289–302, 2018, doi: 10.1016/j.envpol.2018.05.051.

[6] M. Doss, "Linear No-Threshold Model VS. Radiation Hormesis," *Dose Response,* vol. 11, pp. 480–97, 2013, doi: 10.2203/dose-response.13-005.Doss.

[7] K. Ozasa *et al.*, "Studies of the mortality of atomic bomb survivors, Report 14, 1950–2003: an overview of cancer and noncancer diseases." *Radiat Res,* vol. 177, no. 3, pp. 229–43, 2012, doi: 10.1667/rr2629.1.

[8] "TV NEWS: Doctor's Mistake Kills Child at Mary Bridge Hospital." www.youtube.com/watch?v=K6oicECeWW0

[9] P. B. Zanzonico, "Benefits and Risks in Medical Imaging," *Health Phys,* vol. 116, no. 2, pp. 135–137, 2019, doi: 10.1097/HP.0000000000001038.

[10] J. A. Siegel, C. S. Marcus, and M. G. Stabin, "Licensee over-reliance on conservatisms in NRC guidance regarding the release of patients treated with 131I," *Health Phys,* vol. 93, no. 6, pp. 667–77, 2007, doi: 10.1097/01.Hp.0000270300.34270.44.

[11] J. A. Siegel, S. Kroll, D. Regan, M. S. Kaminski, and R. L. Wahl, "A practical methodology for patient release after tositumomab and (131)I-tositumomab therapy," *J Nucl Med,* vol. 43, no. 3, pp. 354–63, 2002.

[12] J. Willegaignon *et al.,* "Outpatient radioiodine therapy for thyroid cancer: a safe nuclear medicine procedure," *Clin Nucl Med,* vol. 36, no. 6, pp. 440–5, 2011, doi: 10.1097/RLU.0b013e3182184fa0.

[13] M. Cristy and K. F. Eckerman, *Specific absorbed fractions of energy at various ages from internal photons sources,* Oak Ridge, TN, 1987: Oak Ridge National Laboratory.

[14] M. G. Stabin *et al., Mathematical models and specific absorbed fractions of photon energy in the nonpregnant adult female and at the end of each trimester of pregnancy.* ORNL/TM-12907 Oak Ridge National Lab., Oak Ridge, TN, 1995. https://www.osti.gov/servlets/purl/91944.

[15] M. G. Stabin, X. G. Xu, M. A. Emmons, W. P. Segars, C. Shi, and M. J. Fernald, "RADAR reference adult, pediatric, and pregnant female phantom series for internal and external dosimetry," *J Nucl Med,* vol. 53, no. 11, pp. 1807–13, 2012. doi: 10.2967/jnumed.112.106138.

[16] ICRP, 2002. *Basic Anatomical & Physiological Data for Use in Radiological Protection - Reference Values.* ICRP Publication 89, Ann. ICRP 32 (3–4).

[17] M. Stabin and A. Farmer, "OLINDA/EXM 2.0: The new generation dosimetry modeling code," *J Nucl Med,* vol. 53, no. Supplement 1, p. 585, 2012.

[18] M. G. Stabin and J. A. Siegel, "RADAR Dose Estimate Report: A Compendium of Radiopharmaceutical Dose Estimates Based on OLINDA/EXM Version 2.0," *J Nucl Med,* vol. 59, no. 1, pp. 154–60, 2018, doi: 10.2967/jnumed.117.196261.

[19] M. G. Stabin, "New-Generation Fetal Dose Estimates for Radiopharmaceuticals," *J Nucl Med,* vol. 59, no. 6, pp. 1005–6, 2018, doi: 10.2967/jnumed.117.204214.

[20] M. G. Stabin, T. E. Peterson, G. E. Holburn, and M. A. Emmons, "Voxel-based mouse and rat models for internal dose calculations," *J Nucl Med,* vol. 47, pp. 655–9, 2006.

[21] ICRP, 2009. *Adult Reference Computational Phantoms.* ICRP Publication 110, Ann. ICRP 39 (2).

[22] C. Lee, D. Lodwick, D. Pafundi, S. Whalen, J. Williams, and W. Bolch, "The University of Florida Pediatric Phantom Series," in *Handbook of Anatomical Models for Radiation Dosimetry.* X. G. Xu and K. F. Eckerman, Eds. Boca Raton: CRC Press/Taylor & Francis Group, 2009, pp. 199–220.

8 Monte Carlo Simulation of Photon and Electron Transport in Matter

José M. Fernández-Varea

CONTENTS

DOI: 10.1201/9780429489549-8

8.1 INTRODUCTION

Monte Carlo (MC) methods are a group of numerical techniques that have in common the use of stochastic (i.e., non-deterministic) algorithms to simulate the behaviour of mathematical or physical systems. They are based on the modelling of individual object–object relationships, which offers not only conceptual simplicity but also a large flexibility to tackle complex problems. The implementation of an MC solution to the problem at hand requires the random sampling of a large number of such object–object interactions in order to obtain the average value of some quantity of interest and its associated (type A) uncertainty. Computers are particularly well suited for this repetitive task.

The idea of using randomness as a means to solve mathematical problems can be traced to the early days of probability theory. Here one would cite the names of Cardano, Fermat, Pascal, Huygens, and Laplace, as well as Buffon's famous needle problem. The foundations of modern probability theory were laid by Kolmogorov. In connection with MC methods, important developments were made by William S. Gosset (also known as Student), von Neumann and others. Nowadays, MC methods find application not only in mathematics but also in diverse disciplines spanning from chemistry and physics to social sciences, finance, game theory, and so forth.

Radiation physics is a field where MC techniques are extensively used to model the transport (i.e., propagation and interaction) of ionizing radiation through matter. In the mid-1930s, Fermi pioneered the study of neutron diffusion employing MC methods. Ulam and von Neumann systematized the use of MC tools while working at Los Alamos in the development of nuclear weapons during the late 1940s. The appearance of the first electronic computers and the ever-increasing computational power spurred the widespread application of these techniques.

In the context of radiation transport, MC simulation provides at least two clear advantages over alternative approaches based on the numerical solution of the (deterministic) Boltzmann transport equation. MC codes can readily incorporate more accurate databases of radiation-matter interaction cross sections as they become available, and they can track radiation through complex geometries. On the other hand, the transport equation can only deal, with approximate cross sections, the tracking of radiation through simplified geometries. The success of MC methods is further explained by the current powerful computer resources as well as the availability (and user-friendliness!) of general-purpose MC codes. Therefore, it is not surprising that MC simulation has become essential to address many applications in medical radiation physics, ranging from radiology to radiotherapy and nuclear medicine.

The focus of this chapter is the MC simulation of photons and light charged particles (electrons and positrons), excluding heavy charged particles (protons, alpha particles, etc.) as well as neutrons. The considered energies span from around 1 keV to 100 MeV. In spite of these restrictions, the selected types of ionizing radiations and energy interval allow for tackling many important applications in all areas of medical physics.

The rest of the chapter is structured as follows: Sections 8.2 and 8.3 summarize the interaction processes experienced by photons and electrons, respectively. Multiple scattering of electrons is touched upon in section 8.4. Section 8.5 briefly addresses random numbers and sampling methods, and section 8.6 is devoted to the MC simulation of photon and electron transport. The available general-purpose MC codes are described in section 8.7. Section 8.8 collects bibliography where the interested reader may find relevant applications of MC methods to medical physics. A simple example of MC simulation is presented in section 8.9. Finally, section 8.10 offers a few concluding remarks.

It should here be mentioned that the principles of the Monte Carlo method are also described in chapter 29, Volume I and with focus on photon transport and use of the method to model imaging systems commonly used in nuclear medicine.

8.2 PHOTON–ATOM INTERACTIONS

γ-rays and x-rays with energies between hundreds of eV and hundreds of MeV interact with atoms in various ways. Here we limit ourselves to a brief overview of the most probable processes, elaborating on the content presented in Chapter 3, Volume I. The article by Hubbell [1] is an excellent source of more detailed information on this topic. Another reference that could be consulted is the review paper [2].

8.2.1 PHOTOELECTRIC EFFECT

In the photoelectric effect, the incident photon is absorbed by one of the bound electrons of the target atom, which is ejected into a free state. Photoabsorption is possible whenever the photon's energy E is larger than the binding energy of the atomic (sub)shell from which the photoelectron is ejected. A simple non-relativistic quantum-mechanical description of this process assumes that the wave function of the ejected photoelectron is a plane wave (Born approximation). These radical simplifications lead to a simple formula for the differential cross section (DCS) that can be found in textbooks like that of Bransden and Joachain [3]. In reality, photoabsorption is more complicated, and relativistic effects should be accounted for together with appropriate initial (bound) and final (free) wave functions for the active electron in the atomic potential. The interested reader may consult the monograph by Sabbatucci and Salvat [4] for an updated review of the formalisms and numerical aspects.

8.2.2 Rayleigh (Elastic, Coherent) Scattering

In this type of collision, the incident photon is absorbed, and a photon is emitted with the same energy in a different direction. Hence, the interaction is elastic because the atom remains in the initial state. In the form-factor approximation, the DCS (per atom) for Rayleigh scattering can be written as the product of the Thomson DCS $d\sigma_T/d\Omega$, Eq. (3.9), and the atomic form factor $F(q,Z)$, where the momentum transfer q depends on the photon energy E and the polar scattering angle θ. The Thomson DCS describes the angular distribution of a photon colliding elastically at a free, stationary electron. In turn, the atomic form factor is the Fourier transform of the atomic electron density, thus taking into account that the electron distribution is bound to the atom. Hubbell and his co-workers [5] tabulated $F(q,Z)$ for all atoms.

A more refined description of Rayleigh scattering would start from a relativistic treatment and second-order perturbation theory. Such calculations are extremely difficult, but the ensuing DCSs can be parameterized adding a complex term $f'+if''$ (anomalous form factor) to the usual form factor, see for example [2],

$$\frac{d\sigma}{d\Omega} = \frac{d\sigma_T}{d\Omega}\left|F(q,Z)+f'+if''\right|^2 \tag{8.1}$$

where f' and f' only depend on Z and E.

8.2.3 Compton (Inelastic, Incoherent) Scattering

This is an inelastic process whereby the photon is absorbed by the target atom and another photon is emitted in a different direction with a lower energy. Part of the energy transfer goes to kinetic energy of one of the atomic electrons, which is expelled (Compton recoil electron). The simplest model to describe this collision mechanism assumes the target electron to be unbound and stationary. Then, the angular distribution of the scattered photon is given by the well-known Klein-Nishina DCS $d\sigma_{KN}/d\Omega$, (Eq. 3.14, Volume I). Binding effects can be accounted for in the Waller-Hartree approximation, multiplying the Klein-Nishina DCS with the incoherent scattering function $S(q,Z)$ [6]. In this approximation, the DCS (per atom) is given by Eq. 3.18, Volume I. Tables with the $S(q,Z)$ functions of all atoms can be found in [5].

More advanced formalisms exist to describe Compton collisions. For instance, the relativistic impulse approximation incorporates in a simple way both the binding and the motion of the target electron [7]. The corresponding DDCS for an atomic (sub)shell i is written as

$$\frac{d^2\sigma_i}{dE'd\Omega} \propto \frac{d\sigma_{KN}}{d\Omega} J_i(p_z) \tag{8.2}$$

where E' is the energy of the scattered photon and $J_i(p_z)$ is the so-called Compton profile, which embodies the linear momentum distribution of the active electron. Biggs and colleagues [8] compiled Compton profiles of the occupied (sub)shells of all atoms. In turn, Stutz [9] has analyzed the accuracy of simpler Compton profiles within the relativistic impulse approximation.

8.2.4 Pair and Triplet Production

High-energy photons may decay into an electron-positron pair in the proximity of a massive, charged particle. The photon energy is invested in the creation of the two leptons, which requires $2m_ec^2$, and the rest goes into kinetic energies of the electron and the positron. Linear momentum can be conserved because the massive particle absorbs some linear momentum. When the spectator charged particle is an atomic nucleus the interaction is called pair production, and the threshold energy for this to happen is $2m_e c^2$. On the other hand, if the electron-positron pair is created in the vicinity of one of the atomic electrons, the process is named triplet production, being the threshold $4m_e c^2$. The DCSs for these processes take involved expressions even in the simplest approach, the Born approximation, where the electron and the positron are described as plane waves thus disregarding their electrostatic interaction with the atom. The classical tabulation of Hubbell and colleagues [10] is still the most used source of information on this process. More recently, Hubbell and Seltzer [11] and Hubbell [1] discussed the status of cross-section data for electron-positron pair production.

8.2.5 OTHER INTERACTION PROCESSES

Photons may also experience other types of interactions. For instance, they may be absorbed by a nucleus and eject one of the nucleons (proton or neutron). These (γ,p) and (γ,n) reactions have threshold energies of the order of 1 MeV. The corresponding cross sections depend not only on the energy of the photon and the atomic number of the target atom but also on the mass number of the nucleus. They are around two or more orders of magnitude smaller than those of the previously described interaction mechanisms. Therefore, photonuclear reactions are disregarded in most medical physics applications.

8.2.6 DATABASES OF PHOTON INTERACTION DATA

Photon interaction data are available in the form of cross sections or mass attenuation coefficients, the latter being the preferred option for tabulation purposes as well as in ionizing-radiation dosimetry. The most comprehensive information on this is the Evaluated Photon Data Library EPDL97 [12] from the Lawrence Livermore Laboratory. Alternatively, the National Institute of Standards and Technology (NIST) maintains the XCOM database [13]. Notice that these databases are for *isolated* atoms. The corresponding cross sections for molecules or compounds can be generated by the additivity rule. This approximation is reasonable for photon interactions because aggregation effects do not distort much the single-atom cross sections. Figure 8.1 shows cross sections for the various interaction mechanisms of photons with Al atoms, taken from XCOM [13].

8.3 ELECTRON–ATOM INTERACTIONS

Electrons and positrons interact with atoms in ways that are quite different from those of photons. As in the case of photons, the present section is intended to supplement the more basic introduction of chapter 3, Volume I. A compact survey of this topic was written by Berger and Wang [14] and Seltzer [15]. Again, the review article [2] contains further references.

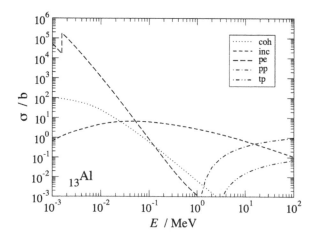

FIGURE 8.1 Cross sections (in barn, 1 b = 10^{-24} cm²) for the interaction of photons with $_{13}$Al atoms. The partial cross sections are Rayleigh (coh), Compton (inc), photoelectric (pe), pair production (pp), and triplet production (tp). The plotted data are from XCOM [13].

8.3.1 ELASTIC SCATTERING

In such interactions the electron merely changes its direction of flight (polar scattering angle θ) while retaining all its kinetic energy E. Classical physics as well as non-relativistic quantum mechanics lead to the famous Rutherford DCS which describes the elastic collision of an electron against a bare nucleus. Screening effects can be easily incorporated within the Born approximation, yielding the screened Rutherford DCS when the projectile–atom interaction is modelled as an exponentially screened Coulomb potential,

$$\frac{d\sigma_{SR}}{d\Omega} \propto \frac{Z^2}{(p\beta)^2} \frac{1}{(2\eta+1-cos\theta)^2} \tag{8.3}$$

where p is the linear momentum of the electron and β is its speed divided by the speed of light in vacuum; η is a small parameter that quantifies the screening. More advanced approaches would circumvent the assumption of plane waves and model screening effects more faithfully within a fully relativistic framework. The elastic DCS then reads

$$\frac{d\sigma}{d\Omega} = |f(\theta)|^2 + |g(\theta)|^2 \tag{8.4}$$

where the scattering amplitudes f and g are expansions in terms of Legendre polynomials and associate Legendre functions, respectively, whose coefficients involve phase shifts. The latter are obtained from the numerical solution of the Dirac wave equation [16]. The ICRU Report 77 [17] contains a comprehensive overview of the various theoretical formalisms employed to describe electron-atom elastic scattering.

8.3.2 INELASTIC SCATTERING

In this case the electron loses part of its kinetic energy E, which is used to excite or ionize the target atom. Simple formulas for the inelastic DCS can be deduced if the collision occurs with a free electron at rest. However, the neglect of binding effects makes these DCSs to diverge as $1/W^2$, where W is the energy loss [15]. The plane-wave Born approximation avoids these simplifications but is numerically cumbersome. And the distorted-wave Born approximation further improves the wave functions of the projectile electron or positron [18]. A summary of various semi-empirical models and *ab initio* formalisms employed to calculate inner-shell ionization by electrons is given in the review by Llovet and colleagues [19]. The review includes a thorough comparison of distorted-wave Born cross sections for the ionization of K, L, and M (sub)shells with existing experimental data. In the case of atoms in condensed phases (solids or liquids), the cross sections for inelastic collisions are strongly affected by aggregation effects.

8.3.3 BREMSSTRAHLUNG EMISSION

Electrons can also lose kinetic energy emitting a photon when they are accelerated close to a massive, charged particle. Electron–nucleus and electron–electron bremsstrahlung refer, respectively, to photon emission if the acceleration is caused by the atomic nucleus or one of the electrons. A simple analytical DCS for electron-nucleus bremsstrahlung can be derived in the non-relativistic case if the electron wave functions before and after the interaction were plane waves (Born approximation). In the relativistic Born approximation case, the analytical formula (Bethe-Heitler DCS) is already quite lengthy. Beyond these simplified approaches the bremsstrahlung DCS must be calculated numerically, but convergence is only achieved for kinetic energies of at most a few MeV. Seltzer and Berger [20] presented a calculation scheme that combines numerical partial-wave DCSs at low energies with Bethe-Heitler DCSs at high energies and suitable interpolation between them. Their bremsstrahlung DCSs are expressed in the form

$$\frac{d\sigma}{d(h\nu)} = \frac{Z^2}{\beta^2} \frac{1}{h\nu} \chi(Z,E,h\nu/E) \tag{8.5}$$

where $h\nu$ is the photon energy. The topic of electron–nucleus bremsstrahlung has been recently revisited by Mangiarotti and his co-workers [21, 22]. In turn, the calculation of electron–electron bremsstrahlung has been addressed by Tessier and Kawrakow [23].

8.3.4 POSITRON ANNIHILATION

Positrons interact with matter as described above, that is, elastic scattering, inelastic scattering, and bremsstrahlung emission. However, a positron may annihilate with one of the atomic electrons, resulting in one or more annihilation photons. The creation of two photons is the predominant process. The analytical DCS for positron annihilation with an electron at rest was deduced by Heitler. Although annihilation may take place while the positron is moving, it happens with a high probability once the positron has slowed down to rest. Then, owing to the conservation of linear momentum and energy, the two photons are emitted "back-to-back" with energies equal to $m_e c^2$.

8.3.5 DATABASES OF ELECTRON INTERACTION DATA

ICRU Report 77 [17] includes a database of elastic scattering DCSs, which has been incorporated in some of the MC codes. Llovet and colleagues [24] prepared tables of inner-shell ionization cross sections by electron and positron impact, which have been endorsed by the NIST. Regarding the DCSs for bremsstrahlung emission, the tabulation by Seltzer and Berger [25] is still the most updated source of information. Cross sections for elastic scattering and bremsstrahlung emission of electrons in Al are displayed in Figure 8.2 along with the ionization cross sections of the K and L (sub)shells; all these cross sections pertain to isolated Al atoms. On the other hand, the cross sections for the inelastic collisions of electrons in metallic Al (not plotted) require careful modelling, in particular to be consistent with the accepted electronic stopping power of this solid.

8.4 MULTIPLE SCATTERING OF ELECTRONS

Photons are absorbed in a medium (by the photoelectric effect or pair production) after at most a few (Rayleigh or Compton) interactions. At variance with this behaviour, electrons may experience a very large number of elastic or inelastic collisions depending on their initial kinetic energy. This is especially true at high energies around and above 1 MeV. Furthermore, at these energies the elastic and inelastic DCSs are large for very small polar scattering angles θ and energy losses W, respectively. In other words, most elastic collisions only produce a small angular deflection, and most inelastic collisions just result in a minute energy loss. Hence, the detailed simulation of all interactions entails a waste of CPU time. Under such circumstances, a macroscopic point of view may be more adequate than a microscopic description to account for the angular deflection and energy loss of electrons after a step length s that is much larger than the elastic and inelastic mean free paths. Such a macroscopic description is the objective of multiple-scattering theories, whose aim is to obtain the 6-dimensional probability density function (PDF) $p(\mathbf{r},\hat{\mathbf{d}},E;s)$ to find an electron around a position $\mathbf{r} = (x,y,z)$, with a direction of flight $\hat{\mathbf{d}} = (\Theta,\Phi)$ and kinetic energy E after a specified path length s; Θ and Φ are the cumulative polar and azimuthal scattering angles, respectively. The unknown function p fulfils the Boltzmann integro-differential equation, which cannot be solved analytically. Simplifications are therefore needed to arrive at partial solutions.

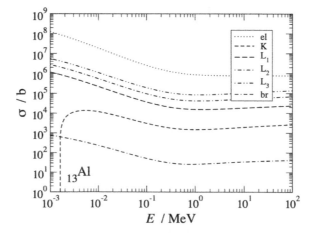

FIGURE 8.2 Cross sections (in barn, 1 b = 10^{-24} cm²) for the interaction of electrons with $_{13}$Al atoms. The partial cross sections are elastic (el), K and L (sub)shell ionization (K, L_1, L_2, L_3), and bremsstrahlung (br). The plotted data are from the PENELOPE database [26].

8.4.1 MULTIPLE ELASTIC SCATTERING

Here we focus on the PDF $p(\Theta;s)$ for the angular deflection of an electron beam after a certain path length s (regardless of the position and energy). Perhaps the simplest approach takes advantage of the central-limit theorem and expresses the PDF as a Gaussian function [27, 28], whose only non-trivial parameter (the variance of the PDF) is related to the mass scattering power T/ρ [29]. This simple model relies on the small-angle approximation.

A more elaborate formalism was developed by Goudsmit and Saunderson. Multiple elastic scattering is viewed as a compound Poisson process: the probability of n elastic collisions along s follows a Poisson distribution $p_n(s)$ whereas the angular PDF $f_n(\Theta)$ after exactly n elastic collisions is the convolution of $f_{n-1}(\Theta)$ and $f_1(\Theta)$, the latter being the single-scattering PDF (i.e., the normalized angular DCS); $f_0(\Theta) = \delta(\Theta)$. Then [30]

$$p(\Theta;s) = \sum_{n=0}^{\infty} p_n(s) f_n(\Theta) \tag{8.6}$$

The Goudsmit-Saunderson expression for the angular distribution is exact for arbitrary elastic DCSs whenever energy loss is negligible, but it is numerically cumbersome. When the DCS is the Rutherford formula, some simplifications can be introduced that yield a more tractable solution known as the Molière theory. On the other hand, Lewis was able to obtain a few spatial moments and spatial-angular correlations of the PDF $p(\mathbf{r},\hat{\mathbf{d}};s)$, and a generalization of Lewis's results was presented in [31]. However, a closed analytical solution for $p(\mathbf{r},\hat{\mathbf{d}};s)$ is not available. The reader interested in multiple-elastic-scattering formalisms may consult ICRU Report 77 [17].

8.4.2 MULTIPLE INELASTIC SCATTERING

Now we consider the PDF $p(\Delta;s)$ for the energy-loss Δ of an electron beam after a certain path length s (ignoring position and angular variables). If all the energy losses were small, $p(\Delta;s)$ would be a Gaussian with its centre displaced to an energy lower than E by an amount related to the mass electronic stopping power [28]. But if the energy-loss PDF of electrons is taken proportional to $1/W^2$ one arrives at the Landau expression for $p(\Delta;s)$. A more general formalism is provided by the Vavilov distribution, which bridges the gap between the Landau and Gaussian limits [32].

In the same vein as for multiple elastic scattering, the PDF for the cumulative energy loss can be regarded as a compound Poisson process [33]:

$$p(\Delta;s) = \sum_{n=0}^{\infty} p_n(s) f_n(\Delta) \tag{8.7}$$

where the energy-loss PDF $f_n(\Delta)$ after n inelastic collisions is the convolution of $f_{n-1}(\Delta)$ and $f_1(\Delta)$, the latter being the energy-loss PDF (the normalized energy-loss DCS); $f_0(\Delta) = \delta(\Delta)$.

8.5 RANDOM NUMBERS AND SAMPLING METHODS

8.5.1 RANDOM AND PSEUDO-RANDOM NUMBERS

The essence of the MC methods is the use of random numbers. Truly random numbers can be generated having recourse to natural phenomena that are intrinsically random, such as the decay of radioactive nuclei or electronic noise. Getting random numbers in this manner is impractical for obvious reasons. An alternative is to use sequences of pseudo-random numbers, which are delivered by a deterministic algorithm, but whose outcome "looks random". Tests have been designed to ensure their quality [34, 35]. These generators are designed to produce pseudo-random numbers ξ uniformly distributed in the interval $(0,1)$.

Among the simplest types of pseudo-random number generators, we have the so-called multiplicative linear congruential generators, based on the algorithm

$$R_n = aR_{n-1} \ (\mathrm{mod}\, m) \qquad \xi_n = R_n / m \tag{8.8}$$

where a and m are suitably selected constants. The R_n are integers, and the sequence for successive n starts from an initial "seed" R_0. A robust choice is $a = 7^5$ and $m = 2^{31}-1$. The main drawback of this family of generators is that their period is less than m-1, insufficient for present-day needs. Other more sophisticated random-number generators are RANLUX, RANECU, and the Mersenne twister [36].

Uniform random numbers ξ in (0,1) have, seemingly, a limited usefulness because in most cases we wish to sample random numbers from PDFs $p(x)$ that are not constant. This can be achieved by various algorithms. Two of them are explained concisely next.

8.5.2 INVERSE-TRANSFORM METHOD

The inverse-transform method is adequate when $p(x)$ has an analytical cumulative distribution function $P(x)$ that, in turn, can be inverted analytically. The equation to sample random values of x is

$$x = P^{-1}(\xi) \tag{8.9}$$

Some of the PDFs incorporated in MC codes are simple enough to allow the straightforward use of this algorithm. For instance, the PDF for the distance s between successive interaction points is $p(s) = \lambda_T^{-1} \exp(-s/\lambda_T)$, where λ_T is the mean free path (see below). The corresponding cumulative distribution function is $P(s) = 1-\exp(-s/\lambda_T)$. Then, imposing $P(s) = \xi = 1-\xi'$ we arrive at the sampling equation $s = -\lambda_T \ln\xi'$ because, if ξ is uniformly distributed in (0,1), so is ξ'. Another example where the inverse-transform method is applicable is the PDF deduced from the screened Rustherford DCS, equation (8.3). Defining $\mu = (1 - \cos\theta)/2$ we have $p(\mu) = A(A+1)/(A+\mu)^2$ so that the sampling formula is $\mu = A\xi/(A+1-\xi)$. The inverse-transform algorithm can also be used to sample from discrete PDFs $p(x) = p_i\,\delta(x-i)$. Specifically, i is the integer that fulfils the conditions $P_i < \xi \leq P_{i+1}$. The procedure is sketched in Figure 8.3.

8.5.3 REJECTION METHODS

Another sampling method that is straightforward to implement is the rejection algorithm. Here we shall just outline the simplest version, when the PDF $p(x) \neq 0$ in a finite interval (a,b). First, we select an (arbitrary) upper bound c such that $p(x) < c$. Then we sample random points (x,y) uniformly distributed in the rectangle $(a,b) \times (0,c)$ by means of the inverse-transform recipe $x = a+(b-a)\xi_1$, $y = c\xi_2$. If $y > p(x)$ we reject the point and sample another one, else the value x is delivered. The sampling efficiency is equal to $[(b-a)c]^{-1}$ if $p(x)$ is normalized to 1. However, the algorithm also works if $p(x)$ is not normalized.

If $p(x)$ is sharply peaked, most sampled (x,y) points are rejected. A more efficient rejection algorithm would be based on an upper bound function $c(x)$ that may be sampled easily using for instance the inverse-transform method to generate random x values that are accepted if $c(x)\xi < p(x)$.

As a pedagogical example of a rejection algorithm with a constant upper bound, Figure 8.4 shows how to sample random kinetic energies of the electrons emitted in the β^- disintegration of ^{90}Y, whose endpoint is 2.281 MeV. The rectangle selected to throw random points uniformly is delimited by $a = 0$, $b = 2.5$ MeV, $c = 0.7$ MeV^{-1}, yielding a sampling efficiency of 57 per cent. The tightest rectangle is achieved with $b = 2.281$ MeV and $c = 0.634$ MeV^{-1}, and the corresponding efficiency would increase to 69 per cent.

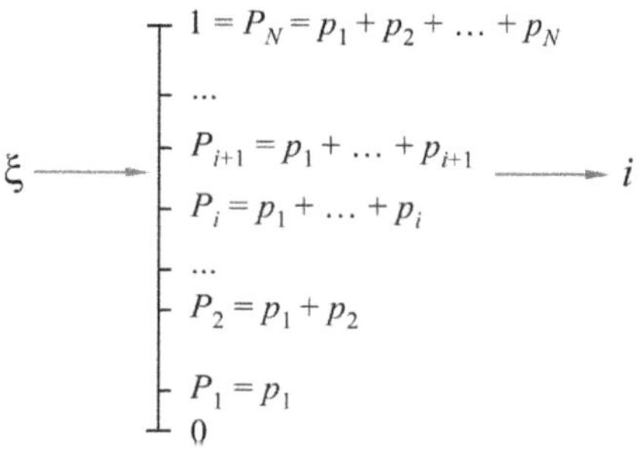

$$\xi \longrightarrow \begin{array}{l} 1 = P_N = p_1 + p_2 + \ldots + p_N \\[4pt] \ldots \\[4pt] P_{i+1} = p_1 + \ldots + p_{i+1} \\[4pt] P_i = p_1 + \ldots + p_i \\[4pt] \ldots \\[4pt] P_2 = p_1 + p_2 \\[4pt] P_1 = p_1 \\[4pt] 0 \end{array} \longrightarrow i$$

FIGURE 8.3   Inverse-transform algorithm to sample the integer index i from a discrete PDF.

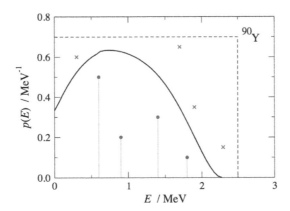

FIGURE 8.4 Rejection algorithm to sample the kinetic energy of the electron emitted in the β⁻ decay of ^{90}Y. The (blue) dashed lines delimitate the adopted $(a,b) \times (0,c)$ rectangle. The (red) crosses and (green) circles represent a few rejected and accepted points, respectively. The vertical lines indicate the kinetic energies delivered by the algorithm. Colour image available at www.routledge.com/9781138593299.

8.6 PHOTON AND ELECTRON TRANSPORT

8.6.1 CROSS SECTIONS AND PROBABILITY DENSITY FUNCTIONS

Consider a particle (photon, electron, or positron) with energy E moving in an infinite, homogeneous, and isotropic medium. Various interactions mechanisms i are possible (photoelectric, ... in the case of photons; bremsstrahlung, ... in the case of electrons and positrons), producing angular deflections and/or energy losses.

As we have summarized above, the theoretical (or experimental) information on radiation-matter interactions is conventionally expressed in the form of DCSs (per target atom or molecule)

$$\frac{\mathrm{d}^2\sigma_i\left(E;W,\theta\right)}{dWd\Omega} \tag{8.10}$$

and the corresponding integrated cross sections

$$\sigma_i\left(E\right) = \int_0^E dW \int_0^\pi 2\pi \sin\theta \, d\theta \frac{\mathrm{d}^2\sigma_i\left(E;W,\theta\right)}{dWd\Omega} \tag{8.11}$$

for each projectile energy E and interaction type i. In the most frequent situation of randomly oriented targets and unpolarized beams, the DCSs do not depend on the azimuthal scattering angle ϕ. The total interaction cross section is

$$\sigma_T\left(E\right) = \sum_i \sigma_i\left(E\right) \tag{8.12}$$

and the corresponding total interaction probability per unit path length, also known as mean free path, is

$$\lambda_T^{-1} = \sum_i \lambda_i^{-1} = N\sigma_T \tag{8.13}$$

N being the number of target atoms or molecules per unit volume.

On the other hand, MC simulation is based on the random sampling from probabilities and PDFs, deduced from the differential and integrated cross sections having recourse to the following relations:

– PDF for the distance between successive interactions (see section 8.5.2)

$$p(s) = \lambda_T^{-1} e^{-s/\lambda_T}$$

(8.14)

– Probability that an interaction is of type i (see Figure 8.3)

$$p_i = \sigma_i / \sigma_T$$

(8.15)

– PDF for the energy loss and polar scattering angle

$$p_i(W, \theta) = \frac{1}{\sigma_i} 2\pi \sin\theta \frac{d^2\sigma_i}{dW d\Omega}$$

(8.16)

– PDF for the azimuthal scattering angle

$$p(\phi) = 1/2\pi \quad \forall i$$

(8.17)

The terminology "radiation transport" refers to the description of the propagation and interaction of ionizing radiation in a medium. The implementation can be done in two ways.

8.6.2 Detailed (Event-by-Event) Simulation

As we have seen, the photoelectric effect and pair and triplet production are interactions wherein the photon is absorbed directly. On the other hand, photons may undergo one or more Rayleigh or Compton scatterings. However, Rayleigh scattering is never a dominant process, and after a few Compton collisions a photon will have lost so much energy that photoabsorption becomes very likely. These features allow for the MC simulation of *all* photon-atom interactions pertaining to a photon history as the required CPU time is small [37]. This detailed or event-by-event simulation strategy can also be adopted for electron transport when their energy is below a few hundred keV so that the number of collisions is not too large.

To generate random tracks, the detailed simulation scheme is implemented in the MC codes as follows. Consider the state of a particle after the n-th interaction. The position, direction of flight and energy are, respectively, $\vec{r}_n, \hat{d}_n, E_n$

i. Sample the distance s to the next interaction point from the exponential PDF by means of the inverse-transform algorithm (see section 8.5.2),

$$s = -\lambda_T \ln\xi$$

(8.18)

The particle is moved to $\vec{r}_{n+1} = \vec{r}_n + s\hat{d}_n$ (provided the new point is inside the same medium as the previous one; otherwise, stop the particle at the interface, update the cross-section tables, and sample a new value of s).

ii. Sample the collision type i (a discrete variable, see section 8.5.2) that occurs at this point.

iii. Sample the energy loss W and the angular deflection θ from the two-dimensional PDF $p_i(W,\theta)$. In the case of unpolarized beams, the azimuthal angle ϕ is uniformly distributed in $(0,2\pi)$, hence $\phi = 2\pi \xi$.
The new energy of the particle is $E_{n+1} = E_n - W$, and the new direction is

$$\hat{d}_{n+1} = R(\theta, \phi)\hat{d}_n$$

(8.19)

where $R(\theta,\phi)$ is a rotation matrix.

iv. Store the initial state (i.e. type of particle, position, direction of flight and energy) of secondary radiations, if any.

The simulation of the track proceeds by repeating steps i-iv until either the particle abandons the material system, or its energy falls below a preselected cutoff E_{abs} and its simulation is discontinued. Then, the simulation of the pending secondary particles is carried out. This completes the simulation of one history. To obtain statistically meaningful results, a large number N of histories must be simulated in the same way with uncorrelated random numbers.

The MC estimate of a requested scalar quantity of interest Q is reported as

$$Q_{MC} = \bar{q} \pm \kappa \sigma(\bar{q}) \qquad (8.20)$$

where the mean (average) of Q is given by

$$\bar{q} = \frac{1}{N} \sum_{i=1}^{N} q_i \qquad (8.21)$$

and the corresponding standard deviation is

$$\sigma(\bar{q}) = \frac{\sigma(q)}{\sqrt{N}} \approx \sqrt{\frac{1}{N} \left[\frac{1}{N} \sum_{i=1}^{N} q_i^2 - \bar{q}^2 \right]} \qquad (8.22)$$

Notice that the MC code has to score the contributions q_i and q_i^2 of each history to the tally. The coverage factor adopted to quote the type A uncertainty is usually $\kappa = 2$ (95% confidence level). It is worth stressing that the relative uncertainty of Q_{MC} decreases as $1/N^{1/2}$.

If the quantity of interest is a continuous distribution (e.g., a depth-dose curve or a photon energy spectrum), it is tallied as a histogram regarding each bin as an independent tally. Similarly, bidimensional distributions are tallied as bidimensional histograms.

8.6.3 Condensed and Mixed Simulation

As already mentioned, at electron kinetic energies exceeding some hundred keV the number of elastic and inelastic collisions is very large and the CPU time per history becomes prohibitive. However, at high energies the angular deflections and energy losses produced in the vast majority of interactions are very small and have a limited influence on the electron tracks. In this scenario, the results of multiple-scattering theories can be utilized to increase the simulation speed. Instead of simulating each individual interaction, one may let the electrons advance in long steps and simulate the global effect of the (many) elastic and inelastic interactions at the end of the step.

As mentioned in section 8.4, we only have limited knowledge of the PDF $p(\mathbf{r},\hat{\mathbf{d}};s)$. Specifically, information on the spatial distribution is only in the form of spatial moments and spatial-angular correlations. Therefore, to select the position $\mathbf{r} = (x,y,z)$ of the electron at the end of the step s one has to make judicious assumptions. Different algorithms, referred to as "transport mechanics" have been proposed to this end and implemented in MC codes. Kawrakow and Bielajew [31] assessed the performance of those electron-transport algorithms, confronting the simulated spatial moments and spatial-angular correlations to Lewis's analytical expressions. Another potential difficulty of some of the algorithms has to do with their accuracy when a boundary between two media (or a medium and vacuum) is crossed.

8.7 MONTE CARLO CODES

MC codes for radiation transport can be classified depending on their generality regarding the materials and energy interval where they can be operated. Some of them implement detailed simulation of relatively low-energy radiations, usually electrons, in just one element or compound. In this group of programs, we highlight the track-structure codes [38]. Liquid water is the substance of primary concern, and the best possible cross sections, which include liquid-phase effects, are adopted for this substance of upmost importance in microdosimetry. Other specialized MC codes simplify the physics models so as to allow the fast simulation in low-atomic-number media, for example, for radiotherapy treatment planning [39], or restrict themselves to photon transport in a limited energy interval, for example, for nuclear medicine imaging [40].

On the other hand, the so-called "general-purpose" codes are able to transport ionizing radiation through arbitrary media (elements, compounds, tissues), in non-trivial geometries, and over a wide energy interval, typically from around 1 keV to 1 GeV in the case of electrons and photons. This generality is achieved assuming the traversed medium to be a "gas" of atoms compressed to the actual mass density. Hence, molecular or aggregation effects on the atomic cross sections are sidelined. This drastic simplification is quite realistic for photons but less so for charged particles.

The majority of general-purpose codes are freely available and are typically well documented. Besides, they are shipped with additional tools, for example to visualize the trajectories of radiation in the simulated setup or to transport charged particles in electromagnetic fields. The main features of three of these programs are outlined in what follows.

8.7.1 GEANT4

Geant4 [41, 42] is a toolkit for the simulation of photons, electrons and positrons, ions (protons, alpha particles, etc.), neutrons and other ionizing radiations in matter. It is developed and maintained by a large international collaboration under the auspices of CERN. The code is open source, written in C++, and it includes powerful visualization software that permits the tracking of photons and particles in very complex geometrical setups. An interesting feature of Geant4 is that the selection of cross sections rests with the user; this may be useful, for instance, to estimate type B uncertainties associated to the chosen physics models, an aspect that is too often left aside.

The learning curve of Geant4 is steep. Part of the intricacies of this toolbox may be circumvented by programs that use Geant4 as the simulation engine but free the user from having to program in C++. For instance, the GATE software is an open-source platform built on top of Geant4 [43, 44]. It was developed originally to deal with nuclear imaging (chapter 29, Volume I), but it has been expanded to external and internal radiotherapy, dosimetry and hadron therapy. GAMOS is another freely available framework for Geant4 geared towards medical physics applications [45]. We may here also cite TOPAS [46], which wraps and extends Geant4 for applications dealing with particle therapy.

8.7.2 EGSNRC

EGSnrc [47] is one of the successors of EGS4, developed by researchers at the National Research Council of Canada. EGSnrc permits the coupled MC simulation of photons and electrons with energies between a few keV and hundreds of GeV in arbitrary media. It includes a class library that can be used to model elaborate geometries and particle sources. The program implements updated physics models. In particular, its multiple-scattering algorithm allows large step sizes minimizing loss of accuracy. It has also been benchmarked at low energies [48]. EGSnrc is distributed with the user codes DOSRZnrc, FLURZnrc, CAVRZnrc, SPRRZnrc for situations where the geometry has cylindrical symmetry. These programs are written in the Mortran language, which is a preprocessor for generating Fortran code and includes a macro functionality that can be very powerful [49]. There is, however, the potential risk of interfering with the underlying EGSnrc code if the Mortran macros are not properly defined. Furthermore, several variance-reduction techniques can be activated to improve simulation efficiency. Owing to these features, EGSnrc has arguably become the gold standard in some branches of medical physics.

8.7.3 PENELOPE

PENELOPE [26, 50] simulates the coupled transport of electrons, positrons, and photons in arbitrary materials. The energy interval spans from 50 eV to 1 GeV. Photon interactions are simulated event-by-event. In turn, a robust mixed simulation algorithm is implemented for electron and positron elastic and inelastic multiple scattering. PENELOPE is written in Fortran, and it is open source. The code has been benchmarked against a large variety of experimental results [51].

PENELOPE incorporates the subroutine package PENGEOM to handle geometries where bodies are defined by quadric surfaces. The bundle comes with the generic steering main program *penmain*. Alternatively, the user may employ the main program *penEasy* [52], which includes a number of tallies intended to facilitate the use of PENELOPE in radiotherapy and medical imaging; *penEasy* also enables radiation transport in voxelized geometries.

8.7.4 OTHER GENERAL-PURPOSE MC CODES

Other MC codes that belong to the general-purpose category and deserve being mentioned are MCNP6 [53], FLUKA [54], and PHITS [55].

8.8 APPLICATIONS OF MONTE CARLO METHODS IN MEDICAL PHYSICS

In medical physics, countless studies have benefited from the possibilities offered by MC methods. The applications encompass radiotherapy, radiology, nuclear medicine, and so forth.

Several review articles on the basics of MC simulation have been published in the main journals devoted to medical physics. Among the classical ones we can mention the introductory accounts by Raeside [56] and Turner and colleagues [57], which contain material that is still valuable as a primer. In 1991, Andreo published a thorough revision of the applications of MC techniques undertaken to that date in all areas of medical physics [58]. The 1990s witnessed the rapid increase in the number of medical physics articles where MC methods played an important part of the reported investigation. By the end of that decade, it became difficult to cover in a single publication all MC applications, and a series of topical review articles appeared that focused on specific areas. For instance, the MC modelling of radiotherapy kV x-ray units [59], electron beams from linacs [60], or external radiotherapy photon beams [61]. Zaidi [62] critically reviewed MC methods for nuclear medical imaging. More recently, Andreo [63] surveyed the use of MC methods in radiotherapy dosimetry.

A number of specialized books have been devoted to MC methods. In the context of medical physics, we may highlight *Monte Carlo Techniques in Radiation Therapy* [64], *Therapeutic Applications of Monte Carlo Calculations in Nuclear Medicine* [65], and *Monte Carlo Calculation in Nuclear Medicine: Applications in Diagnostic Imaging* [66]. These books gather the contributions from many experts in the respective areas and constitute valuable reading if one wishes to deepen one's knowledge.

The issues associated with clinical implementation and experimental verification of MC dose algorithms have been addressed in the AAPM Task Group Report No. 105 [67]. Furthermore, the Report of the AAPM Research Committee Task Group 268 [68] has issued guidelines to improve reporting of MC studies in medical physics research.

8.9 A SIMULATION EXAMPLE WITH PENELOPE

In this section we describe a simple example of a MC simulation. The chosen case is relevant to dosimetry in nuclear medicine when β emitting radionuclides are used. Specifically, in this example we want to simulate the radial distribution of absorbed dose $D(r)$, also known as dose point kernel, produced by 1 MeV electrons in liquid water. To this end, the PENELOPE code with the *penEasy* main program has been adopted. Before running the simulation, one may use the auxiliary program *shower.exe* to quickly display on the computer screen the trajectories of a few electrons and to infer the spatial extension of the energy deposition. The trajectories of 10 simulated electrons are displayed in Figure 8.5. The electron tracks are rather crooked owing to elastic scattering. Also visible is a bremsstrahlung photon that undergoes two Compton interactions before being absorbed.

First, we have to prepare the geometry definition file, *sphere.geo*. In the considered case, we just define a sphere whose centre is at the origin of the lab reference frame and has a radius of 100 cm, and the only body that is declared

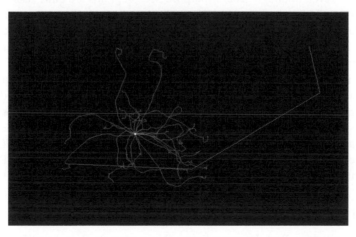

FIGURE 8.5 Ten trajectories of 1 MeV electrons in liquid water (red), simulated with the PENELOPE code [26]. The yellow line corresponds to a bremsstrahlung photon. Colour image available at www.routledge.com/9781138593299.

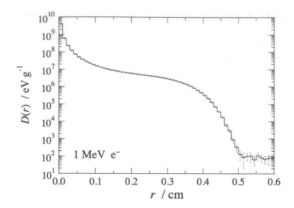

FIGURE 8.6 Dose point kernel of 1 MeV electrons in liquid water simulated with PENELOPE/penEasy. The uncertainty bars correspond to 2 standard deviations.

is located inside the sphere. Next, PENELOPE's preprocessor *material.exe* is employed to produce the file *liquid_water.mat* that contains the cross sections for electron, positron and photon transport in liquid water. Then, the configuration file, *DPK.in*, is edited to define the characteristics of the simulation: type of particle, energy distribution and emission direction of the radiation source (1 MeV electrons emitted isotropically), number of primary particles to simulate (10^5 histories), cutoff energies to discontinue radiation transport (1 keV for all particles), simulation parameters that affect multiple electron scattering (detailed simulation is enforced), indicate the names of the geometry file and the file with the material properties, turn on and customize the tallies that will deliver the requested information (*tallySphericalDoseDistrib*), and activate if needed variance-reduction techniques (none in this example). Finally, the simulation is launched by issuing the command *penEasy.exe < DPK.in* (PC with a Windows 10 Pro operating system). The output file *tallySphericalDoseDistrib.dat* contains a histogram with the simulated dose point kernel and its type A uncertainty, shown in Figure 8.6. Equivalent simulations have been carried out with other MC codes, see e.g. [69].

8.10 CONCLUSIONS AND FINAL REMARKS

MC simulation will continue to play a major role in radiation physics due to the ever-increasing accuracy of the interaction models incorporated in the main MC codes, coupled with their flexibility and the availability of computational resources. Thus, it is realistic to foresee the growing application of MC techniques in a wide range of situations of interest in all areas of medical physics where a faithful description of the propagation and interaction of ionizing radiation in matter is required. However, although general-purpose MC programs are quite user-friendly, one should never use them as black boxes. Instead, one should assess the applicability of the interaction models implemented in the chosen code and estimate the type B uncertainties that originate from the simplifications in the geometry and materials of the simulated setup. For these reasons, a basic understanding of MC methods should be an indispensable part of the background knowledge of medical physicists.

Concerning the physics interaction models, analytical formulas for integrated cross sections have been replaced during the past decades with numerical tables. It is anticipated that MC code developers will dedicate effort to progressively substitute the analytical expressions for at least some of the interaction differential cross sections with databases calculated numerically. The physics models implemented in the updated versions of the codes should be permanently validated against experimental information using statistical analysis tools, see for example [70, 71].

Regarding simulation speed, there has been an impetus to accelerate MC simulation on GPUs, but certain programming issues have only recently been solved [72]; further work along these lines is warranted.

ACKNOWLEDGEMENTS

I would like to express my gratitude to Prof. Francesc Salvat (Universitat de Barcelona) for having kindly shared with me over the years (more than three decades, in fact!) his profound knowledge on radiation physics and MC methods. I have also benefited from many enlightening conversations on these topics with Prof. Josep Sempau (Universitat

Politècnica de Catalunya). Financial support from the Spanish Ministerio de Ciencia, Innovación y Universidades, under grant no. PGC2018-096788-B-I00, is gratefully acknowledged.

REFERENCES

[1] J. H. Hubbell, "Review and history of photon cross section calculations," *Phys Med Biol,* vol. 51, no. 13, pp. R245–62, 2006, doi: 10.1088/0031-9155/51/13/r15.

[2] F. Salvat and J. M. Fernández-Varea, "Overview of physical interaction models for photon and electron transport used in Monte Carlo codes," *Metrologia,* vol. 46, pp. S112–38, 2009.

[3] B. H. Bransden and C. J. Joachain, *Physics of Atoms and Molecules.* 2003.

[4] L. Sabbatucci and F. Salvat, "Theory and calculation of the atomic photoeffect," *Radiation Physics and Chemistry,* vol. 121, pp. 122–40, 2016, doi: 10.1016/j.radphyschem.2015.10.021.

[5] J. H. Hubbell, W. J. Veigle, E. A. Briggs, R. T. Brown, D. T. Cromer, and R. J. Howerton, "Atomic Form Factors, Incoherent Scattering Functions and Photon Scattering Cross Sections," *J Phys Chem Ref Data,* vol. 4, pp. 471–616, 1975.

[6] J. H. Hubbell, "Summary of existing information on the incoherent scattering of photons, particularly on the validity of the use of the incoherent scattering function," *Radiation Physics and Chemistry,* vol. 50, no. 1, pp. 113–24, 1997, https://doi.org/10.1016/S0969-806X(97)00049-2.

[7] R. Ribberfors, "Relationship of the relativistic Compton cross section to the momentum distribution of bound electron states," *Physical Review B,* vol. 12, pp. 2067–74, 1975, doi: 10.1103/PhysRevB.12.2067.

[8] F. Biggs, L. B. Mendelsohn, and J. B. Mann, "Hartree-Fock Compton profiles for the elements," *Atomic Data and Nuclear Data Tables,* vol. 16, no. 3, pp. 201–309, 1975, https://doi.org/10.1016/0092-640X(75)90030-3.

[9] G. E. Stutz, "Compton scattering cross section for inner-shell electrons in the relativistic impulse approximation," *Nuclear Instruments and Methods in Physics Research Section B: Beam Interactions with Materials and Atoms,* vol. 319, pp. 8–16, 2014, doi: 10.1016/j.nimb.2013.11.001.

[10] J. H. Hubbell, H. A. Gimm, and I. Overbo, "Pair, Triplet, and Total Atomic Cross Sections (and Mass Attenuation Coefficients) for 1 MeV-100 GeV Photons in Elements Z=1 to 100," *Journal of Physical and Chemical Reference Data,* vol. 9, no. 4, pp. 1023–1148, 1980, doi: 10.1063/1.555629.

[11] J. H. Hubbell and S. M. Seltzer, "Cross section data for electron–positron pair production by photons: a status report," *Nuclear Instruments and Methods in Physics Research Section B: Beam Interactions with Materials and Atoms,* vol. 213, pp. 1–9, 2004, https://doi.org/10.1016/S0168-583X(03)01524-6.

[12] D. E. Cullen, J. H. Hubbell, and L. Kissel, "EPDL97: The evaluated photon data library `97 version," 1997, doi: 10.2172/295438.

[13] M. J. Berger *et al.* "XCOM: Photon Cross Sections Database." www.nist.gov/pml/xcom-photon-cross-sections database.

[14] M. J. Berger and R. Wang, "Multiple-scattering angular deflections and energy-loss straggling," in *Monte Carlo Transport of Electrons and Photons,* T. M. Jenkins, W. R. Nelson, and A. Rindi, Eds. New York: Plenum Press, 1988.

[15] S. M. Seltzer, "Cross sections for bremsstrahlung production and electron-impact ionization, in Monte Carlo Transport of Electrons and Photons," in *Monte Carlo Transport of Electrons and Photons,* T. M. Jenkins, W. R. Nelson, and A. Rindi, Eds. New York: Plenum Press, 1988.

[16] F. Salvat, A. Jablonski, and C. J. Powell, "ELSEPA—Dirac partial-wave calculation of elastic scattering of electrons and positrons by atoms, positive ions and molecules," *Computer Physics Communications,* vol. 165, p. 190, 2005, doi: 10.1016/j.cpc.2004.09.006.

[17] ICRU, *Elastic Scattering of Electrons and Positrons.* ICRU Report 77, 2007.

[18] D. Bote and F. Salvat, "Calculations of inner-shell ionization by electron impact with the distorted-wave and plane-wave Born approximations," *Physical Review A,* vol. 77, no. 4, p. 042701, 2008, doi: 10.1103/PhysRevA.77.042701.

[19] X. Llovet, C. J. Powell, F. Salvat, and A. Jablonski, "Cross Sections for Inner-Shell Ionization by Electron Impact," *Journal of Physical and Chemical Reference Data,* vol. 43, no. 1, pp. 13–102, 2014, doi: 10.1063/1.4832851.

[20] S. M. Seltzer and M. J. Berger, "Bremsstrahlung spectra from electron interactions with screened atomic nuclei and orbital electrons," *Nuclear Instruments and Methods in Physics Research Section B: Beam Interactions with Materials and Atoms,* vol. 12, no. 1, pp. 95–134, 1985, doi: 10.1016/0168-583X(85)90707-4.

[21] A. Mangiarotti and M. N. Martins, "A review of electron–nucleus bremsstrahlung cross sections between 1 and 10 MeV," *Radiation Physics and Chemistry,* vol. 141, pp. 312–338, 2017, doi: 10.1016/j.radphyschem.2017.05.026.

[22] A. Mangiarotti, M. N. Martins, and V. R. Vanin, "Analytic calculations of electron–nucleus bremsstrahlung cross sections above a few MeV including higher-order corrections and multiple scattering in the target," *Nuclear Instruments and Methods in Physics Research Section B: Beam Interactions with Materials and Atoms,* vol. 446, pp. 58–76, 2019, doi: 10.1016/j.nimb.2019.03.001.

[23] F. Tessier and I. Kawrakow, "Calculation of the electron–electron bremsstrahlung cross-section in the field of atomic electrons," *Nuclear Instruments and Methods in Physics Research Section B: Beam Interactions with Materials and Atoms,* vol. 266, no. 4, pp. 625–34, 2008, doi: 10.1016/j.nimb.2007.11.063.

[24] X. Llovet, F. Salvat, D. Bote, F. Salvat-Pujol, A. Jablonski, and C. J. Powell, "NIST NSRDS 164 NIST Database of Cross Sections for Inner-Shell Ionization by Electron or Positron Impact Version 1. 0 Users Guide," 2016.

[25] S. M. Seltzer and M. J. Berger, "Bremsstrahlung energy spectra from electrons with kinetic energy 1 keV–10 GeV incident on screened nuclei and orbital electrons of neutral atoms with Z = 1–100," *Atomic Data and Nuclear Data Tables,* vol. 35, no. 3, pp. 345–418, 1986, https://doi.org/10.1016/0092-640X(86)90014-8.

[26] F. Salvat, "PENELOPE 2018: A code system for Monte Carlo simulation of electron and photon transport." Issy-les-Moulineaux: OECD, 2019.

[27] E. B. Podgorsak, *Radiation Physics for Medical Physicists,* 3rd ed. Switzerland: Springer, 2016, doi: 10.1007/978-3-319-25382-4.

[28] ICRU, *Stopping Powers for Electrons and Positrons. ICRU Report 37,* 1984.

[29] ICRU, *Radiation Dosimetry: Electron Beams with Energies Between 1 and 50 MeV. ICRU Report 35,* 1984.

[30] X. Ning, L. Papiez, and G. Sandison, "Compound-Poisson-process method for the multiple scattering of charged particles," *Phys Rev E Stat Phys Plasmas Fluids Relat Interdiscip Topics,* vol. 52, no. 5, pp. 5621–33, 1995, doi: 10.1103/physreve.52.5621.

[31] I. Kawrakow and A. F. Bielajew, "On the condensed history technique for electron transport," *Nuclear Instruments and Methods in Physics Research Section B: Beam Interactions with Materials and Atoms,* vol. 142, no. 3, pp. 253–80, 1998, https://doi.org/10.1016/S0168-583X(98)00274-2.

[32] Y. Mejaddem, D. Belkić, S. Hyödynmaa, and A. Brahme, "Calculations of electron energy loss straggling," *Nuclear Instruments and Methods in Physics Research Section B: Beam Interactions with Materials and Atoms,* vol. 173, no. 4, pp. 397–410, 2001, https://doi.org/10.1016/S0168-583X(00)00428-6.

[33] J. McLellan, S. Sawchuk, J. J. Battista, G. A. Sandison, and L. S. Papiez, "A method for the calculation of electron energy-straggling spectra," *Med Phys,* vol. 21, no. 3, pp. 367–78, 1994, doi: 10.1118/1.597383.

[34] P. Hellekalek, "Good random number generators are (not so) easy to find," *Mathematics and Computers in Simulation (MATCOM),* vol. 46, no. 5, pp. 485–505, 1998.

[35] M. Matsumoto, I. Wada, A. Kuramoto, and H. Ashihara, "Common defects in initialization of pseudorandom number generators," *ACM Trans. Model. Comput. Simul.,* vol. 17, p. 15, 2007.

[36] A. Badal and J. Sempau, "A package of Linux scripts for the parallelization of Monte Carlo simulations," *Computer Physics Communications,* vol. 175, no. 6, pp. 440–50, 2006, doi: 10.1016/j.cpc.2006.05.009.

[37] M. Ljungberg and S. E. Strand, "A Monte Carlo program for the simulation of scintillation camera characteristics," *Comput Methods Programs Biomed,* vol. 29, no. 4, pp. 257–72, 1989.

[38] H. Nikjoo, S. Uehara, D. Emfietzoglou, and F. A. Cucinotta, "Track-structure codes in radiation research," *Radiation Measurements,* vol. 41, no. 9, pp. 1052–74, 2006, doi: 10.1016/j.radmeas.2006.02.001.

[39] J. Sempau, S. J. Wilderman, and A. F. Bielajew, "DPM, a fast, accurate Monte Carlo code optimized for photon and electron radiotherapy treatment planning dose calculations," *Phys Med Biol,* vol. 45, no. 8, pp. 2263–91, 2000, doi: 10.1088/0031-9155/45/8/315.

[40] M. Ljungberg, "The SIMIND Monte Carlo Code," in *Monte Carlo Calculation in Nuclear Medicine: Applications in Diagnostic Imaging – 2nd ed,* M. Ljungberg, S. E. Strand, and M. A. King, Eds. Boca Raton: CRC Press/Taylor & Francis Group, 2012, pp. 315–21.

[41] S. Agostinelli *et al.,* "Geant4—a simulation toolkit," *Nuclear Instruments and Methods in Physics Research Section A: Accelerators, Spectrometers, Detectors and Associated Equipment,* vol. 506, no. 3, pp. 250–303, 2003, doi: 10.1016/S0168-9002(03)01368-8.

[42] J. Allison *et al.,* "Recent developments in Geant4," *Nuclear Instruments and Methods in Physics Research Section A: Accelerators, Spectrometers, Detectors and Associated Equipment,* vol. 835, pp. 186–225, 2016, doi: 10.1016/j.nima.2016.06.125.

[43] S. Jan *et al.,* "GATE V6: a major enhancement of the GATE simulation platform enabling modelling of CT and radiotherapy," *Phys Med Biol,* vol. 56, no. 4, pp. 881–901, 2011, doi: 10.1088/0031-9155/56/4/001.

[44] D. Sarrut *et al.,* "A review of the use and potential of the GATE Monte Carlo simulation code for radiation therapy and dosimetry applications," *Med Phys,* vol. 41, no. 6, p. 064301, 2014, doi: 10.1118/1.4871617.

[45] P. Arce *et al.,* "Gamos: A framework to do Geant4 simulations in different physics fields with an user-friendly interface," *Nuclear Instruments and Methods in Physics Research Section A: Accelerators, Spectrometers, Detectors and Associated Equipment,* vol. 735, pp. 304–13, 2014, doi: 10.1016/j.nima.2013.09.036.

[46] J. Perl, J. Shin, J. Schumann, B. Faddegon, and H. Paganetti, "TOPAS: an innovative proton Monte Carlo platform for research and clinical applications," *Med Phys,* vol. 39, no. 11, pp. 6818–37, 2012, doi: 10.1118/1.4758060.

[47] I. Kawrakow, E. Mainegra-Hing, D. W. O. Rogers, F. Tessier, and B. R. B. Walter, "The EGSnrc Code System: Monte Carlo simulation of electron and photon transport," in *Technical Report PIRS-701,* National Research Council Canada: Ottawa, ON, Canada, 2018, http://nrc-cnrc.github.io/EGSnrc/doc/pirs701-egsnrc.pdf

[48] E. S. M. Ali and D. W. O. Rogers, "Energy spectra and angular distributions of charged particles backscattered from solid targets," *Journal of Physics D, Applied Physics,* vol. 41, no. 5, p. 9, 2008, doi: 101088/0022-3727/41/5/055505.

[49] D. Rogers, I. Kawrakow, J. Seuntjens, B. Walters, and E. Mainegra-Hing, "NRC user codes for EGSnrc," NRCC Report PIRS-702 (rev. C), 2003.

[50] J. Sempau, E. Acosta, J. Baro, J. M. Fernández-Varea, and F. Salvat, "An algorithm for Monte Carlo simulation of coupled electron-photon transport," *Nuclear Instruments and Methods in Physics Research Section B: Beam Interactions with Materials and Atoms,* vol. 132, no. 3, pp. 377–90, 1997, doi: 10.1016/S0168-583X(97)00414-X.

[51] J. Sempau, J. M. Fernández-Varea, E. Acosta, and F. Salvat, "Experimental benchmarks of the Monte Carlo code PENELOPE," *Nuclear Instruments and Methods in Physics Research Section B: Beam Interactions with Materials and Atoms,* vol. 207, no. 2, pp. 107–23, 2003, doi: 10.1016/S0168-583X(03)00453-1.

[52] J. Sempau, A. Badal, and L. Brualla, "A PENELOPE-based system for the automated Monte Carlo simulation of clinacs and voxelized geometries-application to far-from-axis fields," *Med Phys,* vol. 38, no. 11, pp. 5887–95, 2011, doi: 10.1118/1.3643029.

[53] C. J. Werner *et al.*, "MCNP Version 6.2 Release Notes," United States, 2018-02-05 2018, www.osti.gov/biblio/1419730

[54] G. Battistoni *et al.*, *Overview of the FLUKA code.* 2015, p. 06005.

[55] K. Niita, T. Sato, H. Iwase, H. Nose, H. Nakashima, and L. Sihver, "PHITS—a particle and heavy ion transport code system," *Radiation Measurements,* vol. 41, no. 9, pp. 1080–90, 2006, doi: 10.1016/j.radmeas.2006.07.013.

[56] D. E. Raeside, "Monte Carlo Principles and Applications," *Phys. Med. Biol.,* vol. 21, pp. 181–97, 1976.

[57] J. E. Turner, H. A. Wright, and R. N. Hamm, "A Monte Carlo primer for health physicists," *Health Physics,* vol. 48, pp. 717–33, 1985.

[58] P. Andreo, "Monte Carlo techniques in medical radiation physics," *Phys. Med. Biol.,* vol. 36, pp. 861–920, 1991.

[59] F. Verhaegen, A. E. Nahum, S. Van de Putte, and Y. Namito, "Monte Carlo modelling of radiotherapy kV x-ray units," *Phys Med Biol,* no. 7, vol. 44, pp. 1767–89, 1999, doi: 10.1088/0031-9155/44/7/315.

[60] C. M. Ma and S. B. Jiang, "Monte Carlo modelling of electron beams from medical accelerators," *Phys Med Biol,* vol. 44, no. 12, pp. R157–89, 1999, doi: 10.1088/0031-9155/44/12/201.

[61] F. Verhaegen and J. Seuntjens, "Monte Carlo modelling of external radiotherapy photon beams," *Phys Med Biol,* vol. 48, no. 21, pp. R107–64, 2003, doi: 10.1088/0031-9155/48/21/r01.

[62] H. Zaidi, "Relevance of accurate Monte Carlo modeling in nuclear medical imaging," *Med Phys,* vol. 26, pp. 574–608, 1999.

[63] P. Andreo, "Monte Carlo simulations in radiotherapy dosimetry," *Radiat Oncol,* vol. 13, no. 1, p. 121, 2018, doi: 10.1186/s13014-018-1065-3.

[64] J. Seco and F. Verhaegen (editors) *Monte Carlo Techniques in Radiation Therapy.* Boca Raton: CRC Press, 2013.

[65] H. Zaidi and G. Sgouros, "Therapeutic applications of Monte Carlo calculations in Nuclear Medicine," Boca Raton: CRC, 2002.

[66] M. Ljungberg, S. E. Strand, and M. A. King, *Monte Carlo Calculation in Nuclear Medicine: Applications in Diagnostic Imaging.* 2nd ed. Boca Raton: Taylor & Francis, 2012.

[67] I. J. Chetty *et al.*, "Report of the AAPM Task Group No. 105: Issues associated with clinical implementation of Monte Carlo-based photon and electron external beam treatment planning," *Med Phys,* vol. 34, no. 12, pp. 4818–53, 2007, doi: 10.1118/1.2795842.

[68] I. Sechopoulos *et al.*, *Records: Improved Reporting of Monte Carlo Radiation Transport Studies: Report of the AAPM Research Committee Task Group 268. Med Phys,* vol. 45, no. 1, pp. e1-e5, 2018, doi: 10.1002/mp.12702.

[69] B. M. Mendes *et al.*, "Calculation of dose point kernel values for monoenergetic electrons and beta emitting radionuclides: Intercomparison of Monte Carlo codes," *Radiat Phys Chem,* vol. 181, p. 109327, 2021, doi: 10.1016/j.radphyschem.2020.109327.

[70] M. Han *et al.*, "Validation of cross sections for Monte Carlo simulation of the Photoelectric Effect," *IEEE T Nucl Sci,* vol. 63, 2016, doi: 10.1109/TNS.2016.2521876.

[71] T. Basaglia, M. Pia, and P. Saracco, "Evolutions in photoelectric cross section calculations and their validation," *IEEE T Nucl Sci,* vol. PP, p. 1, 2020, doi: 10.1109/TNS.2020.2971173.

[72] Y. Liang *et al.*, "A general-purpose Monte Carlo particle transport code based on inverse transform sampling for radio-therapy dose calculation," *Sci Rep,* vol. 10, no. 1, p. 9808, 2020, doi: 10.1038/s41598-020-66844-7.

9 Patient Models for Dosimetry Applications

Michael G. Stabin

CONTENTS

To calculate doses from internal emitters, models of the human body are needed, as doses cannot be measured, only calculated theoretically. A generalized expression for calculating internal dose, is given in the RADAR dose calculation system [1] by the following equation:

$$D = N \times DF \tag{9.1}$$

where N is the number of nuclear transitions that occur in source region S, and DF is a 'dose factor'. The factor DF depends on combining decay data with absorbed fractions (AFs), which are derived generally using Monte Carlo simulation of radiation transport in models of the body and its internal structures (organs, tumours, etc.):

$$DF = \frac{k \sum_i y_i \, E_i \, \phi_i \, w_{R_i}}{m_T}, \tag{9.2}$$

where y_i = number of radiations with energy E_i emitted per nuclear transition
E_i = energy per radiation for the ith radiation (MeV)
$\phi_i(T \leftarrow S)$ = fraction of energy emitted in a source region that is absorbed in a target region
m_T = mass of the target region (kg or g)
w_R = the radiation weighting factor for radiation i, and
k = proportionality constant (Gy-kg/MBq-sec-MeV or rad-g/μCi-hr-MeV)

This equation gives only the dose from one source region to one target region, but they can be generalized easily to multiple source and target regions.

DOI: 10.1201/9780429489549-9

$$D_T = \frac{k \sum_s N_s \sum_i y_i E_i (T \leftarrow S)}{m_T}$$

(9.3)

Computed values of ϕ are most often needed for photons; simple rules apply to alpha and beta emissions, with notable exceptions for hollow organs, bone and marrow and a few other specialized applications.

9.1   SIMPLE BEGINNINGS

For many years, values of ϕ were given by 'considering a spherical human'. The International Commission on Radiation Units and Measurements (ICRU) presented a reference computational phantom, the ICRU sphere, which was a 30 cm diameter sphere composed of 'ICRU tissue' [2]. The earliest radiation regulations in the United States, 10CFR20, used internal dosimetry models that modelled the human body as a similarly sized sphere, with all defined internal organs also defined as spheres [3]. This obviously lacked realism but was computationally easy. Values of ϕ (for self-absorption only) could be calculated simply as $(1 - e^{-\mu R})$, where μ is the photon linear absorption coefficient (for a tissue-equivalent medium), and R is the radius of the sphere representing the object in question.

The Medical Internal Radiation Dose (MIRD) of the Society of Nuclear Medicine (SNM) developed the next generation of computational phantoms, with the 'Fisher-Snyder' anthropomorphic phantom (Figure 9.1) [4]. It used a variety of geometric shapes to model the body and its internal structures; Monte Carlo methods were used to develop absorbed fractions for a couple of dozen source and target regions.

The MIRD Committee also published tables of 'S Values' (identical to 'Dose Factors' defined above) [5] in paper form. Cristy and Eckerman [6] of Oak Ridge National Laboratory (ORNL) developed a series of similar phantoms, representing individuals of different ages from newborns to adults (Figure 9.2).

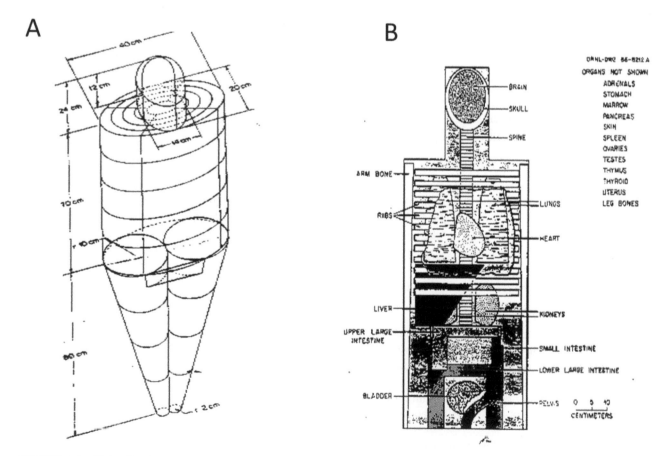

FIGURE 9.1   Fisher-Snyder Anthropomorphic Phantom

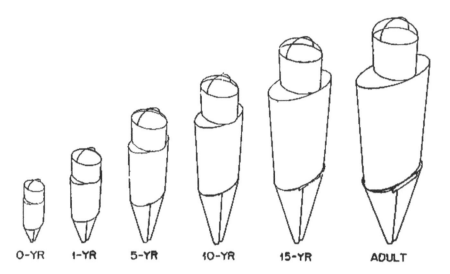

FIGURE 9.2 Cristy-Eckerman adult and pediatric phantom series

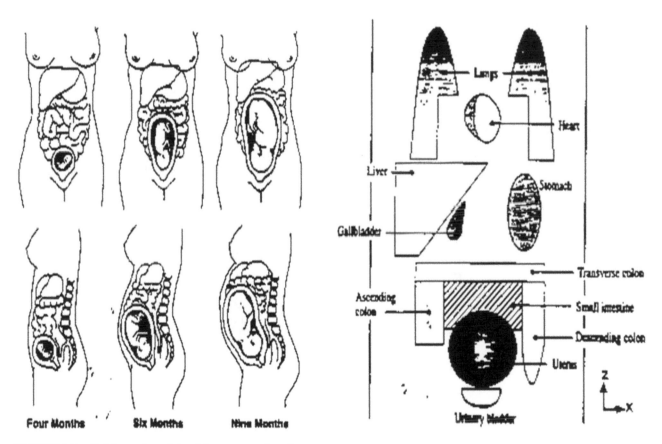

FIGURE 9.3 Stabin *et al.* models of the pregnant female

Stabin and colleagues created a series of three phantoms representing pregnant women at different stages of gestation [7] (Figure 9.3).

Absorbed fractions were published with these two ORNL documents. The MIRD Committee never 'adopted' them and published any Dose Factor tables; but personnel at Oak Ridge Associated Universities (ORAU) developed a personal computer code called 'MIRDOSE' [8] that included all of the ORNL nine phantom-absorbed fractions and implemented them in the MIRD dosimetry system to facilitate dose calculations. The MIRD Committee, however, strongly objected to the use of the name 'MIRDOSE' for the code, as they had not had a direct role in its development. The MIRDOSE code was revised and renamed 'OLINDA', meaning Organ Level INternal Dose Assessment' [9].

Clearly these heterogeneous anthropomorphic phantoms were much better than simple spherical models and were widely adopted by the dosimetry community. For many years, these were the only phantoms available for calculations; in the next generation of phantoms many centres have developed other phantoms, and there is no one, single agreed-upon set of phantoms to use. The key is always which phantoms have been made freely available to the user community, with Dose Factors calculated and easy to use.

9.2 THE PROLIFERATION

A handbook was published by the CRC Press in 2010, summarizing the results of a meeting in the United States in 2005 in which 64 authors from 13 countries and regions presented information on anthropomorphic development [10] based on medical images of actual humans, instead of 'stylized' models, as were developed at ORNL. In addition to this chapter, a comprehensive review paper has been published by Kainz and colleagues [11]. There are now many hundreds of anthropomorphic phantoms that have been developed and used for various dosimetric analyses.

The earliest entrant into the field was the 'VIP-Man' phantom, originally presented by Zubal and colleagues [12] (Figure 9.4).

With the advent of readily available medical images (typically Computed Tomography [CT] scans), many other centres developed realistic phantoms, using a number of mathematical techniques, including simple (and very tedious) manual segmentation of organs, descriptions of organ surfaces by Nonuniform Rational B-Splines (NURBS), polygon mesh, and other technologies. Various Monte Carlo codes have been employed by the authors to develop absorbed fractions for internal and external radiation sources in numerous applications, in medical imaging and therapy, general radiation protection, space exploration and others. In this chapter we will summarize all of the models presented in this symposium and the application areas noted, with emphasis on the models that are having the most impact on routine use.

9.3 THE GSF VOXEL PHANTOMS

A number of phantoms were developed by the GSF (Research Centre for Environment and Health) in Germany, based mostly on CT images of living subjects. There were male and female adults (Figure 9.5), and three other male and six

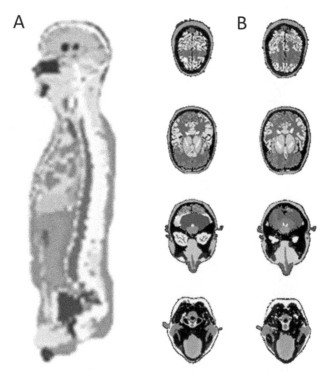

FIGURE 9.4 Zubal *et al.* VIP-Man voxel phantom, right, compared to Fisher-Snyder phantom, left.

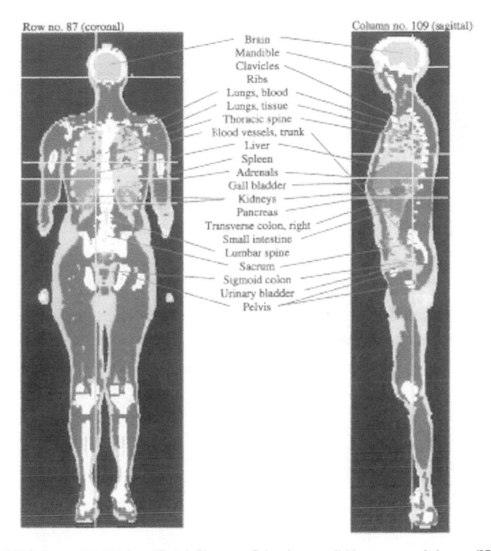

FIGURE 9.5   GSF Reference Adult Male and Female Phantoms. Colour image available at www.routledge.com/9781138593299.

female models, one of whom was pregnant. Most segmentation was performed manually. The two adult models have been adopted by the International Commission on Radiological Protection (ICRP) for use in standard dose calculations for radiation workers [13]. ICRP adoption of models for other ages, likely based on the University of Florida (UF) models, described below, is pending.

9.4   THE RADAR NURBS MODELS

Segars and colleagues developed a series of human and animal models based on NURBS technology. Starting with images of an adult male and female human, two NURBS models were developed, which were actually four-dimensional models – movement due to cardiac or respiratory motion was possible (Figure 9.6) [14]. They also segmented a mouse and rat from micro-CT images (Figure 9.7).

The Radiation Dose Assessment Resource (RADAR) Committee of the Society of Nuclear Medicine scaled the two adult models to conform to the standard organ masses given in ICRP Publication 89 [15], then developed a series of pediatric models by deforming the adult NURBS models – again so that organ masses matched those of ICRP 89 [16]. They used the standard ages defined in the original ORNL documents – newborns, 1-year, 5-year, 10-year and 15-year olds (Figure 9.8).

RADAR also developed NURBS models representing 3 mouse and 5 rat models, again, by deforming the Segars and colleagues MOBY and ROBY basic models [17] (Tables 9.1 and 9.2). Xu and colleagues of the Rensselaer Polytechnic

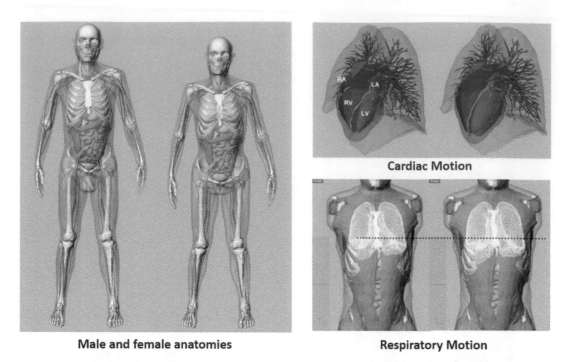

Male and female anatomies   **Respiratory Motion**

FIGURE 9.6   Segars *et al.* NURBS models, adult male and female. Colour image available at www.routledge.com/9781138593299.

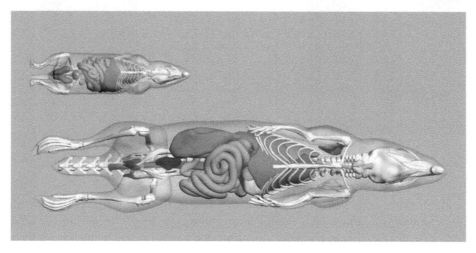

FIGURE 9.7   Segars *et al.* mouse (MOBY) and rat (ROBY) NURBS models. Colour image available at www.routledge.com/ 9781138593299.

Institute developed three realistic models of the pregnant female, to update the Stabin and colleagues ORNL 'stylized' models [18](Figure 9.9).

Absorbed fractions for internal emitters were developed for the twelve adult and pediatric models (male and female at six ages), three pregnant female models, and eight mouse and rat models and incorporated into the (US Food and Drug Administration approved) OLINDA/EXM software [9], to facilitate dose calculations for any of the models, using appropriate input kinetic data. These phantoms now represent the standard dosimetric phantoms for nuclear medicine applications.

As NURBS models are very easy to deform to create new models, RADAR also deformed the reference phantoms (which represent the median, or 50th percentile, individual of a population), to represent children of 10th, 25th, 75th and 90th percentile individuals (Figure 9.10), and added some additional age phantoms to study variations of CT dose with subject body size [19]. Dose estimates for various CT exams were provided as a function of age and body size. All RADAR phantoms are available to the user community for either external or internal dose calculations.

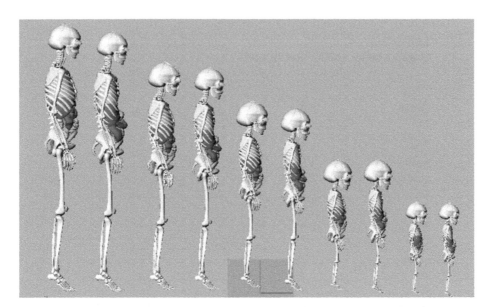

FIGURE 9.8 Sample images from the RADAR reference adult and paediatric phantom series. Colour image available at www. routledge.com/9781138593299.

TABLE 9.1
Organ Masses in Three Mouse Models

Organ	Organ mass (g)		
	25-g mouse	30-g mouse	35-g mouse
Brain	0.466	0.568	0.666
Heart	0.235	0.291	0.342
Stomach	0.055	0.069	0.082
Small intestine	1.74	2.12	2.49
Large intestine	0.583	0.709	0.830
Kidneys	0.302	0.374	0.432
Liver	1.74	2.15	2.57
Lungs	0.087	0.107	0.131
Pancreas	0.305	0.378	0.450
Skeleton	2.18	2.61	3.01
Spleen	0.111	0.136	0.157
Testes	0.160	0.197	0.228
Thyroid	0.014	0.016	0.020
Bladder	0.060	0.075	0.088
Body	24.11	29.80	35.27

9.5 UNIVERSITY OF FLORIDA PHANTOM SERIES

Researchers have also developed a series of adult and pediatric anthropomorphic phantoms, and developed phantoms of different body shape and size (Figure 9.11) [20].

The reference phantoms were also scaled to ICRP 89 reference values, and non-reference phantoms were scaled using published data on variations in human anatomy, as were the RADAR non-reference values. The paediatric phantoms have been adopted by International Commission on Radiological Protection (ICRP) as the international reference for calculations to radiation workers and members of the public, for basic radiation protection studies, but no data are

TABLE 9.2
Organ Masses in Five Rat Models

Organ	Organ mass (g)				
	200-g rat	300-g rat	400-g rat	500-g rat	600-g rat
Brain	1.57	2.32	3.16	3.93	4.54
Heart	1.80	2.64	3.55	4.39	5.28
Stomach	0.941	1.40	1.89	2.37	2.86
Small intestine	10.6	15.5	20.8	25.6	30.8
Large intestine	7.86	11.5	15.5	19.2	231
Kidneys	2.06	3.03	4.09	5.06	6.09
Liver	7.55	11.2	152	18.8	22.8
Lungs	0.594	0.884	1.21	1.50	1.82
Pancreas	0.368	0.535	0.732	0.908	1.10
Skeleton	15.3	22.0	292	35.2	38.7
Spleen	0.607	0.884	1.18	1.45	1.74
Testes	0.174	0.245	0.321	0.386	0.460
Thyroid	0.191	0.275	0.368	0.457	0.549
Bladder	0.475	0.682	0.916	1.12	1.34
Body	226	335	443	547	643

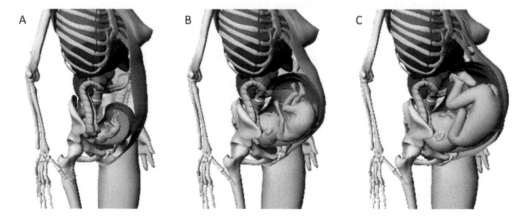

FIGURE 9.9   Sample RPI realistic pregnant female model. Colour image available at www.routledge.com/9781138593299.

currently available. The non-reference phantoms were used to calculate dose coefficients for external sources of radiation, in a collaboration with the National Cancer Institute (Figure 9.12) [21].

9.6   OTHER REALISTIC PHANTOMS

The other phantoms in the CRC handbook will be more briefly covered here, not because the work is not elegant, but because the phantom studies did not obtain international recognition as standard, as have the RADAR and ICRP reference phantoms.

1. Kramer and colleagues described two adult computational phantoms for the adult female and male called 'FAX' and 'MAX' [22]. Manual segmentation was performed to identify about 30 internal organs; dose factors were provided for several external irradiation geometries.
2. A number of studies cited in the CRC handbook describe efforts to produce models of individuals from particular countries:

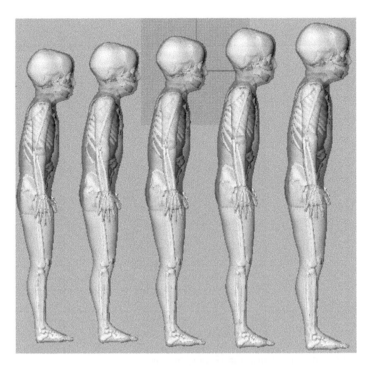

FIGURE 9.10 RADAR phantoms representing children of 10th, 25th, 75th and 90th percentile individuals. Colour image available at www.routledge.com/9781138593299.

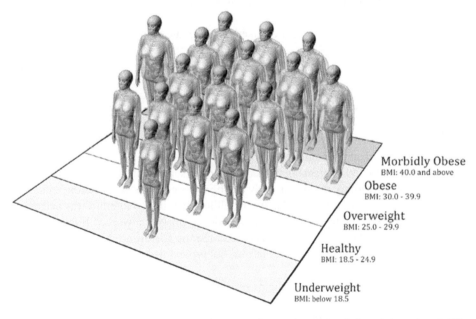

Morbidly Obese
BMI: 40.0 and above

Obese
BMI: 30.0 - 39.9

Overweight
BMI: 25.0 - 29.9

Healthy
BMI: 18.5 - 24.9

Underweight
BMI: below 18.5

FIGURE 9.11 The UF adult and paediatric reference phantom series, and models of the adult male of different body habitus. Colour image available at www.routledge.com/9781138593299.

- Members of the Japanese Atomic Energy Agency computational phantoms for adult males and females, a pregnant woman and several children of various different ages [23]. Absorbed fractions and Dose Factors were calculated.
- Reference Korean phantoms were developed at the Hanyang University for a reference adult male and female Korean individuals [24].
- Voxel phantoms representing three Chinese adult males were developed [25]; dose factors were given for several photon energies for external irradiation geometries.

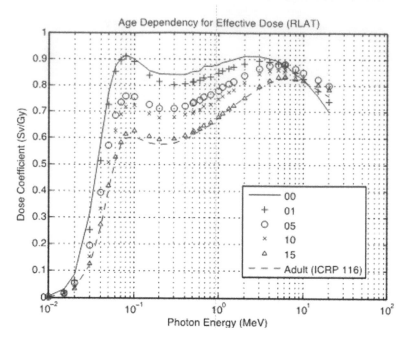

FIGURE 9.12 Sample dose coefficients for external sources of radiation.

3. A teenage voxel phantom called ADELAIDE was developed in a collaborative effort in Australia [26]. Effective doses for some CT examinations were provided.
4. Na and colleagues described the development of a series of female phantoms of differing breast size for use of 'virtual calibration' of lung counters [27].

9.7 APPLICATIONS OF THE PHANTOMS

9.7.1 DOSIMETRIC CALCULATIONS

Even starting with the earliest spherical phantoms, the purpose for their development is to facilitate dose calculations in the human body. In the CRC handbook, Hintenlang and colleagues described the use of physical phantoms for dosimetry, in which a physical object resembling the human body can be exposed to radiation fields, with radiation dosimeters placed within [28]. This is difficult to do for internal emitters, although a limited attempt was performed by Poston and colleagues (reference not available). The use of Monte Carlo codes to provide absorbed fractions for organ doses from internal or external exposures then facilitates generalized calculations for different exposure scenarios and particle types, mostly photon and neutron. Applications are numerous, but typical uses are:

- Calculations of internal dose from nuclear medicine procedures or internal intakes of radionuclides by workers.
- Calculations of external dose from medical irradiations – diagnostic (x-ray or CT) and therapeutic.
- Calculations of external dose to radiation workers or members of the public from industrial uses of radiation.
- Calculation of doses to individuals involved in space exploration.

9.7.2 IMAGE-BASED DOSIMETRY

The XCAT phantom has been widely used for evaluation of nuclear medicine imaging. The present version has 158 parameters that can be changed by the user to define the resultant phantom, the 70 segmented volumes (organs, vessels, fat, bone etc.). This then allow studies of the accuracy and precision in scintillation camera images and related dosimetry procedures [29]. Figure 9.13 shows examples of simulated whole-body images, using the SIMIND code [30, 31], for

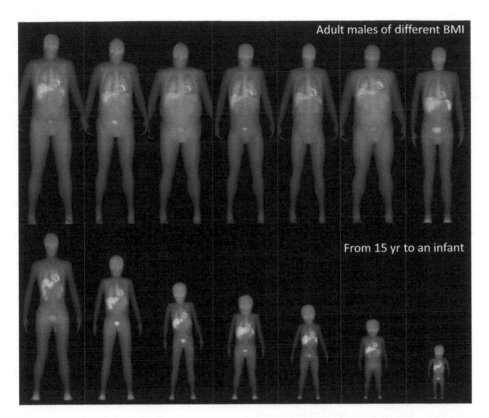

FIGURE 9.13 Monte Carlo simulation of whole-body of a scintillation camera images with a LEHR collimator for different XCAT models. A fictitious ^{99m}Tc activity distribution was defined for visual purposes, where the activity concentration in each organ was kept the same for all simulated cases. Colour image available at www.routledge.com/9781138593299.

TABLE 9.3
Effective Doses for a Variety of Nuclear Medicine Pharmaceuticals Using the 'Old' (Cristy/Eckerman Stylized Phantoms) and 'New' (RADAR NURBS) Phantoms

		Adult	15 year	10 year	5 year	1 year
^{18}FDG	Old	1.86×10^{-2}	2.39×10^{-2}	3.58×10^{-2}	5.29×10^{-2}	8.90×10^{-2}
	New	1.73×10^{-2}	2.21×10^{-2}	3.26×10^{-2}	4.76×10^{-2}	7.83×10^{-2}
	Ratio	9.30×10^{-1}	9.25×10^{-1}	9.11×10^{-1}	9.00×10^{-1}	8.80×10^{-1}
^{11}C Acetate	Old	3.03×10^{-3}	3.77×10^{-3}	5.70×10^{-3}	8.60×10^{-3}	1.59×10^{-2}
	New	2.88×10^{-3}	3.72×10^{-3}	5.41×10^{-3}	8.20×10^{-3}	1.38×10^{-2}
	Ratio	9.50×10^{-1}	9.87×10^{-1}	9.49×10^{-1}	9.53×10^{-1}	8.68×10^{-1}
^{99m}Tc MAA	Old	1.17×10^{-2}	1.64×10^{-2}	2.35×10^{-2}	3.54×10^{-2}	6.56×10^{-2}
	New	1.10×10^{-2}	1.40×10^{-2}	2.21×10^{-2}	3.31×10^{-2}	5.85×10^{-2}
	Ratio	9.40×10^{-1}	8.54×10^{-1}	9.40×10^{-1}	9.35×10^{-1}	8.92×10^{-1}
^{111}In Octeotate	Old	5.15×10^{-2}	6.76×10^{-2}	1.01×10^{-1}	1.49×10^{-1}	2.42×10^{-1}
	New	5.09×10^{-2}	6.34×10^{-2}	9.19×10^{-2}	1.30×10^{-1}	2.02×10^{-1}
	Ratio	9.88×10^{-1}	9.38×10^{-1}	9.10×10^{-1}	8.72×10^{-1}	8.35×10^{-1}
^{123}I BMIPP	Old	1.51×10^{-2}	1.92×10^{-2}	2.94×10^{-2}	4.44×10^{-2}	8.05×10^{-2}
	New	1.49×10^{-2}	1.94×10^{-2}	2.79×10^{-2}	4.08×10^{-2}	7.13×10^{-2}
	Ratio	9.87×10^{-1}	1.01	9.49×10^{-1}	9.19×10^{-1}	8.86×10^{-1}

FDG=Fluorodeoxyglucose, MAA=Macroaggregated Albumin, BMIPP= β-methyl-p-iodophenyl-pentadecanoic acid a standard 3/8-inch NaI(Tl) camera, equipped with a LEHR collimator and with ^{99m}Tc distributed in fourteen different XCAT phantom ranging from seven male adult models with different Body-Max Index to youth models down to an infant. A fictious activity distribution was used with the purpose to make major organs visible.

9.8 SUMMARY

It is difficult to imagine future phantom developments that can produce models more detailed or elegant than we have at present but, of course, scientists are always looking for challenges to improve the present state of the art. Models to address the issue of electron and alpha dose to bone and marrow are still developing; this is a topic outside the scope of this chapter.

Obviously, it was a huge leap in improvement moving from the simple 'body is a sphere' to the first heterogeneous stylized phantoms. In the ICRP 2 calculations [3], the organs were simplified spheres, but also no cross-irradiation from one organ to another was possible. So, the newer dose estimates were clearly better. Interestingly, however, the move from stylized phantoms to sophisticated image-based phantoms did not result in a marked change in overall dosimetry. The organs are closer together and overlap more, but, for example, for effective doses in nuclear medicine procedures, the changes were modest (Table 9.3).

REFERENCES

[1]   M. G. Stabin and J. A. Siegel, "Physical models and dose factors for use in internal dose assessment," *Health Phys,* vol. 85, no. 3, pp. 294–310, 2003, doi: 10.1097/00004032-200309000-00006.

[2]   A. McNair, "ICRU Report 33 - Radiation Quantities and Units Pub: International Commission on Radiation Units and Measurements, Washington D.C. USA issued 15 April 1980, pp.25," *Journal of Labelled Compounds and Radiopharmaceuticals,* vol. 18, no. 9, pp. 1398–98, 1981, doi: 10.1002/jlcr.2580180918.

[3]   "Report of Committee II on permissible dose for internal radiation (1959)," *Annals of the ICRP/ICRP Publication,* vol. OS_2, no. 1, pp. i-v, 1960, doi: 10.1016/s0074-27406080001-3.

[4]   W. Snyder, M. Ford, and G. Warner. *MIRD Pamphlet No 5: Estimates of specific absorbed fractions for photon sources uniformly distributed in various organs of a heterogeneous phantom.* (1978). Society of Nuclear Medicine. New York.

[5]   W. Snyder, M. Ford, G. Warner, and S. Watson. *MIRD Pamphlet No 11: "S," absorbed dose per unit cumulated activity for selected radionuclides and organs.* (1975). Society of Nuclear Medicine. New York.

[6]   M. Cristy and K. F. Eckerman, *Specific Absorbed Fractions of Energy at Various Ages from Internal Photon Sources. Report ORNL/TM-8381/V1-V7.* Oak Ridge National Laboratory, Oak Ridge, TN, 1987.

[7]   M. G. Stabin *et al.,* "Mathematical models and specific absorbed fractions of photon energy in the nonpregnant adult female and at the end of each trimester of pregnancy," ORNL/TM-12907. Oak Ridge National Lab., TN, 1995, www.osti.gov/servlets/purl/91944.

[8]   M. G. Stabin, "MIRDOSE: Personal computer software for internal dose assessment in nuclear medicine," *J Nucl Med,* vol. 37, pp. 538–46, 1996.

[9]   M. G. Stabin, R. B. Sparks, and E. Crowe, "OLINDA/EXM: The Second-Generation Personal Computer Software for Internal Dose Assessment in Nuclear Medicine," *J Nucl Med,* vol. 46, pp. 1023–27, 2005.

[10]   X. G. Xu and K. F. Eckerman, Eds. *Handbook of Anatomical Models for Radiation Dosimetry.* CRC Press/Taylor & Francis Group, 2009.

[11]   W. Kainz *et al.,* "Advances in Computational Human Phantoms and Their Applications in Biomedical Engineering – A Topical Review," *IEEE Transactions on Radiation and Plasma Medical Sciences,* vol. 3, no. 1, pp. 1–23, 2019, doi: 10.1109/TRPMS.2018.2883437.

[12]   I. G. Zubal and C. R. Harrell, "Computerized three-dimensional segmented human anatomy," *Med Phys,* vol. 21, pp. 299–302, 1994.

[13]   ICRP, 2009. *Adult Reference Computational Phantoms.* ICRP Publication 110, Ann. ICRP 39 (2).

[14]   W. Segars and B. Tsui, "The MCAT, NCAT, XCAT and MOBY computational human and mouse phantoms," in *Handbook of Anatomical Models for Radiation Dosimetry,* X. G. Xu and K. F. Eckerman, Eds. Boca Raton: CRC Press/Taylor & Francis Group, 2009, pp. 150–34.

[15]   ICRP, 2002. *Basic Anatomical & Physiological Data for Use in Radiological Protection - Reference values.* ICRP Publication 89, Ann. ICRP 32 (3–4).

[16]   M. Stabin, M. Emmons-Keenan, W. Segars, and M. Fernald, "The Vanderbilt University Reference Adult and Pediatric Phantom Series," in *Handbook of Anatomical Models for Radiation Dosimetry,* X. G. Xu and K. F. Eckerman, Eds. Boca Raton: CRC Press/Taylor & Francis Group, 2009, pp. 337 46.

[17]   M. A. Keenan, M. G. Stabin, W. P. Segars, and M. J. Fernald, "RADAR realistic animal model series for dose assessment," *J Nucl Med,* vol. 51, no. 3, pp. 471–76, 2010, doi: 10.2967/jnumed.109.070532.

[18] X. Xu, C. Shi, M. Stabin, and V. Taranenko, "Pregnant Female/Fetus Computational Phantoms and the Latest RPI-P Series Representing 3, 6, and 9-month Gestational Periods," in *Handbook of Anatomical Models for Radiation Dosimetry*, X. G. Xu and K. F. Eckerman Eds. Boca Raton: CRC Press/Taylor & Francis Group, 2009, pp. 305–36.

[19] S. D. Kost *et al.*, "Patient-specific dose calculations for pediatric CT of the chest, abdomen and pelvis," *Pediatr Radiol,* vol. 45, no. 12, pp. 1771–80, 2015, doi: 10.1007/s00247-015-3400-2.

[20] C. Lee, D. Lodwick, D. Pafundi, S. Whalen, J. Williams, and W. Bolch, "The University of Florida Pediatric Phantom Series," in *Handbook of Anatomical Models for Radiation Dosimetry*, X. G. Xu and K. F. Eckerman, Eds. Boca Raton: CRC Press/Taylor & Francis Group, 2009, pp. 199–220.

[21] C. Lee, K. P. Kim, W. E. Bolch, B. E. Moroz, and L. Folio, "NCICT: A computational solution to estimate organ doses for pediatric and adult patients undergoing CT scans," *J Radiol Prot,* vol. 35, no. 4, pp. 891–909, 2015, doi: 10.1088/0952-4746/35/4/891.

[22] R. Kramer *et al.*, "The FAX06 and the MAX 06 Computational Voxel Phantoms," in *Handbook of Anatomical Models for Radiation Dosimetry*, X. G. Xu and K. F. Eckerman, Eds. Boca Raton: CRC Press/Taylor & Francis Group, 2009, pp. 163–98.

[23] K. Saito, K. Sato, S. Kinase, and T. Nagaoka, "Japanese Computational Phantoms: Otoko, Onago, JM, JM2, JF, TARO, HANAKO, Pregnant Woman and Deformable Child," in *Handbook of Anatomical Models for Radiation Dosimetry*, X. G. Xu and K. F. Eckerman, Eds. Boca Raton: CRC Press/Taylor & Francis Group, 2009, pp. 221–54.

[24] C. Lee and C. Kim, "Korean Computational Phantoms: KMIRD, KORMAN, KORWOMAN, KTMAN-1, KTMAN-2 and HDRK-Man," in *Handbook of Anatomical Models for Radiation Dosimetry*, X. G. Xu and K. F. Eckerman Eds. Boca Raton: CRC Press/Taylor & Francis Group, 2009, pp. 255–78.

[25] B. Zhang, J. Ma, G. Zhang, Q. Liu, R. Qiu, and J. Li, "Chinese Voxel Computational Phantoms: CNMAN, VCH, and CVP," in *Handbook of Anatomical Models for Radiation Dosimetry*, X. G. Xu and K. F. Eckerman, Eds. Boca Raton: CRC Press/Taylor & Francis Group, 2009, pp. 279–304.

[26] M. Caon, G. Bibbo, and J. Pattison, "The ADELAIDE Teenage Female Voxel Computational Phantom," in *Handbook of Anatomical Models for Radiation Dosimetry*, X. G. Xu and K. F. Eckerman, Eds. Boca Raton: CRC Press/Taylor & Francis Group, 2009, pp. 87–104.

[27] Y. Na, J. Zhang, A. Ding, and X. Xu, "Mesh-based and Anatomically Adjusted Adult Phantoms and a Case Study in Virtual Calibration of a Lung Counter for Female Workers," in *Handbook of Anatomical Models for Radiation Dosimetry*, X. G. Xu and K. F. Eckerman, Eds. Boca Raton: CRC Press/Taylor & Francis Group, 2009, pp. 347–76.

[28] D. Hintenlang, W. Moloney, and J. Winslow, "Physical Phantoms for Experimental Radiation Dosimetry," in *Handbook of Anatomical Models for Radiation Dosimetry*, X. G. Xu and K. F. Eckerman, Eds. Boca Raton: CRC Press/Taylor & Francis Group, 2009, pp. 389–412.

[29] J. Gustafsson, G. Brolin, M. Cox, M. Ljungberg, L. Johansson, and K. S. Gleisner, "Uncertainty propagation for SPECT/CT-based renal dosimetry in (177)Lu peptide receptor radionuclide therapy," *Phys Med Biol,* vol. 60, no. 21, pp. 8329–46, 2015, doi: 10.1088/0031-9155/60/21/8329.

[30] M. Ljungberg, "The SIMIND Monte Carlo Code," in *Monte Carlo Calculation in Nuclear Medicine: Applications in Diagnostic Imaging, 2nd ed.*, M. Ljungberg, S. E. Strand, and M. A. King, Eds. Boca Raton: CRC Press/Taylor & Francis Group, 2012, pp. 315–21.

[31] M. Ljungberg and S. E. Strand, "A Monte Carlo program for the simulation of scintillation camera characteristics," *Comput Methods Programs Biomed,* vol. 29, no. 4, pp. 257–72, 1989.

10 Patient-specific Dosimetry Calculations

Manuel Bardiès, Naomi Clayton, Gunjan Kayal, and Alex Vergara Gil

CONTENTS

10.1 INTRODUCTION

The absorbed dose calculation is one of the last steps of the clinical dosimetric workflow, after activity determination, time activity curve fitting and determination of time-integrated activity (TIA).

Historically, it was difficult to model radiation transport, especially in heterogeneous media. This explains why pre-computed, model-based dosimetric parameters such as the S values (absorbed doses in a target volume per disintegration in a source volume), designed for risk assessment of diagnostic procedures, were used in dosimetric approaches for several decades, even in a context of therapy where more specific approaches would have been more appropriate [1].

Whenever patient-specific calculations were looked for, some adjustments to S values were made for self-absorbed dose calculation ($S_{Source \leftarrow Source}$). For cross irradiation, the adjustment is difficult due to the inverse square law and is usually not performed.

The explicit modelling of radiation transport was only possible using complex Monte Carlo codes, usually coming from the world of high-energy particle physics and mostly only available in nuclear research centres.

The development of absorbed dose calculation codes accessible to a wider audience was rendered possible by access to ever-growing computing power. For the type of situations encountered in clinical nuclear medicine (type of radiation, energy, volumes of interest), it is now possible to perform detailed absorbed dose computations (including Monte Carlo modelling of radiation transport and energy deposition) on personal computers. This explains why a large number of approaches, most of them involving Monte Carlo modelling, are now reported in the literature [2–5]. In addition,

DOI: 10.1201/9780429489549-10

absorbed dose calculation algorithms, based on patient-specific pharmacokinetics and geometry, are included in dosimetry workstations which are becoming widely commercially available.

In fact, this rapid evolution leads to the conclusion that the hardest part of the dosimetric workflow, or at least which leads to the largest uncertainties and limitations, is the quantitative imaging or pharmacokinetic assessment, whereas absorbed dose calculation is now considered not especially challenging: in only a few decades, the absorbed dose calculation step has evolved from being restricted to a limited number of specialized centres to being widely available in the clinical environment.

10.2 RADIATION RANGE AND IMPACT ON ABSORBED DOSE DETERMINATION

The main parameter that impacts the selection of an absorbed dose calculation approach is the relationship between the radiation range, which is fixed for a given isotope, and the spatial sampling of activity and/or the density of the medium that depends on the application. For clinical applications, the spatial sampling of SPECT images is in the order of 0.44 to 0.48 cm for 128 × 128 images, whereas preclinical imaging uses a much finer sampling of about 1 mm. This is why it is important to have a preliminary idea of how the energy is deposited at a distance of the emission source. The following examples, which will illustrate this, are made for some of the most commonly used isotopes in nuclear medicine therapy: ^{90}Y, ^{131}I and ^{177}Lu.

The first example presented in Figure 10.1 considers point sources emitting isotropically in a homogeneous medium (water). The energy deposited at a distance from the point source only depends on the distance to the emission point. The *cumulated* energy deposited per disintegration (MeV·Bq^{-1}·s^{-1}) was scored in spheres of growing radii. The calculations were based on an analytical approach equivalent to that proposed in Bardiès and Chatal (1994) [6], using Berger absorbed dose point kernels [7] and considering the full beta energy spectra. The results illustrate the impact of radiation range on dosimetric results.

The energy deposited at a given distance from the point source varies between the 3 isotopes:

1. At distance very close to the emission point (~200 μm), the energy absorbed per decay is very similar in magnitude for the 3 isotopes: 114.9 keV, 110.0 keV and 105.8 keV for ^{131}I, ^{177}Lu and ^{90}Y, respectively.
2. As the distance from the emission point increases, the difference between the energy deposited for the three radionuclides tends to vary in proportion to the emitted energy per decay. The fact that ^{90}Y emits beta electron with higher energies (per decay) compared to ^{131}I or ^{177}Lu could be compensated by a larger number of emissions,

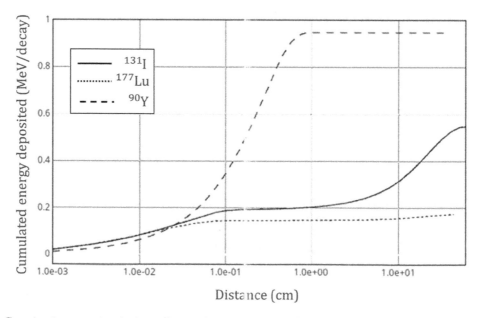

FIGURE 10.1 Cumulated energy absorbed at a distance from a point source in water. The mean energy of electron (monoenergetic and ß) and photon emissions are 0.146 and 0.030 MeV·Bq^{-1}·s^{-1}, respectively, for ^{177}Lu, 0.192 and 0.375 MeV·Bq^{-1}·s^{-1} for ^{131}I and the mean beta energy for ^{90}Y is 0.949 MeV·Bq^{-1}·s^{-1} (MB personal data).

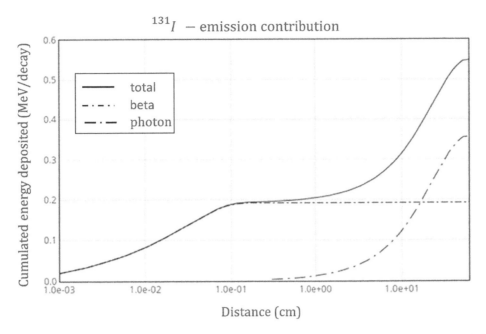

FIGURE 10.2 Cumulated energy absorbed at a distance of a point source in water for ^{131}I: contribution of beta and photon emissions.

but the important feature to consider in Figure 10.1 is that it displays the *energy deposition pattern*, that is, how energy is deposited at a distance from the emission point:

3. For ^{131}I, the electron/beta component is absorbed within the first mm. This limit corresponds to a threshold after which this radiation can be considered as non-penetrating (i.e., locally absorbed). Interestingly, the gamma contribution only becomes significant after 1 cm (Figure 10.2), meaning that between 1 mm and 1 cm the cumulated energy per decay remains relatively constant (i.e., no energy is delivered to the medium).

4. As far as the particulate emissions (electrons/beta) are concerned, ^{131}I and ^{177}Lu behave in a rather similar manner: even though the emitted energies are different, the energy deposition pattern is quite close for these 2 isotopes (especially when compared to ^{90}Y). It can be seen from the figure that the cumulated energies deposited at 2 mm are different (194.4 versus 146.3 keV/decay for ^{131}I and ^{177}Lu respectively, but again this relative difference of 25 per cent could easily be compensated by increasing the number of decays.

5. The main differences are in the contribution of photons. That of ^{131}I only becomes visible after 1 cm, but is considerable, whereas that of ^{177}Lu remains very low, even at larger distances.

These observations are relevant, as they orient the choice of the algorithm implemented to perform absorbed dose calculations. The various possibilities will be described later.

In the example above we only considered electrons (or beta) and photon radiation. The situation of alpha is slightly different in the sense that all alpha emitters considered so far in nuclear medicine emit particles with a range inferior to 100 μm in water. This means that alpha particles can be safely considered as non-penetrating radiation at the clinical scale, where activity is at best assessed with a spatial sampling of some mm (and an even larger spatial resolution).

It must be noted that the definition of non-penetrating radiation does not consider the above geometry. Non-penetrating radiation is usually defined by assessing how the energy emitted within a volume (not from a point source) is absorbed in the volume itself.

According to the MIRD nomenclature [8], this means considering the absorbed fractions $\phi_{Target \leftarrow Source}$ when source and targets coincide.

Non-penetrating emissions are defined by:

$$\phi_{Target \leftarrow Source} = 1 \text{ when Source volume} = \text{Target volume, and}$$
$$\phi_{Target \leftarrow Source} = 0 \text{ when Source volume} \neq \text{Target volume}$$

In addition, penetrating emissions are defined by:

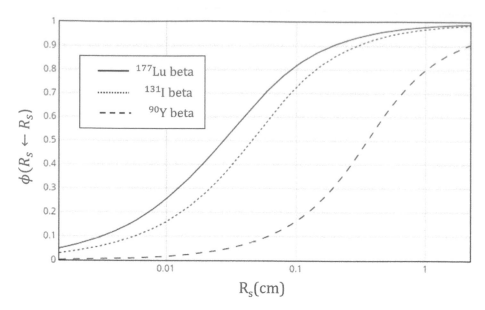

FIGURE 10.3 Absorbed fraction in a sphere of radius Rs homogeneously filled with radioactivity. Plot created using data from Bardiès and Chatal 1994 [6].

$\phi_{Target \leftarrow Source}$ < 1 when Source volume = Target volume, and
$\phi_{Target \leftarrow Source}$ ≠ 0 when Source volume ≠ Target volume

Yet, penetrating/non-penetrating radiation must be defined not only by radiation type or energy, but also in relation to the volume of interest. This is a major point to consider: a given radiation can be penetrating for one geometry, and non-penetrating for another on a different scale.

An example can be extracted from Bardiès and Chatal (1994) [6]. Figure 10.3 considers the absorbed fraction of energy deposited in spherical sources of varying radii Rs. The difference compared with the previous example is that here the radioactive sources are homogeneously distributed within a sphere as opposed to a single point source. As can be seen, all the absorbed fractions eventually converge towards 1, thereby defining the conditions for non-penetrating radiation. It can be noted that the Rs value at which the absorbed fractions converge towards 1 are higher than would be obtained from Figure 10.1, thereby highlighting the difference between the consideration of only point sources or spherical sources.

In fact, the geometry selected for the first example (Figure 10.1) is mostly relevant in the context of the development of absorbed dose calculation software, as it considers the energy deposited at a distance from point sources. This is adapted to form the situation where source volumes can be considered as a collection of point sources (principle of superposition): the knowledge of how energy is deposited at a distance from a point source enables the calculation of energy deposition for more complex geometries. This is the basis of absorbed dose point kernel approaches, one of the different absorbed dose calculation algorithms described in the next section.

10.3 ABSORBED DOSE ALGORITHMS

Clinical dosimetry can be separated into model-based and patient-specific dosimetry:

1. In the first technique, precomputed S values, in $Gy \cdot Bq^{-1} \cdot s^{-1}$ are obtained from an anthropomorphic model, representing a population of humans and used to compute the absorbed dose to the model rather than to a specific patient. That approach is mainly useful for risk estimates regarding stochastic radiation effects (at a population level).
2. In the second, the absorbed dose is directly calculated from the number of radioactive decays, obtained from quantitative SPECT studies, and the density distribution, obtained from a CT study, for the volumes of interest (the patient). Patient-specific dosimetry is preferably implemented in targeted radiotherapy.
3. An amalgamated approach can be considered where precomputed S values are adjusted for a patient-specific geometry. This is done for self-absorbed dose calculations only ($D_{Source \leftarrow Source}$), using a mass ratio for non-penetrating radiation, and another adjustment for penetrating radiation (power ⅔) [9].

Regardless of the approach taken, the absorbed dose calculation can be performed using only a limited number of algorithms, which are presented here.

10.3.1 LOCAL ENERGY DEPOSITION

Local energy deposition is an analytical method based on the assumption that all the kinetic energy of the charged particles emitted is absorbed locally within the source volume. The simplicity of this assumption makes this algorithm the fastest computationally as it is only a scaling of the SPECT values to energy considering the mass of a SPECT voxel volume. It also provides an upper limit for the absorbed energy in a given source volume because no particle will carry released energy outside the volume.

The mean free path of charged particles, emitted from radionuclides that are typically used in nuclear medicine procedures, is often less than one centimetre in water (the maximum range of the most energetic electrons emitted by ^{90}Y is 1.1 cm in water, but as can be seen in Figure 10.1, most of the emitted energy is absorbed before that distance). Therefore, the kinetic energy of the charged particles is deposited mostly inside the emitting voxel. Depending on the isotope maximum beta energy, the amount of self-absorbed energy is likely to vary. Yet assuming local energy deposition allows calculating the absorbed dose at a voxel level (D_{voxel}), considering a self-absorbed fraction $\phi_{Source \leftarrow Source} = 1$.

$$D_{voxel} = \frac{E^{e^-}_{kinetic}}{m_{voxel}} \qquad (10.1)$$

where $E^{e^-}_{kinetic}$ is the average kinetic energy per disintegration [J·Bq^{-1}·s^{-1}] of the full electron spectrum emitted within the voxel and m_{voxel} is the voxel mass in [kg].

To calculate the absorbed dose rate $\dot{D}_{i,j,k}(t)$ [Gy·s^{-1}] in every voxel, given a density map $\rho_{i,j,k}$ [$kg \cdot m^{-3}$] and an activity map $A_{i,j,k}(t)$ [Bq], the following equation can be used

$$\dot{D}_{i,j,k}(t) = A_{i,j,k}(t) \cdot \frac{E^{e^-}_{kinetic}}{\rho_{i,j,k} \cdot V_{voxel}} \qquad (10.2)$$

where V_{voxel} [m^3] is the voxel volume.

To calculate the absorbed dose rate in a volume of interest or an organ, the procedure is similar.

$$\dot{D}_{organ}(t) = \frac{E^{e^-}_{kinetic}}{m_{organ}} \cdot \sum_{i,j,k} A_{i,j,k} \qquad (10.3)$$

where the sum covers all voxels belonging to the organ.

This approach only considers the charged particle contribution to the self-absorbed dose in source regions (voxels or volumes of interest) and neglects the gamma contribution. The cross absorbed dose (when source and target are different) is not considered.

Last, we put in perspective here the spatial sampling (voxel dimensions) versus radiation range. The voxel size of SPECT images is around 5 mm. In addition, the spatial resolution of SPECT images is usually 2–3 times larger than voxel size, and even with resolution recovery techniques cannot be reduced to less than a centimetre. This questions the relevance of determining the activity – and therefore to compute the absorbed dose – at the voxel level. In addition, this also questions the relevance of more refined absorbed dose calculation approaches in that context [10].

10.3.2 CONVOLUTION (HOMOGENEOUS MEDIUM)

In situations where particle emissions (electrons, beta) cannot be assumed to be locally absorbed, or if the gamma contribution to the irradiation cannot be neglected, it is necessary to evaluate how emitted energy is absorbed at a distance from the emission point. In a homogeneous medium, and for isotropic emission, energy deposition is a function of the distance to the emission point. This defines the absorbed dose point kernels (DPK) that can be expressed in spherical coordinates as:

$$DPK(r) = \frac{dE}{\rho \cdot r^2 dr} \tag{10.4}$$

where dE is the energy deposited per disintegration in the volume $dV(r) = r^2 dr$ with density ρ. This is usually expressed with the radial energy deposition function (J) as [11]:

$$J(r) = \frac{dE}{dr} = \rho \cdot r^2 \cdot DPK(r) \tag{10.5}$$

Equation 10.2 can be rewritten for a voxelized geometry in terms of a convolution as:

$$\dot{D}_{i,j,k}(t) = \sum_{m,n,o} A_{m,n,o}(t) \cdot S_{i,j,k \leftarrow m,n,o}(t) \tag{10.6}$$

This operation, when made as a matrix convolution, can be time-consuming. Early attempts at this method used a direct Fourier convolution of the activity map with the DPK in order to reduce the computational burden [12].

10.3.3 Generation of DPK

Originally, the generation of DPK initially was done analytically, or based on measurements [13–16]. In the literature, most authors provide DPK for several media using direct Monte Carlo simulation [17–19] (Figure 10.4). Some use concentric spherical shells and calculate the absorbed dose in a 3D voxel map, as shown in Figure 10.5.

Another approach described by Janicki [20] is to compute the absorbed dose directly in each spherical shell and derive the deposited energy as a function of the radial distance by using the effective shell radius ($R_{D,i}$), as shown in Equation 10.7:

$$R_{D,i} \approx \sqrt{\frac{1}{3} \cdot \frac{R_{i+1}^3 - R_i^3}{R_{i+1} - R_i}} \tag{10.7}$$

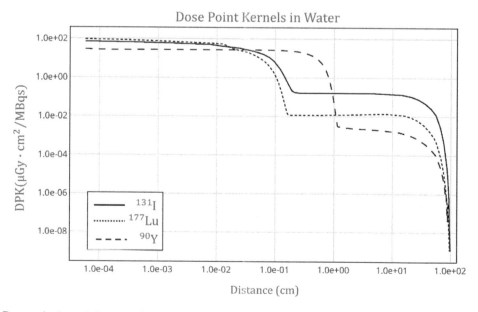

FIGURE 10.4 Dose point kernels in water for selected radionuclides created using GATE Monte Carlo code.

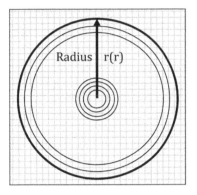

Radius $r(r)$

FIGURE 10.5 DPK simulation schema.

Then, the energy deposited in the shell per disintegration ($E_{D,i}$) is divided by the shell mass ($M_{D,i}$), to obtain an absorbed dose as a function of effective shell radius.

$$DPK\left(R_{D,i}\right) = \frac{E_{D,i}}{M_{D,i}} \tag{10.8}$$

As Monte Carlo modelling is now the default mode of calculation of DPK, they can be generated directly for different media. Yet, it is also possible to use DPK pre-calculated in water and extrapolate to other materials using the formalism proposed by Cross [11].

$$DPK(r) = \eta_w^3 \cdot \left(\frac{\rho}{\rho_w}\right)^2 \cdot DPK_w\left(\eta_w \cdot r\right) \tag{10.9}$$

where DPK_w is the pre-calculated DPK in water, ρ and ρ_w are the densities of the new material and water respectively and η_w is the relative attenuation of the material with respect to water.

10.3.4 FROM DPK TO VDK: DIFFERENT APPROACHES

DPK are defined for point sources. However, in a geometry defined by voxels as is the case in clinical nuclear medicine dosimetry, it is important to generate voxel sources.

The DPK can be converted to a voxel dose kernel (VDK) map:

$$VDK\left(O \leftarrow A\right) = \iint DPK\left(R_{O \leftarrow A}\right) dV_A dV_O \tag{10.10}$$

where the contribution of voxel A to voxel O is integrated over both volumes. With this definition it is now possible to write:

$$\dot{D}_{i,j,k}(t) = F^{-1}\left(F(A) \times F(VDK)\right)(i,j,k) \tag{10.11}$$

where both, **A** and **VDK**, are matrices with the same voxel size (but different dimensions, as a patient image, for example, covers a wider range than the VDK). The convolution can be made in matrix mode or using discrete Fourier convolution.

Another possibility is to calculate the **VDK** matrix directly using a Monte Carlo (MC) simulation. This may provide more realistic results but require longer calculation times. It is possible to interpolate VDK obtained at various scales to resample at a different voxel dimension [21, 22]. Databases of pre-calculated VDK for selected voxel sizes, materials, and isotopes are currently available for absorbed dose calculation purposes [19, 23].

10.3.5 CONVOLUTION IN HETEROGENEOUS MEDIA

Even though the convolution of DPK (or VDK) applies by principle to homogeneous media, approaches have been proposed to correct for heterogeneous densities present in patient organs/tissues. Different methods have been proposed to correct for density heterogeneity.

The conventional approach is to correct the absorbed dose to water using a density map [11].

$$\dot{D}_{i,j,k}\left(m,t\right)=\frac{\rho_m}{\rho_w}\cdot\dot{D}_{i,j,k}\left(w,t\right) \tag{10.12}$$

Here, the correction is made voxel by voxel, although this can be extended to organ level. Since the correction is made after the absorbed dose rate calculation, it effectively corrects for target voxels only. Therefore, the assumption that radiation interacts in the same way with different materials, and that the number of interactions per emission is constant, represents a significant flaw in this approach.

A second possibility is the Pencil Beam and Pathlength Scaling [24]. The average density along the linear path taken by the radiation between each combination of source/target voxels is calculated and used in Equation 10.11 as matrix convolution. This way the number of interactions per emission becomes more realistic as it is averaged over all the materials traversed by the radiation. However, the practical implementation of this algorithm for internal dosimetry is too slow to compete with more advanced methods such as Monte Carlo simulation.

A third possibility is the collapsed cone convolution [25]. In this method the energy depositions in the source/target path are discretized. Each deposition considers the materials at each point therefore correcting for heterogeneity in the process. This method is widely used in external beam radiotherapy, where the photon interactions are the main contribution to the absorbed dose. In this situation, where the majority of photons interacting with the patient originate from a single external source and therefore traverse very similar paths, the collapsed cone algorithm works well. However, in the case of charged particle interactions, this method underestimates scatter. The application to internal dosimetry is even more complex as it involves charged particles emitted isotropically inside the patient volume. Therefore, a full simulation for every combination source–target must be done, and the practical implementation of this algorithm becomes protracted when compared to more sophisticated Monte Carlo methods.

10.3.6 FULL MONTE CARLO SIMULATION

The explicit modelling of radiation transport by Monte Carlo simulation can be used directly to deal, in principle, with any kind of radiation and media. This method implements the full simulation of possible interactions of every emitted particle as it propagates through a medium. In the past this was a very time-consuming process, but with the improved computing power now available results can be produced within a reasonable timeframe. As with all approaches, the results are only as good as the input information. In nuclear medicine, where SPECT voxel dimensions are usually larger than the mean free path of the emitted electrons, the advantages of this method are reduced due to the poor definition of the propagating media, meaning that the increased computation requirements of the Monte Carlo approaches are not always justified in a clinical setting.

Codes used for absorbed dose calculations are usually generic Monte Carlo codes, initially from the high energy physics, but adapted to energies that can be encountered in nuclear medicine [26–32].

10.3.7 CHOOSING THE RELEVANT ABSORBED DOSE CALCULATION APPROACH

Due to the relationship between radiation range and spatial sampling of the geometry, absorbed dose calculation approaches can conveniently be sorted out according to the scale of the problem studied [33]. Depending on the scale, non-penetrating radiation can become penetrating, and the algorithms of choice may be different. Small animal (mouse) dosimetry is a good example in that respect: as the range of most beta radiation is of the order of magnitude of organs/

tissue dimensions, it is not possible to assume that beta radiation is locally absorbed. Furthermore, the mass scaling as applied in the clinics to take account of differences between patient and model geometries is no longer applicable [34].

Still, scale is not the only parameter to consider when differentiating between dosimetric approaches. Another relevant way is to consider the intended purpose, as this conditions the degree of accuracy required for the calculations, and therefore the calculation speed. A first order estimate of the irradiation delivered (almost) in real time in selective radiotherapy will necessitate accepting some compromise in accuracy and assuming only local energy deposition of ^{90}Y beta radiation in the liver. However, the generation of reference-specific absorbed fractions and S values will require more refined approaches to be implemented, with the emphasis put on uncertainties associated with S value generation [35].

10.3.8 REFERENCE DOSIMETRY

Reference dosimetry is intended to provide reference values for a type of procedure, or a radiopharmaceutical. Reference dosimetry makes a systematic use of reference human models, as proposed in IRCP reports [36, 37], and uses reference dosimetric models, built for the purpose of absorbed dose calculation [38–40] combined with reference pharmacokinetics obtained for each radiopharmaceutical.

Obviously, the objective of a dosimetric approach in a context of reference dosimetry should be to provide results with a high degree of accuracy. Even though the S values presented in MIRD 11 [1] and Cristy and Eckerman ORNL reports [41] for mathematical models suffer from the computing limitations of their time (MC modelling was performed with a number of particles that probably would not be accepted nowadays), the average S values obtained are actually close to those obtained more recently using an incomparably large computing power [35].

The accuracy associated with absorbed dose calculation (S values) is currently higher than that associated with activity and pharmacokinetics assessment. In addition, the absorbed dose estimates used for risk assessment in the context of diagnostic imaging represent a compromise between the ease of use, the traceability associated with model-based dosimetry, and the fact that the objective is not to derive the absorbed dose delivered to a specific patient. Yet, if reference dosimetric parameters (S values) are generated, it is usually done with the best possible accuracy and the best available computational means at the time.

Recent evolutions have seen the generation of a range of computational models [42] adapted to various morphology or even ethnic models. The objective is sometimes to generate a range of models easily adapted to provide a timely answer in the event of radiation accidents (selecting the closest model to the irradiated individual). Although this can be accepted for radiation safety purposes, it must be noted that this is contradictory with the objective of establishing *reference* models for the comparison of medical procedures. The traceability of results obtained using variable models (or "hybrid" NURBS- or MESH-based models) is harder to establish. Yet the availability of such models – and their endorsement by the ICRP [40] – enables their implementation in multiscale dosimetry where relevant.

10.3.9 PATIENT-SPECIFIC DOSIMETRY

Patient-specific dosimetry is a domain that covers a whole range of approaches, characterized by the way activity/cumulated activity are obtained and how, and for which organs/tissues, the absorbed doses are calculated. A usual complaint, and an excuse for not implementing clinical dosimetry in practice, is the supposed lack of standardization of the approaches. This has been often accepted by physicists as a flaw in the dosimetry status, but should in fact be considered with a variable perspective:

- Every absorbed dose calculation should generate associated uncertainties [43], should be traceable and compliant with basic metrology principles. The efforts undertaken by several national metrology institutes to improve these aspects should be acknowledged [44, 45]. SPECT reconstruction, ML-EM/OS-EM approaches, and CT-based attenuation/scatter correction can be standardized. Yet, the clinical workflow as a whole is still highly variable from one centre to another [46].
- Since dosimetry is always performed with a medical objective, the definition of the volumes where absorbed doses should be calculated is a medical responsibility, and so are the levels of accuracy required (or the degree of inaccuracy accepted).

In every clinical dosimetry situation, two factors should be considered – accuracy and speed – with an understanding of how the requirement for one will affect the other. It is a clinical decision whether a fast result is preferable to a more accurate one. Obviously, this means that every approach offered should have at least an estimate of associated uncertainty, and this is the responsibility of the physicist.

The desired clinical endpoint will always influence the dosimetric approach required. It has been demonstrated that even some very simple dosimetry can enable a considerable modulation of administered activity [47], leading to an immediate impact on patient care. The dosimetry protocols needed to adequately define toxicity limits will have different requirements from those investigating efficacies. More refined methodologies have to be implemented to observe clearly the absorbed dose–biological effectiveness relationship.

This means that there is not – and there will never be – a standard unique approach to clinical dosimetry. With that in mind, documentation and traceability of every dosimetry procedure is of major importance [48].

10.4   EXAMPLE OF CALCULATION APPROACHES

In order to illustrate the impact of the calculation scheme, presented here are the results of a calculation performed on one patient dataset, but using different available software that covers a range of approaches. Pharmacokinetic parameters and patient geometry were obtained from a study performed within the IAEA CRP E2.30.05 [49]. In this case, activity was quantified in kidneys, liver, lungs, spleen, and the remainder of the body. A tumour present in the liver was also considered for its high contrast versus normal liver. Table 10.1 presents the residence times (h) obtained after administration of 6848 MBq of Lutathera.

Three different dosimetric approaches were considered: model-based dosimetry based on mathematical (OLINDA V1) or voxel-based (OLINDA V2) models, and direct Monte Carlo modelling of radiation transport (GATE).

Calculations were made for the previously mentioned 3 isotopes of interest in nuclear medicine therapy (^{177}Lu, ^{131}I and ^{90}Y). The average kinetic energy of the beta electron spectra emitted by the selected isotopes are presented in Table 10.2, and Figure 10.6 presents the emission spectra for these isotopes. The residence times were kept constant for all isotopes, as the objective of the exercise is to compare the impact of changing algorithms or isotopes, but the clinical irrelevancy of the situation should not impact the discussion of the results obtained.

TABLE 10.1
Mass (kg) and Residence Times (h) for the Volumes of Interest Defined in the Clinical Example

Organ/Tissue	Mass (kg)	Residence time (h)
Whole FOV	17.90	*8.33
Lungs	0.55	0.40
Liver	1.35	4.45
Kidneys	0.39	2.11
Spleen	0.12	1.18
Tumour	0.25	8.12

* For the whole field of view, the value for the residence time corresponds to the remainder.

TABLE 10.2
Average Kinetic Energy of Emitted Electrons per Disintegration Calculated Using the MIRD Database for Selected Isotopes [50]

	^{177}Lu	^{131}I	^{90}Y
$E_{kinetic}^{e-}$	148.23 keV	191.97 keV	931.81 keV

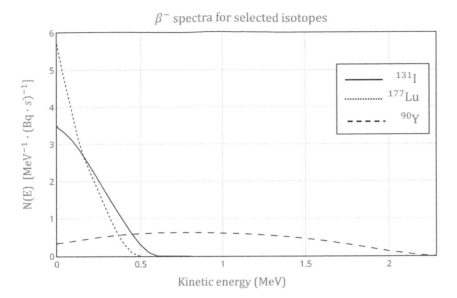

FIGURE 10.6 Beta electron spectra for selected radionuclides created using MIRD reference values [50].

TABLE 10.3
Mean Absorbed Doses Delivered to the Volumes of Interest for ^{177}Lu

Organ/Tissue	Mean absorbed doses (Gy) for ^{177}Lu		
	OLINDA V1	OLINDA V2	GATE
Lungs	4.51E-01	3.86E-01	4.76E-01
Liver	2.00E+00	1.99E+00	2.19E+00
Kidneys	3.23E+00	3.62E+00	3.31E+00
Spleen	5.84E+00	5.68E+00	5.88E+00
Tumour	1.94E+01	1.81E+01	2.22E+01

TABLE 10.4
Mean Absorbed Doses Delivered to the Volumes of Interest for ^{131}I

Organ/Tissue	Mean absorbed doses (Gy) for ^{131}I		
	OLINDA V1	OLINDA V2	GATE
Lungs	8.42E-01	7.81E-01	1.10E+00
Liver	3.37E+00	3.40E+00	4.27E+00
Kidneys	4.98E+00	5.51E+00	5.30E+00
Spleen	8.77E+00	8.49E+00	8.72E+00
Tumour	3.05E+01	2.86E+01	3.33E+01

Tables 10.3 to 10.5 present the mean absorbed doses to the organs/tissues of interest for the various approaches and for the 3 isotopes of interest.

The analysis of the results shows that the mean absorbed doses to the organ/tissue do not vary markedly with the approach chosen: model-based (mathematical or voxel) and direct Monte Carlo modelling give results usually within 10 per cent and often better.

TABLE 10.5
Mean Absorbed Doses Delivered to the Volumes of Interest for ^{90}Y

Organ/Tissue	Mean absorbed doses (Gy) for ^{90}Y		
	OLINDA V1	OLINDA V2	GATE
Lungs	2.63E+00	2.16E+00	2.77E+00
Liver	1.22E+01	1.16E+01	1.29E+01
Kidneys	1.95E+01	2.11E+01	1.85E+01
Spleen	3.51E+01	3.28E+01	3.23E+01
Tumour	1.12E+02	1.12E+02	1.25E+02

An interesting situation is that of the liver tumour: as model-based dosimetry does not consider the cross absorbed dose (tumour absorbed doses are calculated using the same sphere module in OLINDA V1 and V2), the tumour absorbed dose is systematically higher when computed with Monte Carlo. Yet the differences lie in the range of what is observed for other organs/tissues.

A conclusion regarding these results is that whenever a tissue/organ contains radioactivity, it is likely to become the main source of its irradiation. In other words, the self-irradiation, when present, almost always dominates cross irradiation. This has consequences because, as already mentioned, self-absorbed doses can be mass corrected: one needs to have the reference model organ mass and S value and an evaluation of the patient organ mass. The first two are easy to find in published tables, whereas the third is usually available via CT imaging. This means that clinical dosimetry is feasible in most clinical departments without having to implement complex absorbed dose calculation algorithms.

The dosimetry of non-source organs/tissues, where the cross irradiation is most often delivered by photons, is more challenging. This means that in principle the propagation ranges are higher than for electrons or beta, and therefore radiation transport algorithms should cover larger ranges. Therefore, radiation propagation over large distances in a patient should most often consider the heterogeneous composition of patient tissues, thereby orienting towards Monte Carlo modelling. Yet, for large distances – say the impact of radioactivity present in the brain to the gonads – the solid angles from the source to the target are such that the number of primaries that need to be generated to reach acceptable statistics may become unmanageable in an appropriate time frame. In addition, the scaling from a model to patient-specific geometry is difficult, as not all organs and tissues vary in the same way from one patient to another. Even though the specific absorbed fractions are not considerably impacted by mass changes, geometry changes and source/target distances are pertinent due to the inverse square law. This means that computing absorbed doses, in a context of reference dosimetry or if a high degree of accuracy is required, may become difficult for non-sources. Yet the situation is not necessarily that problematic because, as mentioned above, the absorbed doses delivered in that context are most frequently low when compared to self-absorbed doses.

The fact is that most codes designed for radiopharmaceutical dosimetry tend to consider essentially the dosimetry of source organs/tissues. Studying how they may fail in a context of absorbed dose assessment in diagnostic procedures, where it is predominantly target organs that are of interest, is interesting – but is finally more of a mind game than a real clinical issue [51].

10.5 CONCLUSION

The evolution of computing capabilities in the past few decades has triggered important changes in the way absorbed dose calculations are addressed. It is currently possible, if needed, to implement refined absorbed dose computation approaches (including Monte Carlo simulation) that used to not be accessible to most clinical departments. Furthermore, commercial solutions are appearing, with CE marking or FDA approval, that allow the implementation of dosimetry as a matter of routine in a clinical environment. Some integrate most, if not all, of the steps that lead from activity determination to absorbed dose calculation. This comprehensive approach to clinical dosimetry is relevant in the sense that global absorbed dose uncertainty will be limited by the least accurate step. Observation of this evolution shows that, contrary to the not so distant past, the absorbed dose calculation step is less and less likely to be the weak link of the dosimetric chain. This still leaves many domains in need of improvement in the dosimetric workflow (quantitative imaging, registration, segmentation, to name a few). Reproducibility, standardization of acquisitions in a multicentric context, and robustness appear to be the next frontiers of clinical dosimetry.

Still, the growing awareness of the relationship between the clinical objectives and required methodologies is probably the most essential development, proving that the collaboration between medical physicists and clinicians is more vital than ever before.

REFERENCES

[1] W. Snyder, M. Ford, G. Warner, and S. Watson. *MIRD Pamphlet No 11: "S," absorbed dose per unit cumulated activity for selected radionuclides and organs.* (1975). Society of Nuclear Medicine. New York.

[2] S. Chiavassa *et al.*, "Dosimetric comparison of Monte Carlo codes (EGS4, MCNP, MCNPX) considering external and internal exposures of the Zubal phantom to electron and photon sources," *Radiat Prot Dosimetry,* vol. 116, no. 1–4 Pt 2, pp. 631–35, 2005, doi: 10.1093/rpd/nci063.

[3] J. Lehmann *et al.*, "Monte Carlo treatment planning for molecular targeted radiotherapy within the MINERVA system," *Phys Med Biol,* vol. 50, no. 5, pp. 947–58, 2005, doi: 10.1088/0031-9155/50/5/017.

[4] S. Marcatili *et al.*, "Development and validation of RAYDOSE: A Geant4-based application for molecular radiotherapy," *Phys Med Biol,* vol. 58, no. 8, pp. 2491–508, 2013, doi: 10.1088/0031-9155/58/8/2491.

[5] S. D. Kost, Y. K. Dewaraja, R. G. Abramson, and M. G. Stabin, "VIDA: A voxel-based dosimetry method for targeted radionuclide therapy using Geant4," *Cancer biotherapy & radiopharmaceuticals,* vol. 30, no. 1, pp. 16–26, 2015, doi: 10.1089/cbr.2014.1713.

[6] M. Bardies and J. F. Chatal, "Absorbed Doses for Internal Radiotherapy from 22 Beta-Emitting Radionuclides – Beta-Dosimetry of Small Spheres," *Phys. Med. Biol.,* vol. 39, pp. 961–81, 1994.

[7] M. J. Berger, "Improved point kernels for electron and beta-ray dosimetry," NBSIR. Commerce Department, National Institute of Standards and Technology (NIST). 1973,

[8] R. Loevinger, T. F. Budinger, and E. E. Watson, "MIRD primer for absorbed dose calculations. Revised Edition," 1991.

[9] M. G. Stabin, R. B. Sparks, and E. Crowe, "OLINDA/EXM: The second-generation personal computer software for internal dose assessment in nuclear medicine," *J Nucl Med,* vol. 46, no. 6, pp. 1023–7, 2005.

[10] M. Ljungberg and K. Sjogreen-Gleisner, "The accuracy of absorbed dose estimates in tumours determined by quantitative SPECT: A Monte Carlo study," *Acta Oncol,* vol. 50, no. 6, pp. 981–9, 2011, doi: 10.3109/0284186X.2011.584559.

[11] W. G. Cross, N. O. Freedman, and P. Y. Wong, "Tables of beta-ray dose distributions in water," Canada, 1992, http://inis.iaea.org/search/search.aspx?orig_q=RN:23047981.

[12] H. B. Giap, D. J. Macey, J. E. Bayyouth, A. L. Boyer, "Validation of a dose-point kernel convolution technique for internal dosimetry," *Phys Med Biol,* vol. 40 Mar, no. 3, pp. 365–81, 1995, doi: 10.1088/0031-9155/40/3/003.

[13] M. J. Berger, *Distribution of Absorbed Dose Around Point Sources of Electrons and Beta Particles in Water and other Media: MIRD Pamphlet no. 7. J Nucl Med,* vol. 12, pp. 5–23, 1971.

[14] M. J. Berger, *Energy Deposition in Water by Photons from Point Isotropic Sources: MIRD Pamphlet no. 2, J Nucl Med,* vol. 9, pp. 15–25, 1968.

[15] W. G. Cross, "Empirical Expressions for Beta Ray Point Source Dose Distributions," *Radiation Protection Dosimetry,* vol. 69, no. 2, pp. 85–96, 1997, doi: 10.1093/oxfordjournals.rpd.a031898.

[16] M. J. Berger, "Beta-Ray Dosimetry calculations with the use of point kernels," National Bureau of Standards, Washington, DC and Tennessee, 1970, www.osti.gov/biblio/4105457.

[17] N. Lanconelli *et al.*, "A free database of radionuclide voxel S values for the dosimetry of nonuniform activity distributions," *Phys Med Biol,* vol. 57, no. 2, pp. 517–33, 2012, doi: 10.1088/0031-9155/57/2/517.

[18] P. Papadimitroulas, G. Loudos, G. C. Nikiforidis, and G. C. Kagadis, "A dose point kernel database using GATE Monte Carlo simulation toolkit for nuclear medicine applications: Comparison with other Monte Carlo codes," *Med Phys,* vol. 39, no. 8, pp. 5238–47, 2012, doi: 10.1118/1.4737096.

[19] S. A. Graves, R. T. Flynn, and D. E. Hyer, "Dose point kernels for 2,174 radionuclides," *Med Phys,* vol. 46, no. 11, pp. 5284–93, 2019, doi: 10.1002/mp.13789.

[20] C. Janicki and J. Seuntjens, "Accurate determination of dose-point-kernel functions close to the origin using Monte Carlo simulations," *Med Phys,* vol. 31, no. 4, pp. 814–8, 2004, doi: 10.1118/1.1668393.

[21] A. Dieudonné, R. F. Hobbs, W. E. Bolch, G. Sgouros, and I. Gardin, "Fine-resolution voxel S values for constructing absorbed dose distributions at variable voxel size," *J Nucl Med,* vol. 51, no. 10, pp. 1600–7, 2010, doi: 10.2967/jnumed.110.077149.

[22] M. Fernández *et al.*, "A fast method for rescaling voxel S values for arbitrary voxel sizes in targeted radionuclide therapy from a single Monte Carlo calculation," *Med Phys,* vol. 40, no. 8, p. 082502, 2013, doi: 10.1118/1.4812684.

[23] N. Lanconelli *et al.*, "A free database of radionuclide voxel S values for the dosimetry of nonuniform activity distributions," *Physics in Medicine and Biology,* vol. 57, no. 2, pp. 517–33, 2012, doi: 10.1088/0031-9155/57/2/517.

[24] S. E. Davidson, G. S. Ibbott, K. L. Prado, L. Dong, Z. Liao, and D. S. Followill, "Accuracy of two heterogeneity dose calculation algorithms for IMRT in treatment plans designed using an anthropomorphic thorax phantom," *Med Phys,* vol. 34, no. 5, pp. 1850–7, 2007, doi: 10.1118/1.2727789.

[25] A. Ahnesjo, "Collapsed cone convolution of radiant energy for photon dose calculation in heterogeneous media," *Med Phys,* vol. 16, no. 4, pp. 577–92, 1989, doi: 10.1118/1.596360.

[26] M. Bardies and M. Ljungberg, "Monte Carlo codes in radionuclide therapy," in *Dosimetry of Radionuclide Therapy* vol. Report 104, A. Nicol and W. Waddington, Eds., York: Institute of Physics and Engineering in Medicine, 2011, pp. 116–133.

[27] S. Agostinelli *et al.*, "Geant4 – a simulation toolkit," *Nuclear Instruments and Methods in Physics Research Section A: Accelerators, Spectrometers, Detectors and Associated Equipment,* vol. 506, no. 3, pp. 250–303, 2003, doi: 10.1016/S0168-9002(03)01368-8.

[28] D. Sarrut *et al.*, "A review of the use and potential of the GATE Monte Carlo simulation code for radiation therapy and dosimetry applications," *Med Phys,* vol. 41, no. 6, p. 064301, 2014, doi: 10.1118/1.4871617.

[29] I. Kawrakow, E. Mainegra-Hing, D. Rogers, F. Tessier, and B. Walter, "The EGSnrc Code System: Monte Carlo simulation of electron and photon transport," in *Technical Report PIRS-701,* National Research Council Canada: Ottawa, ON, 2015, http://nrc-cnrc.github.io/EGSnrc/doc/pirs701-egsnrc.pdf.

[30] F. Salvat, J. Fernández-Varea, and J. Sempau, "Penelope. A code system for Monte Carlo simulation of electron and photon transport," *NEA Data Bank, Workshop Proceeding, Barcelona,* pp. 4–7, 2007.

[31] T. T. Böhlen *et al.*, "The FLUKA Code: Developments and Challenges for High Energy and Medical Applications," *Nuclear Data Sheets,* vol. 120, pp. 211–14, 2014, doi: 10.1016/j.nds.2014.07.049.

[32] L. Waters *et al.*, "The MCNPX Monte Carlo radiation transport code," *AIP Conference Proceedings,* vol. 896, pp. 81–90, 2007, doi: 10.1063/1.2720459.

[33] M. Bardies and M. J. Myers, "Computational methods in radionuclide dosimetry," *Phys Med Biol,* vol. 41, no. 10, pp. 1941–55, 1996, doi: 10.1088/0031-9155/41/10/007.

[34] T. Mauxion, J. Barbet, J. Suhard, J. P. Pouget, M. Poirot, and M. Bardiès, "Improved realism of hybrid mouse models may not be sufficient to generate reference dosimetric data," *Med Phys,* vol. 40, no. 5, p. 052501, 2013, doi: 10.1118/1.4800801.

[35] M. Chauvin *et al.*, "OpenDose: Open-Access Resource for Nuclear Medicine Dosimetry," *J Nucl Med,* vol. 61, no. 10, pp. 1514–19, 2020, doi: 10.2967/jnumed.119.240366.

[36] ICRP, 2002. *Basic Anatomical and Physiological Data for Use in Radiological Protection – Reference Values.* ICRP Publication 89, Ann. ICRP 32 (3–4).

[37] ICRP, 1975. *Report of the Task Group on Reference Man.* ICRP Publication 23, Pergamon Press.

[38] ICRP, 2009. *Adult Reference Computational Phantoms.* ICRP Publication 110, Ann. ICRP 39 (2).

[39] ICRP, 2020. *Paediatric Reference Computational Phantoms. Publication.* ICRP Publication 143, Ann. ICRP 49 (1).

[40] ICRP, 2020. *Adult mesh-type reference computational phantoms.* ICRP Publication 145, Ann. ICRP 49 (3).

[41] M. Cristy and K. F. Eckerman, *Specific Absorbed Fractions of Energy at Various Ages from Internal Photon Sources. Report ORNL/TM-8381/V1-V7,* Oak Ridge National Laboratory, Oak Ridge, TN, 1987.

[42] X. G. Xu, "An exponential growth of computational phantom research in radiation protection, imaging, and radiotherapy: A review of the fifty-year history," *Phys Med Biol,* vol. 59, no. 18, pp. R233–302, 2014, doi: 10.1088/0031-9155/59/18/R233.

[43] J. I. Gear *et al.*, "EANM practical guidance on uncertainty analysis for molecular radiotherapy absorbed dose calculations," *Eur J Nucl Med Mol Imaging,* vol. 45, no. 13, pp. 2456–74, 2018, doi: 10.1007/s00259-018-4136-7.

[44] "MRTDosimetry Project." http://mrtdosimetry-empir.eu.

[45] "MetroMRT Project." http://projects.npl.co.uk/metromrt.

[46] M. Bardies and J. I. Gear, "Scientific Developments in Imaging and Dosimetry for Molecular Radiotherapy," *Clin Oncol (R Coll Radiol),* vol. 33, no. 2, pp. 117–24, 2021, doi: 10.1016/j.clon.2020.11.005.

[47] S. E. Buckley, S. J. Chittenden, F. H. Saran, S. T. Meller, and G. D. Flux, "Whole-body dosimetry for individualized treatment planning of 131I-MIBG radionuclide therapy for neuroblastoma," *J Nucl Med,* vol. 50, no. 9, pp. 1518–24, 2009, doi: 10.2967/jnumed.109.064469.

[48] M. Lassmann, C. Chiesa, G. Flux, and M. Bardiès, "EANM Dosimetry Committee guidance document: Good practice of clinical dosimetry reporting," *Eur J Nucl Med Mol Imaging,* vol. 38, no. 1, pp. 192–200, 2011, doi: 10.1007/s00259-010-1549-3.

[49] IAEA. "Dosimetry in Molecular Radiotherapy for Personalized Patient Treatments." IAEA. www.iaea.org/projects/crp/e23005.

[50] K. Eckerman and A. Endo, *MIRD: Radionuclide Data and Decay Schemes,* 2nd Edition. 2008.

[51] S. Marcatili, D. Villoing, T. Mauxion, B. J. McParland, and M. Bardies, "Model-based versus specific dosimetry in diagnostic context: Comparison of three dosimetric approaches," *Med Phys,* vol. 42, no. 3, pp. 1288–96, 2015, doi: 10.1118/1.4907957.

11 Whole-body Dosimetry

Jonathan Gear

CONTENTS

11.1 INTRODUCTION

Potentially the greatest advantage of the MIRD schema is its flexibility for application in a wide range of scenarios, from the very simple to the highly complex. Arguably, the simplest scenario where dosimetry is commonly used is referred to as whole-body (WB) dosimetry. Unlike organ-based dosimetry no measure of the in-vivo activity distribution is made, and the uptake and distribution of the radiopharmaceutical is assumed to be uniform within the body. Whilst this assumption may seem simplistic, whole-body dosimetry has been successful in a variety of clinical applications and, as will be discussed later, shown to correlate very well with measurable response and toxicity.

11.2 METHOD

As with any dosimetry method based on the MIRD schema, the calculation of absorbed dose can be considered in two parts, the estimation of the S-value and the measurement of time-integrated activity (TIA). Given the assumption that the activity is uniformly distributed throughout the body, it is unnecessary to perform a complex calculation to ascertain a patient specific S-value; rather it is sufficient to use an age-appropriate model for S and scale according to patient mass.

$$S_{patient} = S_{model} \frac{m_{model}}{m_{patient}} \qquad\qquad (11.1)$$

Where $S_{patient}$ is the radionuclide-specific quantity representing the mean absorbed dose to a patient of mass, $m_{patient}$ per unit time-integrated activity and S_{model} is the equivalent for a model of mass, m_{model}. S-values for various models are available from a number of resources, including MIRD, RADAR and ICRP. Alternatively, an analytical function can be derived by plotting the published S-values for different radionuclides against model mass. A power function of the form,

$$S_{patient} = a.m^{-b}, \qquad\qquad (11.2)$$

can be fitted to the data and used to calculate a more patient-specific calculation. This approach is recommended by EANM guidance for mIBG dosimetry [1] and generated by interpolating data from the newborn, 1-year-old, 5-year-old and adult phantoms [2, 3] yielding the formula

$$S_{patient} = 1.34 \cdot \times 10^{-4} m^{-0.921} \left(Gy\,MBq^{-1}h^{-1} \right) \qquad\qquad (11.3)$$

Plots for other radionuclides are given in Figure 11.1. In most cases the fitting parameter b, will take a value very close to 1, which is not surprising when one considers the definition of the S-value (see Chapter 2 and Chapter 8). The reason why the power term of Eq. 11.3 does not take a perfect value of unity is that the fraction of energy absorbed in the body will vary slightly between the different models. The appropriateness of an analytical equation fitted to model data should always be considered with care, as a newborn model may offer no useful information when deriving an S-value for an adult patient and vice versa. Interpolation over a smaller range of models can also be considered.

Having established the method of determining the S-value, the only real challenge for whole-body dosimetry is the estimation of time-integrated activity. To determine this, the activity remaining within the patient should be measured periodically post administration.

11.2.1 Equipment

As activity is assumed to be uniformly distributed, there is no requirement for imaging. Although whole-body activity data can be obtained using whole-body gamma camera imaging if necessary. This may be useful if similar imaging is being undertaken for other reasons, such as organ or lesion dosimetry (see Chapter 15 in Volume I). However, it is often more straightforward and reliable to monitor the activity remaining in a patient using a simple radiation-detector system. These have the advantage that a large number of data points may be acquired without imposition on a busy nuclear medicine department. Suitable monitors include

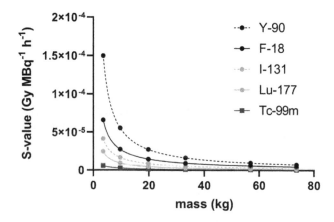

FIGURE 11.1   A plot of whole-body S-values verses mass for different radionuclides.

- An energy compensated Geiger-Muller counter connected to a rate meter;
- A sodium iodide gamma probe connected to a multi-channel analyser;
- A sodium iodide gamma probe connected to a calibrated single-channel analyser;
- A dose rate meter (provided the output is sufficiently precise for the expected range).

A system with the functionality to average or integrate over a set period is also advantageous for fluctuating measurements at low activities. All of the above systems will be sensitive to position and geometry between detector and patient, so care must be taken to ensure that this is reproduced for each measurement. To reduce effects of positioning errors it is recommended to monitor the count rate at a distance of at least 2 meters from the patient, this can be with the patient standing, sitting, or lying down. A system using a ceiling-mounted counter that enables the patient to lie down in a reproducible position, has been described by Chittenden and colleagues [4]. For systems designed for therapeutic monitoring, positioning such a device inside the treatment facility will reduce radiation exposure to staff, as patients do not need to be transported through the hospital.

The steps required to perform accurate whole-body dosimetry using this method are as follows: Readings from ceiling-mounted counters should be acquired with patients lying in the same position. If possible, the bed should be lowered to a horizontal position and supporting pillows should be removed. Particular care should be taken with paediatric patients to ensure that they are in the same position on the bed for each measurement, and the bed should not be moved between readings. In the case of using a hand-held counter, it is essential to ensure that the patient-counter geometry is reproduced as accurately as possible, as the inverse square law effect can significantly impair the accuracy of calculations. Patient positioning using a spacer, against a wall, or with feet positions drawn on the floor can help improve reproducibility.

11.2.2 BACKGROUND READINGS

A measure of environmental background should be acquired prior to measuring the patient. For systems that integrate detected events over time, a sufficient number of counts (> 500) should be obtained to maintain the Poisson statistics. Where possible during the course of measurement, or if contamination or background fluctuations are expected, background readings should be obtained to properly correct each sequential measurement. Sources of variable background are typically from contaminated bed linen, clothing, the bathroom, or other patients in nearby rooms without sufficient shielding.

11.2.3 FIRST MEASUREMENT

Radiation detectors do not directly measure activity and, therefore, a conversion from the system readout to activity is required. Whilst a direct calibration of the system could be made, due to the sensitivity of the system to geometrical changes (patient weight, height, size, position, etc.) it is conventional to use the initial measurement of the patient as a means of calibration. The first patient reading should therefore be acquired immediately following administration and before the first void to obtain a baseline to which further measurements will be normalized. It is recommended to acquire multiple measurements at each time point to obtain an average reading. Where feasible, the geometric mean of the count rate from anterior and posterior positions can be also acquired.

11.2.4 SUBSEQUENT READINGS

Readings should ideally be taken as often as possible, and commensurate with the biological half-life of the pharmaceutical. As a general rule a minimum of 3 measurements are required to characterize an exponential function. However, whole-body monitoring systems based on radiation detectors located in a patient treatment room or a mobile system, can facilitate many more measurements with very little burden to the patient or technical staff. The more measurements taken, the lower the uncertainty in the dose calculation. For a time-activity curve (TAC) that can be described by a single exponential function, the timing of each measurement should ideally be chosen to cover a period greater than 3 half-lives. For more complex retention curves, a useful measure to test that the TAC is adequately characterized is to calculate the time-integrated activity up to the last measurement. It is recommended that the fraction of the time-integrated activity between measurements should be greater than 80 per cent of the total time-integrated activity when extrapolated from zero to infinity [5]. As the activity in the patient decreases over time it may be necessary to increase the measurement period to record sufficient events at later time points. An appropriate scaling for the measurement period should therefore be made when normalizing against the first measurement.

11.2.5 Time-activity Curve (TAC) and Data Fitting

After determining the activity residing in the patient at each time point it is conventional to plot these in the form of a time-activity curve. The time-integrated activity (TIA) is determined from the area under this curve, or the integral of the function fitted to the data. Provided there is sufficient sampling, linear or exponential interpolation between data points can be used as an easy method to determine the area under the curve, to a reasonable accuracy. In this instance the time-integrated activity is taken as a sum of the trapezoidal areas between data points, shown in the diagram of Figure 11.2b.

$$\tilde{A} = \frac{1}{2}\sum_{i=0}^{n}\frac{A_i - A_{i+1}}{t_{i+1} - t_i} + f\left(A_n\right) \tag{11.4}$$

Where A_i is activity measure at the ith time point, at time t_i post administration and $f\left(A_n\right)$ is a function that described the TIA after the last point and will depends on how the activity is extrapolated beyond this time. This could be based on an extrapolation of the last two time points, assuming physical decay, or set to zero.

A potentially more robust method to determine the TIA is to fit a function to the activity data, usually based on a sum of exponential functions:

$$f\left(t\right) = \sum_{s=1}^{N} A_{s,0} e^{-\lambda_s t} \tag{11.5}$$

Selection of an appropriate function to the data may be user-defined, based on statistical tests such as the F-test, or based on known physiological processes and pharmacokinetic models [6]. When determining fit parameters for the model a least squares approach with a non-linear regression techniques can be used to minimize the objective function,

$$\chi^2 = \sum_{i=1}^{n}\left[A_i - f\left(t\right)\right]^2 \tag{11.6}$$

Example fits to the data of Figure 11.2a are given in Figure 11.3, for a single and bi- exponential function. In this example a significant improvement in the fit is observed with the bi-exponential function, conformed by a reduction in χ^2 of 95 per cent. An extra-sum-of-squares F test further confirms the significance of this result with a F statistic of $F(n,p) = 30.23$ (2, 3) and p-value = 0.01.

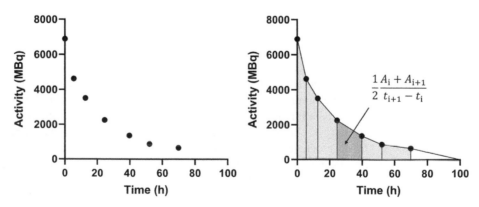

FIGURE 11.2 Example time activity data (a) fitted using linear interpolation and highlighting the trapezoidal method for integration (b).

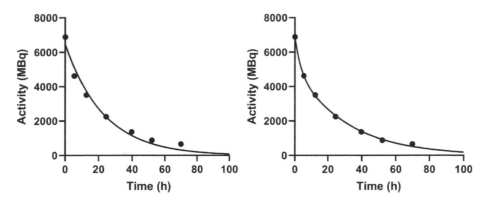

FIGURE 11.3 Example time activity data fitted using a single (a) and bi-exponential function (b).

11.2.6 Uncertainty Analysis

Since radioactive decays are random and emitted at an average rate, the events arriving at the detector are also random. Thus, the probability of measuring a certain counting rate is described by a Poisson distribution, centred on some mean value, $\mu(C)$ with a standard deviation, $\sigma(C)$. Due to the nature of Poisson statistics, the statistical uncertainty in detecting a number of Poisson counts, C_i is given by:

$$u(C_i) = \sqrt{C_i} \tag{11.7}$$

These uncertainties can be used in the fitting algorithm to weight the data according to the total number of events recorded at any time point. In addition, as each measurement is background corrected and scaled according to that recorded immediately following administration, the uncertainty in an activity measurement $u(A_i)$ is described by:

$$u^2(A_i) = \left(\frac{\partial}{\partial A_{adm}}\right)^2 u^2(A_{adm}) + \left(\frac{\partial}{\partial C_0}\right)^2 u^2(C_0) + \left(\frac{\partial}{\partial C_{BG}}\right)^2 u^2(C_{BG}) + \left(\frac{\partial}{\partial C_i}\right)^2 u^2(C_i) \tag{11.8}$$

Where A_{adm} is the administered activity, C_0 is the count measurement recorded immediately after administration, C_{BG}, is the background count measurement taken prior to administration and C_i is the ith count measurement, $u^2(A_{adm})$, $u^2(C_0)$, $u^2(C_{BG})$ and $u^2(C_i)$ are the associated variances of these respective parameters. A weighting to the least squares minimization can then be obtained using;

$$\chi^2 = \sum_{i=1}^{n} \frac{[A_i - f(t)]^2}{u^2(A_i)}.$$

Methods to determine the uncertainties in TAC fit parameters and how to propagate these to that associated with TIA are described by Flux and colleagues [7] and Gear and colleagues [8]. For TACs with multiple sets of parameters it is easiest to estimate uncertainties using matrix algebra,

$$V_p = \frac{\chi^2}{n-q} \left[J_p^\mathsf{T} J_p \right]^{-1} \tag{11.9}$$

Where V_p is a covariance matrix of fit parameters, J_p is a matrix of first-order partial derivatives of the TAC model with respect to the parameters evaluated at each time point, n is the number of data points and q is the number of parameters. For the case of a single exponential function,

$$V_p = \begin{bmatrix} u^2(A_0) & u(A_0, \lambda) \\ u(A_0, \lambda) & u^2(\lambda) \end{bmatrix} \tag{11.10}$$

and

$$J_p = \begin{bmatrix} \dfrac{\partial A_1}{\partial A_0} & \dfrac{\partial A_1}{\partial \lambda} \\ \vdots & \vdots \\ \dfrac{\partial A_n}{\partial A_0} & \dfrac{\partial A_n}{\partial \lambda} \end{bmatrix} = \begin{bmatrix} e^{-\lambda t_1} & -A_0 t_1 e^{-\lambda t_1} \\ \vdots & \vdots \\ e^{-\lambda t_n} & -A_0 t_n e^{-\lambda t_n} \end{bmatrix}. \tag{11.11}$$

Where, A_0 is activity extrapolated from the TAC to $t = 0$ and $u(A_0, \lambda)$ is the covariance between A_0 and λ which described the correlation between the parameters. As all data points are scaled to the first measurement point, a systematic uncertainty in the data is present. Total uncertainty in TIA is therefore a combination of the parameter uncertainties and that associated with the first measurement,

$$\left[\frac{u(\tilde{A})}{\tilde{A}} \right]^2 = \left[\frac{u(A_0)}{A_0} \right]^2 + \left[\frac{u(\lambda)}{\lambda} \right]^2 - 2 \frac{u(A_0, \lambda)}{A_0 \lambda} + \left[\frac{u(C_0)}{C_0} \right]^2 + \left[\frac{u(A_{admin})}{A_{admin}} \right]^2 \tag{11.12}$$

In cases of a single exponential fit, $A_0 \approx A_{admin}$ or potentially fixed by the operator to be equal, in which case the number of fitting parameters in the TAC reduces to 1 and the expression simplifies to

$$\left[\frac{u(\tilde{A})}{\tilde{A}} \right]^2 = \left[\frac{u(\lambda)}{\lambda} \right]^2 + \left[\frac{u(C_0)}{C_0} \right]^2 + \left[\frac{u(A_{admin})}{A_{admin}} \right]^2 \tag{11.13}$$

Note, that in both expression 12 and 13, uncertainties related to background counts have been omitted. As the background count rate is generally significantly lower than that at the initial measurement, it is reasonable to assume a negligible contribution to uncertainty in this instance.

11.3   ACCEPTANCE TESTING AND QUALITY CONTROL

When designing and commissioning a counting system for whole-body measurements, it is important that the equipment is shown to be fit for purpose and, as with any other medical device, a quality assurance program should be considered to ensure consistent and reliable results throughout the life of the equipment.

11.3.1   LINEARITY

Count rate linearity is tested to ensure a predictable detector response across the potential counting rates for which the system will be used. For therapeutic purposes activities could vary from a few megabecquerel to tens of gigabecqueral, these high activities will almost certainly result in count losses due to dead time effects [Chapter 6, Volume 1]. Whilst most detectors have in-build corrections, validation of the system correction should still be undertaken. If energy discrimination is being used it is important to characterize dead time effects under similar scatter conditions to that observed in patients. This is because dead-time effects are a condition of the total radiation flux incident on the detector, which will include scattered events rejected by the energy discriminator. For systems without energy window discrimination, such as Geiger counters, it is not necessary to simulate the scatter conditions; indeed, a different isotope could even be used. This is particularly useful if measuring dead time using a decaying source, an isotope with a shorter half-life can then be used to reduce the interval between measurements.

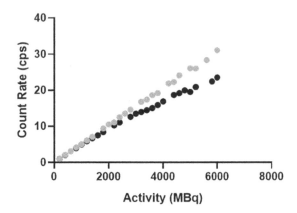

FIGURE 11.4 Example count rate data, acquired at different activities to test linearity. The light grey data demonstrates good linearity. The black data points demonstrate the effect of dead-time.

Count rate linearity is assessed by placing a source of known activity in front of the detector and periodically recording the count rate as the source decays. Alternatively, multiple sources of different activities can be used to enable a wider range of count rates to be observed without waiting for the source to decay. For a perfectly corrected system the count rate will increase linearly with activity. Any deviation from linearity indicates dead-time effects and should be appropriately modelled and patient data corrected accordingly. Example linearity data are given in Figure 11.4 for a detection system with and without dead-time correction applied. Methods for modelling and correcting for dead time are described in more detail in Chapter 19 in Volume 1.

11.3.2 Sensitivity and Cross Talk

There is no pre-requisite to measure the sensitivity of the detector if a patient baseline calibration is to be used. However, it may be useful to ascertain the suitability of the detector prior to use and also evaluate the impact of potential cross talk from nearby sources. Detector sensitivity will vary depending on isotope, position, and source geometry. Therefore, an appropriate source and geometry should be selected to simulate that expected in a patient. A large cylindrical phantom uniformly filled with activity is usually sufficient. As with patient data, sensitivity measurements should be performed with background correction.

Cross talk is the increase in count rate due to the presence of activity in an adjacent room or area. It is particularly important to characterize cross-talk effects when commissioning a new detector system to ensure activity in neighbouring rooms will not significantly affect patient measurements. For measurements at very low activities, this may require the system to be located outside of the main nuclear medicine department or for the case of therapy ensuring adequate shielding and collimation is available around the room or detector. Figure 11.5 is a diagram of a therapy suite containing two treatment rooms, with ceiling mounted counting systems located above the patient beds.

Position of the detectors are indicated with a red cross. Background measurements were first performed for 600 s, without any sources in the suite. Further measurements were then taken with a 500 MBq ^{131}I source positioned at a – d, as indicated in the diagram. Table 11.1 gives the events recorded at each source position for a measurement period of 600 s. Detector sensitivity, s, for each room can then be determined using,

$$s = \frac{C_{a,c}}{A.t}.$$ (11.14)

Where $C_{a,c}$ represents the background, corrected counts recorded with the source positioned directly under the detectors at a or c over a measurement period, t, and A is the activity in the source. For this example, a sensitivity of 0.44 and 0.48 cps/MBq was determined for the detectors in room 1 and 2, respectively. Cross talk from sources present in the adjoining rooms is described as the percentage increase in background corrected counts per unit activity for a source located outside the room. It is important to consider different source positions as patients are likely to move around the room, and shielding may not be consistent throughout the walls. This is particularly evident with the source located in

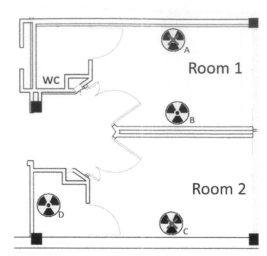

FIGURE 11.5 A diagram of a therapy suite, indicating positions of the WB detectors (red crosses) and positions used to measure sensitivity and cross talk (trefoils). Colour image available at www.routledge.com/9781138593299.

TABLE 11.1
Measured Counts from an ^{131}I Source Placed at Different Positions within Therapy Suite of Figure 11.5

	Counts	
Position	Room 1	Room 2
a	133056	2334
b	–	2564
c	2370	144504
d	2874	–
BG	2293	2030

the bathroom of room 2. Cross talk from a source positioned in the bathroom is 7 times higher than when the source is positioned on the bed.

Table 11.2 demonstrates the influence of cross talk for a scenario of patients in each room located on their respective beds in positions A and C. Provided that activity within each patient is similar, cross-talk effects will be negligible (0.25%). However, if the activity of a patient is significantly higher than the other then WB retention measurements could be greatly affected.

11.3.3 FIELD UNIFORMITY

A measure of field uniformity is useful to determine the sensitivity of the detector to changes in position. In many cases an approximation can be made by modelling an inverse square relationship. In general, it is advised to perform WB measurements at the greatest distance possible to reduce effects of positioning errors. For example, a 10 cm lateral positioning error can cause a 1 per cent reduction in intensity measured at a counter 1 m from the patient, yet the error for a detector placed at 2 m would only be 0.2 per cent. The relative error from a change in distance between patient and detector is much larger, with a 10 cm miss-positioning giving rise to a 23 per cent relative error at 1 m and 11 per cent at 2 m. These errors will potentially vary further depending on the type of collimation used around the detector. A check of position sensitivity can be made by performing repeat measurements of a source at different offset locations from the iso-centre of the detector. Figure 11.6a shows the field uniformity maps from a ceiling-mounted detector system in two adjacent detector rooms. An 800 MBq Tc99m source was placed at different positions around the room,

TABLE 11.2
Effect of Cross Talk to Patient WB Measurements due to Second Patients in an Adjoining room.
Measurements Are Shown for a Range of ^{131}I Activities in Each Patient and Assumes Both Patients Are
Situated on the Bed During Readings

		Secondary source (MBq)							
		100	**500**	**1000**	**2000**	**3000**	**4000**	**5000**	**6000**
Primary source	100	0.25%	1.24%	2.48%	4.95%	7.43%	9.91%	12.38%	14.86%
(MBq)	500	0.05%	0.25%	0.50%	0.99%	1.49%	1.98%	2.48%	2.97%
	1000	0.02%	0.12%	0.25%	0.50%	0.74%	0.99%	1.24%	1.49%
	2000	0.01%	0.06%	0.12%	0.25%	0.37%	0.50%	0.62%	0.74%
	3000	0.01%	0.04%	0.08%	0.17%	0.25%	0.33%	0.41%	0.50%
	4000	0.01%	0.03%	0.06%	0.12%	0.19%	0.25%	0.31%	0.37%
	5000	0.00%	0.02%	0.05%	0.10%	0.15%	0.20%	0.25%	0.30%
	6000	0.00%	0.02%	0.04%	0.08%	0.12%	0.17%	0.21%	0 25%

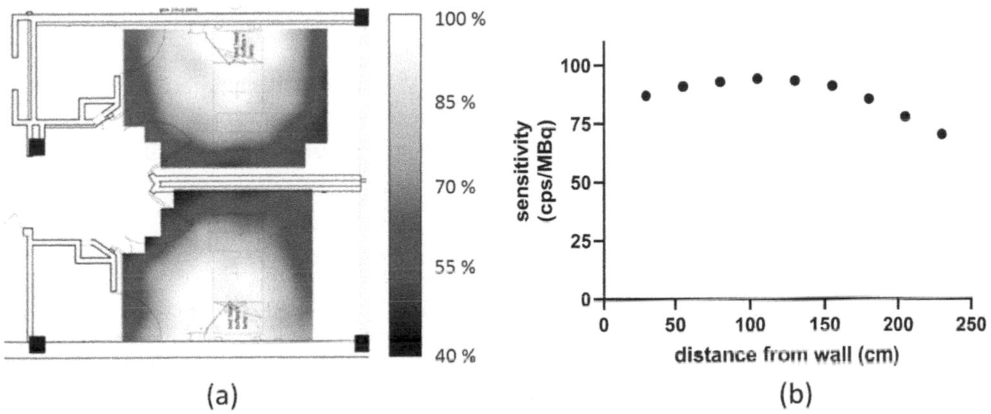

FIGURE 11.6 A diagram showing the change in detector sensitivity throughout the therapy suite (a) for a ceiling mounted Geiger system. The change in detector sensitivity down the length of the bed for a ceiling mounted sodium iodine detector. Colour image available at www.routledge.com/9781138593299.

and 60 s measurements acquired in each source position. Measurements at each position were corrected for decay and normalized. Data between the location intervals were linearly interpolated to produce a 16x16 sensitivity matrix. The sensitivity matrix for each room was then scaled for distance and overlaid onto a floor plan of the therapy suite. Results from similar measurements are shown in Figure 11.6b for a sodium iodine detector. Measurements are shown for a source measured at intervals down the length of the bed. The figures demonstrate the importance of maintaining a consistent bed position throughout the measurement period, and for small and paediatric patients the need to position them reproducibly on the bed.

11.3.4 QUALITY CONTROL

Regular quality tests to detect any changes in sensitivity or drift are vital to ensure the reliability of the detector. For simple counting systems without any energy discrimination, it is sufficient to take period measurements from a long-lived reference source positioned in front of the detector and compare results over time. Reliable positioning of the QC source is paramount for accurate results and therefore a jig or stand with which to position the source is useful.

For scintillation-based systems a similar check is required. However, the peak and width of the photopeak should also be recorded, to check for any drift in PMT gain. As some systems are sensitive to external factors such as temperature and humidity, it is useful to also record these values when performing the QC. Figure 11.7a and Figure 11.7b give example

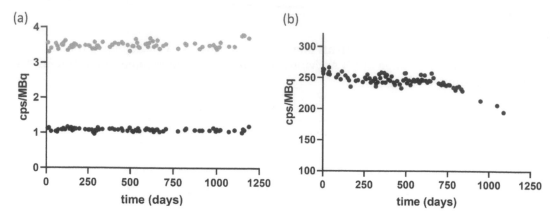

FIGURE 11.7   Quality assurance results for a Geiger (a) and Sodium Iodide detector (b) covering a period of 3.5 years.

QC data for a system comprising two energy compensated Geiger counters and a scintillator-based system, respectively. Weekly sensitivity measurements from the Geiger-based system is given over a period of 3.5 years. Although the two Geiger counters show markedly different sensitivities, each detector is consistent over time, and the different sensitivity is irrelevant provided a patient baseline calibration is used and the same monitor is used throughout a patient measurement period. With a similar source and geometry, the scintillation-based system is significantly more sensitive than the Geiger system and displayed reasonable stability over a period of 2 years. After this time a clear decrease in sensitivity is evident as PMT gains began to drift and recalibration of the energy spectra were required. Despite the change in sensitivity, it may still be possible to use such a system provided the detector does not drift to such an extent that sensitivity changes during the course of a set of patient measures. Such changes may also be an indication of early tube failure, and future replacement of the equipment may be necessary.

11.4   CLINICAL EXAMPLES AND METHODOLOGIES

11.4.1   WHOLE-BODY DOSIMETRY FOR TREATMENT PLANNING

A hugely successful application of whole-body dosimetry is that to ^{131}I-mIBG therapy for which the organ that limits the activity to be administered is mainly the red marrow. Red-marrow dosimetry can be performed by measuring the activity within blood samples taken from the patient [5]. However, direct blood withdrawal is time consuming, difficult in many patients, and requires prolonged repeated contact with radioactive patients. Thus, whole-body dosimetry is often performed as a surrogate for red-marrow dosimetry [1]. Lashford and colleagues [9] showed one of the first correlations between whole-body dose and haemotoxicity, demonstrating 80 per cent of patients developed grade 3 or 4 thrombocypenia at whole-body doses of 2.5 Gy. This reduced to 25 per cent at dose of 2.0 Gy (Figure 11.8).

This observation has led to a treatment regimen based on a maximum tolerated whole-body doses of 2 Gy. To maximize treatment efficacy, a multicycle administration was proposed [10]. Initial treatment activity is determined by patient body weight, 444 MBq/kg and the activity of the second cycle chosen to deliver an average whole-body dose of 2 Gy across the two cycles. Figure 11.9a shows the whole-body absorbed doses for the 8 patients treated during this pilot study. The mean whole-body absorbed dose delivered to the patients over the two fractions was 4.20 Gy with a mean variance from the prescribed dose of 7.7 per cent (range -6.7 to 16.5%). For comparison, the absorbed doses from a repeat weight-based administration are shown in Figure 11.9b. In this example, the range of absorbed doses is significantly higher, with patient receiving between 3.3 and 5.8 Gy.

Buckley and colleagues [11] further confirmed these findings for a larger set of patients, determining that in 70 per cent of patients a whole-body absorbed dose could be prescribed to within 10 per cent. Compared with a fixed or weight-based radioactivity administration, the whole-body absorbed dose allowed higher activities of ^{131}I-mIBG to be administered within the confines of bone marrow toxicity and thus enabled a personalization of therapy.

11.4.2   WHOLE-BODY ACTIVITY RETENTION MEASUREMENTS FOR PERSONALIZED RADIATION PROTECTION ADVICE

In addition to calculation of absorbed doses to patients, whole body activity measurements can also play a key role in evaluating effective doses to persons coming into contact with the patient. When a patient receiving molecular

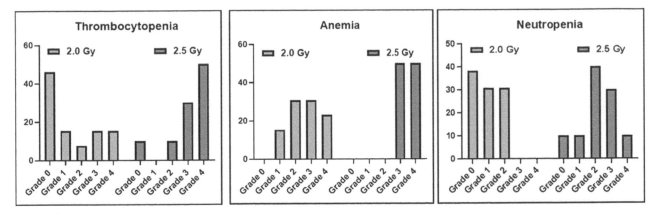

FIGURE 11.8 Summary of results reported by Lashford et al [9] showing different grades of blood toxicity for patient treated to whole body doses of 2.0 Gy and 2.5 Gy.

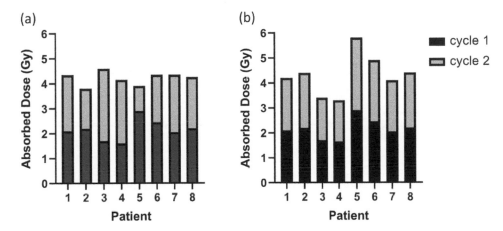

FIGURE 11.9 Whole body doses delivered to patients following a dosimetry guided mIBG administration (a) and estimated doses if a purely weight-based administration had been given (b).

radiotherapy is discharged from hospital, advice should be given informing them of how they need to restrict contact with people to ensure against radiation exposure to members of the public, and members of the household are constrained. All doses should be kept as low as reasonably practicable, and below any dose limits set by the legislative body. Very often generic advice may be given, with identical restrictions imposed on all patients. However, dose rates and activities retained within a patient will vary depending on a number of factors, such as BMI, tumour load, kidney function, or metabolism. Figure 11.10a shows time activity data for two patients, both treated with 7400 GBq of Lu-177 DOTATATE. The retained activity over the 24 hours of measurement clearly demonstrates a significant difference between patients. Dose rate at discharge from patient A were 5 times higher than for patient B. Applying similar contact restrictions on both patients will either be overly constrictive or insufficient depending on how they are determined. Personalized contact restrictions can be generated based on the activity or dose rate at discharge and the rate of excretion after leaving hospital. A dose calculation can essentially be performed where the source is the patient, and the target is the member of the public. An S-value is perhaps inappropriate in the situation as source and target distance will vary. However, in a practical sense, doses can be considered proportional to the TIA determined from this data.

The period over which whole-body measurements are performed will therefore affect the decisions made regarding contact restrictions and potential public exposures. In many cases, there are strong arguments for performing such therapies as a day case administration, notably regarding resourcing and cost implications. However, from Figure 11.10b, it is evident in both examples the TAC did not fully characterize solely on the data gathered on the first day. This can result in an underestimation of public exposure if insufficient contact restrictions are given based on this poorly sampled data. A similar result occurs if insufficient data is acquired over the measurement period. Figure 11.10c demonstrates the underestimation when the retention curve is only based on a single measurement taken at discharge rather than fully

TABLE 11.3
Variation in Time-integrated Activity for Different
Patient Datasets and when Fitted Using Different
Subsets of Data as Described in Figure 11.10

Fit	Normalized TIA (to A1)
A1	100%
B1	21%
A2	26%
B2	3%
A3	46%
B3	7%

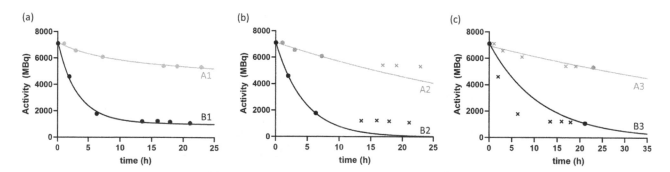

FIGURE 11.10 Whole body time activity data, fitted to all data points (a), the first 8 hours of data (b) and only the first and last data points (c).

characterizing the TAC during therapy. Normalized values for TIA are given in Table 11.3 for both patients and each of the TAC fitting scenarios. It can be seen that TIA can vary considerably, not only depending on the patient, but also how the data is acquired.

11.4.3 Whole-body Dosimetry Following Pregnancy after Radioiodine Therapy

Whole body activity and dosimetry measurements can also play a pivotal role when a treatment or protocol does not go according to plan. Treatment with radioactivity during pregnancy is contraindicated, and for most patients, pregnancy or fathering a child is discouraged for a period of time post therapy. For ^{131}I NaI therapies for thyroid carcinoma it is recommended to avoid fathering a child for a period of 4 months after treatment. This period is suggested as it is longer than the sperm regeneration cycle. It is also prudent to postpone pregnancy for at least several months after ^{131}I therapy to allow sufficient time for repair of any genetic damage which may have occurred. In addition, as the foetal thyroid gland is known to concentrate radioiodine avidly during the second and third trimesters of pregnancy; to avoid the risk of ^{131}I crossing the placenta and being taken up by an embryonic thyroid gland, the quantity of radioactivity within the pregnant patient should not exceed 30 kBq. The effect of exposure to radiation of the conceptus depends on the time of exposure. For radiation within a couple of weeks the effect of damage to the cells will likely result in a failure to implant or undetectable death. During the rest of the period of major organogenesis, taken from the third week onwards, malformations may be caused, usually at a dose threshold of 100–200 mGy [12]. In cases of early pregnancy, the foetal dose can be taken as the uterus dose.

In this example a dose calculation is made based on WB data for a hypothetical scenario but, based on real patient data, the example deals with the potential of a patient becoming pregnant within the first three weeks following ^{131}I radioiodine therapy. In this example the conception would have occurred within the standard 4 month recommended restriction period. However, as WB retention data were gathered, further calculations can be made to ascertain if any dose limits were breached and used to inform any potential action or intervention. Figure 11.11 is a time-activity curve

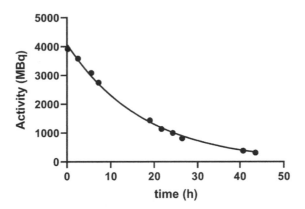

FIGURE 11.11 Time activity data for a patient treated with ^{131}I NaI for thyroid ablation.

TABLE 11.4
Time Activity Parameters for the Data Shown in Figure 11.11

Parameter	Value
A_0	3919 MBq
λ	12.10 h
t_{eff}	0.0573 h^{-1}
$A_{discharge}$	314 MBq

---

for a patient treated with 3700 MBq of ^{131}I for ablation for papillary Thyroid Carcinoma. Activity measurements were obtained using a ceiling mounted WB counter for a period of 48 hours post administration. The patient was discharged from hospital with a residual activity of 314 MBq.

As is the case for many patients, iodine retention is dominated by biological excretion and the TAC is well characterized with a single exponential function.

$$A(t) = A_0 e^{-\lambda t} \tag{11.15}$$

Fit parameters to the TAC are given in Table 11.4.

The activity in the patient at the time of conception (20 days post administration) can be estimated by extrapolating the TAC to the start of pregnancy. Using the fit parameters of Table 11.4 for a value of t = 480, the activity in the patient is estimated to be less than 1 Bq at conception, and no further intervention would be required. However, for radiation protection purposes, it may be prudent to estimate activities and doses based on a worst-case scenario. In this case, once the patient has been discharged from hospital there is no further information regarding radiation retention. A calculation could therefore be performed assuming only physical decay of the isotope from this point on. Based on this estimate the maximum activity that could be present in the body would be 66 MBq at conception and 27 kBq at the start of the second trimester.

Absorbed dose to the uterus can be calculated by estimating the time-integrated activity within the body. This is achieved by integrating the TAC from t = 480 to infinity, yielding:

$$\tilde{A} = \frac{A_{t=480}}{\lambda_{phys}} = \frac{66}{0.0036} = 18333.3 \text{MBq.h} \tag{11.16}$$

Where $A_{t=480}$ is the activity in megabecquerels within the patient at conception and λ_{phys}, is the physical decay constant for ^{131}I in units h^{-1}. An appropriate value of S, is a uterine target organ and whole-body source volume. The activity is assumed uniformly distributed. S-values for selected radionuclides and organs are given for multiple sources and targets in MIRD pamphlet 11 [13]. For whole body to uterus, $S_{uterus \leftarrow WB} = 4.07 \times 10^{-5}$ rad/µCi.h which, converting to more appropriate units is equal to 1.10×10^{-5} Gy/MBq.h. The maximum potential absorbed dose to the uterus is therefore,

$$\bar{D}_{uterus} = \tilde{A}_{WB} \cdot S_{uterus \leftarrow WB} \tag{11.17}$$

$$\bar{D}_{uterus} = 18333.3 \times 4.07 \times 10^{-2} = 201 \text{mGy} \tag{11.18}$$

This value is potentially approaching doses where deterministic effects may be observed. However, given that time-integrated activity was overly exaggerated by assuming physical decay, and given that the activity in the mother will still be below the 30 kBq limit during the second and third trimester, there is still little evidence to cause concern over this pregnancy. Were such a situation to occur in reality, it may be appropriate to have the patient return to hospital once pregnancy is confirmed to re-measure the activity retention and re-evaluate the time-integrated activity rather than extrapolating or assuming physical decay.

REFERENCES

[1] J. Gear et al., "EANM Dosimetry Committee series on standard operational procedures for internal dosimetry for I-131 mIBG treatment of neuroendocrine tumours," *Ejnmmi Phys,* vol. 7, no. 1, 2020.

[2] M. G. Stabin and M. W. Konijnenberg, "Re-evaluation of absorbed fractions for photons and electrons in spheres of various sizes," *J Nucl Med,* vol. 41, no. 1, pp. 149–60, 2000.

[3] M. G. Stabin and J. A. Siegel, "Physical models and dose factors for use in internal dose assessment," *Health Phys,* vol. 85, no. 3, pp. 294–310, 2003.

[4] S. J. Chittenden et al., "Optimization of equipment and methodology for whole-body activity retention measurements in children undergoing targeted radionuclide therapy," *Cancer Biother Radio,* vol. 22, no. 2, pp. 243–49, 2007, doi: 10.1089/ cbr.2006.315.

[5] C. Hindorf, G. Glatting, C. Chiesa, O. Linden, and G. Flux, "EANM Dosimetry Committee guidelines for bone marrow and whole-body dosimetry," *Eur J Nucl Med Mol I,* vol. 37, no. 6, pp. 1238–50, 2010, doi: 10.1007/s00259-010-1422-4.

[6] G. Glatting, P. Kletting, S. N. Reske, K. Hohl, and C. Ring, "Choosing the optimal fit function: Comparison of the Akaike information criterion and the F-test," *Med Phys,* vol. 34, no. 11, pp. 4285–92, 2007.

[7] G. D. Flux, M. J. Guy, R. Beddows, M. Pryor, and M. A. Flower, "Estimation and implications of random errors in whole-body dosimetry for targeted radionuclide therapy," *Phys Med Biol,* vol. 47, no. 17, pp. 3211–23, 2002, doi: 10.1088/0031-9155/47/17/311.

[8] J. I. Gear et al., "EANM practical guidance on uncertainty analysis for molecular radiotherapy absorbed dose calculations," *Eur J Nucl Med Mol I,* vol. 45, no. 13, pp. 2456–74, 2018.

[9] L. S. Lashford et al., "Phase I/Ii Study of I-131 Metaiodobenzylguanidine in Chemoresistant Neuroblastoma – a United-Kingdom Children's Cancer Study-Group Investigation," *J Clin Oncol,* vol. 10, no. 12, pp. 1889–96, 1992, doi: 10.1200/ Jco.1992.10.12.1889.

[10] M. N. Gaze, Y. C. Chang, G. D. Flux, R. J. Mairs, F. H. Saran, and S. T. Meller, "Feasibility of dosimetry-based high-dose (131)I-meta-iodobenzylguanidine with topotecan as a radiosensitizer in children with metastatic neuroblastoma," *Cancer Biother Radio,* vol. 20, no. 2, pp. 195–99, 2005, doi: 10.1089/cbr.2005.20.195.

[11] S. E. Buckley, S. J. Chittenden, F. H. Saran, S. T. Meller, and G. D. Flux, "Whole-Body Dosimetry for Individualized Treatment Planning of I-131-MIBG Radionuclide Therapy for Neuroblastoma," *J Nucl Med,* vol. 50, no. 9, pp. 1518–24, 2009, doi: 10.2967/jnumed.109.064469.

[12] ICRP, 2000. "Pregnancy and Medical Radiation." ICRP Publication 84. Ann. ICRP 30 (1).

[13] W. S. Snyder, M. R. Ford, G. G. Warner, and W. S. B. *"S," Absorbed Dose per Unit Cumulated Activity for Selected Radionuclides and Organs.* (1975). New York: Society of Nuclear Medicine.

12 Personalized Dosimetry in Radioembolization

Remco Bastiaannet and Hugo W.A.M. de Jong

CONTENTS

12.1 INTRODUCTION

Radioembolization is an established treatment for chemo-resistant and unresectable liver cancers. The treatment consists of the administration of microspheres that are loaded with a beta-emitter into the arterial hepatic vasculature. As a result of a differential vasculature of the healthy liver and tumour tissue, the microspheres preferentially accumulate in the tumour tissue, resulting in a local radiation dose to the tumour whilst sparing healthy liver tissue.

DOI: 10.1201/9780429489549-12

Currently, two types of microspheres are approved for clinical use by the FDA and are CE-marked: resin microspheres (SIR-spheres; SirTex Medical) and glass microspheres (TheraSphere; BTG International), both of which are loaded with ^{90}Y. A third type consists of ^{166}Ho-loaded poly-lactate spheres, called QuiremSpheres, which is yet to receive FDA approval, but has been CE-marked.

Radioembolization treatment planning is currently based on semi-empirical methods, which are designed to yield acceptable toxicity profiles and have enabled the large-scale application in a palliative setting. The addition of radioembolization with SIR-spheres to first-line treatments for metastatic colorectal cancer was investigated in three large randomized controlled trials SIRFLOX [1], FOXFIRE [2], and FOXFIRE-global. The combined analyses of these three trials did not show a significant improvement in either progression-free survival [3] or overall survival [4]. Similarly, the SARAH and SIRveNIB Phase III studies failed to show an improvement in overall or progression-free survival after the treatment of advanced hepatocellular carcinoma with SIR-spheres versus sorafenib [5], [6].

One reason for this might be that the current activity planning methods often result in underdosing (and in some cases overdosing) in patients [1], [2], [7–9]. Fortunately, a recent survey amongst European institutes has shown that some form of absorbed dose-based prescription was used by 64 per cent and 96 per cent of the respondents for the use of resin and glass microspheres, respectively [10]. The lack of biological clearance of the microspheres simplifies dosimetry compared to most other molecular radiotherapies. In order to further increase the adoption of absorbed dose-based prescription, the package inserts of both manufacturers could be improved by placing more emphasis on this type of activity prescription. Furthermore, there is mounting evidence for clear dose-effect relationships (see Table 12.1). However, the estimated absorbed dose needed to elicit a reliable tumour response or complication varies between studies. As such, reliable absorbed dose targets and limits are yet to be established.

This review aims to investigate the current state-of-the-art of dosimetry in relation to this discussion from a physics perspective, elaborating on technical difficulties and providing an overview of the relevant hiatuses in the current knowledge.

12.2 CURRENT ACTIVITY PLANNING METHODS

12.2.1 PRE-TREATMENT SAFETY PROCEDURE

Before the infusion of the therapeutic dose, an angiographic work-up is performed in which the hepatic vessel anatomy is explored, and an infusion site is selected. As per EANM guidelines, this is followed by the administration of 75–150 MBq of the surrogate particle ^{99m}Tc macroaggregated albumin (^{99m}Tc-MAA) [11]. These imageable protein aggregations aim to simulate the expected distribution of the subsequent therapeutic microspheres. There are three main reasons for the use of a simulation procedure using ^{99m}Tc-MAA [12].

First, extrahepatic depositions can be detected. This used to be done using planar scintigraphy, however SPECT/CT has been shown to be superior for this goal [13].

Second, the lung shunt fraction (LSF) is estimated. This fraction is used as a proxy for the absorbed lung dose and is subsequently used to adjust the prescribed activity, as described in the next sections. The microsphere manufacturers specify that this estimation should be performed on planar scintigraphic imaging [14], according to the formula

$$LSF = \frac{C_{lungs}}{C_{lungs} + C_{liver}},\qquad(12.1)$$

where C_{lungs} indicates the total counts in the lungs and C_{liver} the total counts in the liver. Usually, the number of counts in these regions-of-interest (ROIs) is determined on the geometric mean of the anterior and posterior views. However, the validity method has been questioned as it does not include proper compensation for differences in attenuation between the liver and the lungs, resulting in a systematic overestimation of LSF estimated on planar images relative to LSF estimated on SPECT/CT images [15–17].

Third, by using the ^{99m}Tc-MAA distribution as a predictor for the subsequent ^{90}Y distribution, it may be used for multi-compartment dosimetry (see the section Multi-compartment Dosimetry) [18].

The type of planning method used in clinical practice depends on the type of microsphere. For resin microspheres, the most commonly used method is the body surface area-based (BSA) method [14]. For glass microspheres and holmium-loaded microspheres, a commonly used method is the MIRD mono-compartment method [19–21]. Collectively, these methods are referred to as semi-empirical methods.

12.2.2 BSA-based Method for Resin Microspheres

The BSA-based method was developed to overcome the clinically observed high toxicity of a previous method, used in early clinical studies [22]. The prescribed activity using this previous method ranged between 2 and 3 GBq, depending on tumour load only and not on liver size [23]. Conversely, the BSA-based method is based on the observation that BSA correlates with liver volume in the healthy population [24]. As such, the planned activity is adjusted to an individual patient's liver volume. The activity is calculated according to the following relationship [14]:

$$A[GBq] = \left(BSA[m^2] - 0.2\right) + \frac{V_{tumor}}{V_{tumor} + V_{normal\ liver}}, \tag{12.2}$$

where V_{tumor} and $V_{normal\ liver}$ indicate the volumes of the tumour and the healthy parenchyma, respectively. For lobar or super-selective treatment, the activity is reduced in proportion to the size of the liver volume being treated.

The prescribed activity is reduced by 20 per cent or 40 per cent if there is an LSF between 10–15 per cent or 15–20 per cent, respectively. An LSF higher than 20 per cent is a contraindication for the treatment [14].

A modified BSA method was used for the SIRFLOX, FOXFIRE and FOXFIRE-global studies, where activity was reduced relative to the BSA method, based on LSF and tumour involvement [1].

12.2.3 MIRD Mono-compartment for Glass Microspheres

For glass microspheres the activity calculation is based on the desired mean absorbed dose to the target liver mass (independent of tumour burden), following:

$$A[GBq] = \frac{Desired\ dose[Gy] \times M_{target}[kg]}{50[J/GBq]}. \tag{12.3}$$

The desired absorbed dose is set assuming a completely homogeneous distribution of the microspheres over the target volume. The target mass may be determined using either CT, MRI, PET or ^{99m}Tc-MAA SPECT [21].

The recommended absorbed dose ranges from 80 to 150 Gy, depending on the judgment of the treating physician. The estimated total activity shunting to the lungs should not exceed 610 MBq, which equates to approximately 30 Gy in 1 kg lung tissue [21].

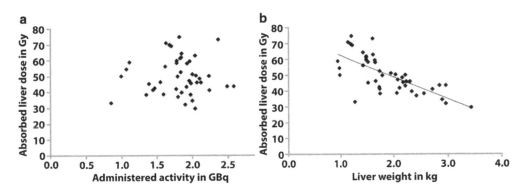

FIGURE 12.1 Adapted from [35]. Absorbed dose to the whole liver was not correlated to the administered activity (a). However, liver weight was negatively correlated with whole liver absorbed dose (r = –0.723, P < 0.001), leading to patients with small liver being relatively over-dosed and patients with larger liver under-dosed (b).

12.2.4 MIRD Mono-compartment Method for Holmium Microspheres

For the administration of holmium microspheres, a methodology akin to the MIRD mono-compartment method for glass microspheres was used in a phase I absorbed dose-escalation study [25]. The administered activity was calculated according to:

$$A[GBq] = \frac{Liver\,dose[Gy] \times M_{liver}[kg]}{15.9[J/GBq]}, \tag{12.4}$$

where the liver mass was determined on contrast-enhanced CT. The absorbed dose was escalated from 20 to 80 Gy in four steps. The maximum tolerated absorbed dose was established to be 60 Gy. However, it has been demonstrated that these holmium microspheres may be used for a scout procedure as well [26], which provides a prediction of the microsphere biodistribution, which is superior in accuracy to MAA [27]. This, in combination with the absorbed dose-response relationship that was published in 2019 [28], the expectation is that this will enable a scout dose-based personalized dosimetry, based on multi-compartment dosimetry.

12.2.5 Limitations of Current Methods

An obvious limitation of these methods is that the actual spatial dose distribution of an individual patient is neglected. In general, these methods seek to prevent overdosing to the parenchyma (and lungs), minimizing the occurrence of radioembolization-induced liver disease [29–31]. As a consequence, the resultant prescribed activities are likely curbed by toxicity limitations of the most vulnerable patients and the occurrence of patients with a highly unfavourable absorbed-dose distribution. This is thought to result in under-dosing in some patients [32–34].

For the BSA method, an added limitation is that the estimated liver volume is based on a healthy population. As such, this relation might not hold for patients with liver tumours. Indeed, it has been shown that absorbed liver dose does not correlate with prescribed activity, using the BSA method [35]. This results in patients with relatively small livers that are more likely to be overdosed, and patients with larger livers are more likely to be under-dosed (see Figure 12.1) [33], [35], [36]. An illustration of this is given in [35] where, based on the BSA method, a patient received 1.82 GBq (BSA 1.78 m², tumour involvement 15%), resulting in a high liver absorbed dose of 74.7 Gy, due to its relatively low mass of 1.22 kg. In the same study, another patient received a similar activity of 1.85 GBq (BSA 1.50 m², tumour involvement 45%), but that patient had a larger liver of 2.33 kg, resulting in a much lower average liver absorbed dose of 39.7 Gy. Furthermore, there are currently no guidelines regarding activity prescription after prior resection [37].

12.3 MULTI-COMPARTMENT DOSIMETRY

A different approach to activity prescription from the homogenous, single compartment models of the BSA and MIRD mono-compartment methods is the partition model (PM). It postulates three compartments with potentially different activity uptakes: tumour, normal liver and lung tissue [18]. As such it allows for the selection of a prescribed activity that maximizes the absorbed dose to the tumour tissue, whilst not exceeding toxicity thresholds for the other two compartments. The expected activities in each compartment are usually based on the distribution of ^{99m}Tc-MAA on the safety scan. However, there is some discussion in the literature about the predictive value of these particles for the subsequent ^{90}Y microsphere distribution [39–42].

The respective compartments are usually segmented on an anatomical imaging modality (e.g. contrast-enhanced CT) or a functional modality (e.g. SPECT thresholding) and registered to the reconstructed ^{99m}Tc-MAA distribution. The activity distribution over the compartments is described by the tumour-to-normal tissue ratio (TN ratio), expressed as:

$$TN = \frac{A_T[MBq]/M_T[kg]}{A_{NL}[MBq]/M_{NL}[kg]} \tag{12.5}$$

where A and M indicate the activity in, and the mass of, the tumour (T) and normal liver tissue (NL) compartments.

Using some algebra, the following relation can be derived for the prescribed activity, given a certain TN ratio, LSF, and compartment masses [43]:

$$A[GBq] = D_{NL}[Gy]\frac{TN \times M_T[kg] + M_{NL}[kg]}{50[J/GBq] \times (1 - LSF)}, \tag{12.6}$$

where D_{NL} indicates the absorbed dose to the parenchyma. Implicit in this equation is the assumption that dose is deposited locally in the compartment that contains the activity, which is a simplification. This is discussed in further detail in the section Dosimetric models.

Multi-compartment dosimetry is claimed to be more 'scientifically sound' than the BSA-based or MIRD mono-compartment method [33]. However, besides being more labour intensive to work with in clinical practice, there are several technical caveats to using the PM.

12.3.1 Different Methods to Calculate TN Ratio

When multiple lesions are present, each may have a different microsphere uptake, leading to errors in the subsequent individual tumour-absorbed dose estimates, due to averaging of the TN ratio. Mikell and colleagues have shown this effect by comparing the silver standard Monte Carlo-based dose estimates with the MIRD mono-compartment based dosimetry and the PM model in realistic patient data [44]. In the case of multiple tumours, there can be large discrepancies between the methods for the estimated tumour-absorbed dose. For example, the variability between PM-based and Monte Carlo-based tumour absorbed dose estimates was higher by a factor five in cases where there were multiple tumours present, compared to single tumour samples.

However, there is currently no consensus on how to calculate the TN ratios for individual tumours for the use in the PM model. Some authors use the entire normal liver volume for this calculation [45], whilst others opt for a smaller sample volume, placed near the tumour-of-interest [41]. Although this simplification makes the use of the PM model more feasible in clinical practice, it also inevitably leads to larger uncertainty ($\approx$2.5x) in the TN ratio estimations when the microspheres are not strictly homogenously distributed in the healthy liver tissue [44].

12.3.2 Definition of Compartments on Anatomical Imaging

When diagnostic (contrast-enhanced) CT or MRI is used for the delineation of the tumour compartments, these delineations subsequently need to be transferred to the SPECT/CT reconstructions. This can be achieved by copying the volume-of-interest (VOI) delineation to the SPECT/CT data or by using (non-rigid) co-registration. However, mismatches are likely to occur, causing a misalignment between the anatomical delineations and the SPECT reconstruction. A common cause is differences in patient positioning between both anatomical scans. For instance, different arm positioning (above the head versus lying next to the body) or body position (e.g. different placement on the table).

Another issue for co-registration is breathing during the CT acquisition. The acquisition of the liver volume is usually much faster than an entire respiratory period, resulting in a 'snapshot' of a random respiratory phase. As the SPECT or PET activity reconstruction is a superposition of all respiratory phases, this can result in mismatches of > 1 cm between the anatomical delineations and the reconstructed activity [46]. Using CTs acquired during breath-holding for coregistration might mitigate this effect, but breath-holds are shown to have a limited reproducibility between acquisitions, resulting in different relative respiratory states between scans [47]. A viable solution might be the use of so-called 'time-averaged 3D mid-position CT scans' in this context, often used in radiotherapy [48].

Besides leading to mismatches in co-registration, respiratory motion also results in activity reconstructions that are 'smeared out'. This leads to an underestimation of the local activity concentration, especially in tumour tissue, which has a smaller volume compared to the motion amplitude than the background compartment. The effect of motion blurring is well-known in general [49], [50], but the impact of respiratory motion in the context of radioembolization has recently been shown for both PET [51] and SPECT [52].

Furthermore, defining the boundaries of the tumour compartment on anatomical modalities may be non-trivial in the case of morphologically diffuse or infiltrative tumours [33]. Tumours with substantial necrosis pose a similar problem. A possible solution to this might be the use of FDG PET for the demarcation of vital tumour tissue in the case of FDG-avid tumours.

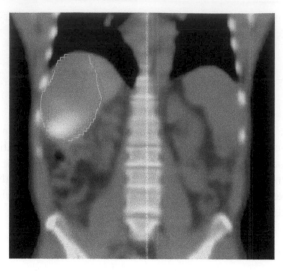

FIGURE 12.2 Exemplar case where a VOI delineation based on SPECT thresholding only (dark contour) does not match the CT-based anatomical tumour definition (bright contour). The mismatch results in a difference in tumour volume and mean tumour uptake. *Image originally published in* [38] *and reprinted according to Creative Common CC BY license (creativecommons.org).* Colour image available at www.routledge.com/9781138593299.

12.3.3 DEFINITION OF COMPARTMENTS USING PHYSIOLOGICAL INFORMATION

Similarly, the uptake information in SPECT reconstructions (e.g. when using MAA for absorbed dose prediction) could be used to indicate vital tumours. However, as delineations drawn directly on SPECT will generally result in errors in the estimated volume [53–55] (Figure 12.2), Garin and colleagues have developed a hybrid method in which the SPECT reconstruction and CT information are presented in conjunction, integrating functional and anatomical information and aiding manual delineation [56], [57]. This has been shown to work well for both phantom and patient studies, in which anatomical borders are readily discernible. However, this type of method does not have a well-defined contouring guideline, which reduces reproducibility.

A more fundamental approach to this segmentation problem was proposed in a study by Lam and colleagues [58], in which directly after the normal ^{99m}Tc-MAA SPECT scan, the participating patients were injected with ^{99m}Tc-sulfur colloid (SC) and another SPECT was acquired after 5 minutes. This compound specifically accumulates in functional (non-tumour) liver tissue and as such will act as a negative template for the tumour compartments. By taking the difference between the MAA and SC SPECT reconstructions, voxel maps for healthy parenchyma and tumour tissue are automatically obtained, providing a 'physiology-based segmentation'.

12.4 VOXEL-BASED DOSIMETRY

In voxel-based dosimetry, the reconstructed voxel is taken as the smallest independent spatial unit for activity. This allows for the expression of (estimated) absorbed dose gradients and non-homogeneities on a small spatial scale, somewhat similar to external beam radiotherapy (EBRT). This contrasts with multi-compartment models, where absorbed dose estimates are averaged over each compartment. By including this spatial dimension, voxel-based dosimetry potentially provides a link to the rich EBRT literature on dose-effect relationships, which could potentially be used for both therapy planning and post-therapy outcome assessment. However, in contrast to image-guided absorbed dose planning for EBRT, voxel-based dosimetry for radioembolization is based on nuclear medicine images, which are generally noisy and of low resolution, prohibiting a direct translation of EBRT concepts to the radioembolization paradigm.

12.5 USING SPATIAL DOSE INFORMATION

To aid assessment and comparison between individual cases, the spatial dose information can be combined into a (cumulative) dose-volume histogram (cDVH). These graphs express the fraction of the total VOI (be it a tumour, normal tissue, or entire liver) receiving a certain minimum absorbed dose. This expresses in a single graph how the absorbed

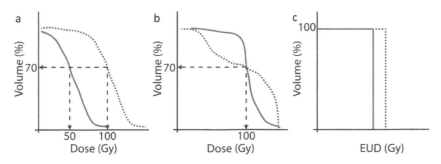

FIGURE 12.3 Hypothetical cDVHs illustrating key concepts in voxel-based dosimetry, which may be used for outcome prediction. In panel A the situation of the solid absorbed dose distribution may be expected to have a smaller impact on the tissue under consideration (less toxic or less tumour kill). This is also reflected in the D_{70} and V_{100} being lower for the solid than the for the dashed curve. Due to highly heterogeneous absorbed dose distributions, which is typical for radioembolization, two different cases with cDVHs as depicted in panel B might occur. Which of these cDVHs may be expected to have a larger effect on the tissue, is ambiguous (same D_{70} and V_{100}) and might depend on the tissue type. Panel C depicts the hypothetical differences in equivalent uniform doses (EUD), derived from the situation in panel B, potentially resolving the ambiguity. *Image originally published in* [38] *and reprinted according to Creative Common CC BY license (creativecommons.org).*

dose is distributed over the volume (Figure 12.3). The concept of cDVHs also enables the introduction of spatially-dependent measures of absorbed dose such as D_{70} (minimum absorbed dose to 70% of VOI) and V_{100} (percentage of VOI receiving at least 100 Gy) that might be expected to be good predictors of treatment effect [59], [60]. For example, it is clear from Figure 12.3A that the blue absorbed dose distribution clearly delivers a higher absorbed dose to more of the tumour volume (or conversely, red is less toxic when this is a cDVH of normal tissue). These metrics are widely used for the comparison between EBRT plans and are gaining some traction within the radioembolization dosimetry community to help better explain clinical outcomes [59], [61–64].

Due to the typical heterogeneous distribution of the microspheres, comparing cDVHs of, for instance, two patients, is not always trivial (as is the case in Figure 12.3a). Ambiguity can occur and an example of such a case is shown in Figure 12.3b, where the cDVH curves are crossing. In such cases, it is completely dependent on the specific organ (e.g. parallel organ or not) which cDVH would lead to the highest tumour kill or least amount of toxicity.

This ambiguity is a well-known phenomenon in EBRT, and efforts have been undertaken to create radiobiological models that aim to quantify the biological effect of any treatment plan and enable the comparison of plans based on expected outcome [65]. The premise of most of these models is that an irradiated tumour exhibits a binary response (control or survival), which is determined by the surviving fraction (SF) of a population of cells after irradiation. This SF is modelled as a function of absorbed dose and may include any additional clinically relevant parameters, such as repopulation between treatments, clonogen radioresistance and dose rate effects. Subsequently, the parameters of these models are retrospectively fitted on clinical data and can then be used to predict treatment outcome. As such, these radiobiological models provide a link between physical quantities such as spatial dose distribution and expected clinical outcome. The potential importance of radiobiological modeling is illustrated with a clinical example Figure 12.4.

Importantly, two such models have been adapted from EBRT for the context of radioembolization [61], [66]. First, the effect of dose rate and cell repair mechanisms can be modeled with the Biologically Effective Dose (BED), such that $\ln(SF) = -\alpha BED$. BED can be calculated for a unit volume i (e.g. a voxel) according to

$$BED_i = D_i \left(1 + \frac{D_i \cdot T_{rep}}{\left(T_{rep} + T_{phys}\right) \cdot \alpha / \beta} \right), \tag{12.7}$$

with D_i the locally absorbed dose, T_{rep} and T_{phys} the halftimes for cell repair after damage and the physical halftime of ^{90}Y, respectively. α and β denote the so-called intrinsic radio sensitivity and potential sparing capacity [67].

Furthermore, spatial non-uniformities can be normalized to a single number, called Equivalent Uniform Biologically Effective Dose (EUBED), see also Figure 12.3C. This number is the same for different absorbed dose distributions that have the same biological effect [68]. EUBED can be defined as

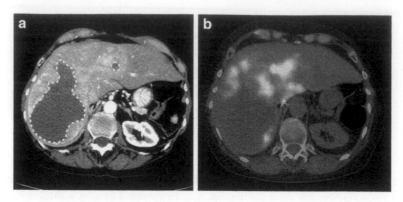

FIGURE 12.4 Example of a large neuroendocrine tumour, which was treated with glass microspheres. Activity was prescribed according to the MIRD mono-compartment method to reach 120 Gy. According to the PM model, the average absorbed dose to the tumour was 150 Gy. The patient has shown no response after treatment (RECIST, mRECIST, and EASL). The contrast-enhanced CT shows the tumour as a large enhanced area (solid line) and necrosis (dashed line) (A). A strong absorbed dose inhomogeneity can be observed (B). Voxel-based dosimetry and radiobiological models may account for such absorbed dose inhomogeneities. *Image originally published in* [38] *and reprinted according to Creative Common CC BY license (creativecommons.org).* Colour image available at www. routledge.com/9781138593299.

$$EUBED = -\frac{1}{\alpha} \ln\left(\frac{\sum_i e^{-\alpha BED_i}}{n_{voxel}} \right), \tag{12.8}$$

Where α is the radiosensitivity (1/Gy) of the local tissue, n_{voxel} the number of voxels of the current VOI and i denotes the voxel index [66]. A reasonable simplification for radioembolization is to neglect quadratic effects (i.e. $\beta = 0$) and BED, in which case BED_i is substituted with D_i in equation 12.8, which then yields Equivalent Uniform Dose (EUD).

In theory, this approach will aid physicians to optimally weigh risks and benefits of an individual absorbed dose distribution, as clinical outcomes can be linked to a single number such as BED and EUBED. However, the existence and robustness of such dose-effect relationships in the context of radioembolization are currently still under investigation.

12.6 TIMING OF DOSIMETRY-BASED TREATMENT PLANNING

Pre- and post-treatment are not the only time points for dosimetry, as Bourgeois and colleagues report on intra-procedural PET/CT in a case study [69]. They used a three-step protocol wherein the first step ^{90}Y microspheres with a total activity determined by the BSA model was administered to the patient. For the second step, the patient was transferred for PET/CT imaging. The maximum absorbed dose by normal hepatic parenchyma and the average absorbed dose by the tumour were determined. For one out of the six patients in this study, the absorbed dose by the tumour was below the assumed tumouricidal absorbed dose of 100–120 Gy for HCC (the other five patients reached this threshold with the first infusion, which was based on the BSA model). For this single, undertreated patient the third step of the protocol was performed which was a repeated infusion of ^{90}Y microspheres with an optimized activity determined from the quantitative PET/CT data to reach the target tumour absorbed dose. Although the initial treatment planning was based on the suboptimal BSA method, the dosimetry based on the intra-procedural PET/CT scan allowed for activity delivery based on patient-specific physiology at the time of the procedure. A downside of this three-step protocol is the increased time, costs and access to equipment and personnel.

This last disadvantage might be partly solved by imaging in the intervention room. Walrand and colleagues describe a camera dedicated to bremsstrahlung SPECT of ^{90}Y [70]. They suggested mounting the gamma camera on a robotic arm to allow SPECT acquisition within a few minutes in the intervention room during the catheterization procedure to optimize the ^{90}Y activity to inject.

Another option for imaging in the intervention room is proposed by Beijst and colleagues [71]. The authors propose a hybrid imaging system, consisting of an X-ray c-arm combined with gamma imaging capabilities, for simultaneous real-time fluoroscopic and nuclear imaging. A slightly modified version of this prototype [72] was shown to be able to accurately estimate LSF of a ^{99m}Tc-MAA scout dose in an interventional setting [73]. When this hybrid imaging modality becomes available in the angiography room it may be possible to move towards one-day procedures by combining scout and therapy dose in one session.

Using microspheres labeled with a paramagnetic element, like ^{166}Ho, will provide contrast on MRI. It has been shown that the absorbed dose by the tumour and healthy liver can be accurately quantified using a post-treatment MRI scan [74], [75]. Since MRI provides excellent soft tissue contrast it would be a well-suited modality for radioembolization guidance as well as evaluation of therapy. The feasibility of fully MR-guided real-time navigation of hepatic catheterization was demonstrated in an animal model [76]. Drawbacks of MR-guided radioembolization are the potentially limited availability of MR scanners and MR-compatible catheters and guide wires and the relatively high costs.

12.7 QUANTITATIVE IMAGE RECONSTRUCTION

Besides the above-mentioned factors concerning dosimetry, differences in outcome between these studies may in part also be explained by the wide range in technical scan parameters used and the measurement variance inherent to nuclear medicine images. An overview of the current topics in nuclear image acquisition and reconstruction is therefore desired.

In quantitative image reconstruction, all relevant interactions between the radionuclide, the patient, and the imaging system need to be accounted for during reconstruction. The current state-of-the-art consists of iterative reconstruction algorithms that incorporate models for all such image-degrading effects (e.g. attenuation, scatter, nuclide decay, detector uniformity, etc.) [77–79].

From its inception, PET was considered a quantitative modality, in contrast to SPECT. This is due to the high signal-to-noise ratio of PET and the relative simplicity of the physics of coincidences, which enables a straight-forward method for attenuation correction. This was available in early generations of PET scanners. However, with the advent of inherently coregistered CT in SPECT/CT, attenuation and scatter correction are now common practice and some authors have claimed that modern clinical SPECT systems can now be considered quantitative as well [80], [81]. Furthermore, vendors are currently implementing calibration routines and inherently quantitative reconstruction software in their machines [82], [83], which enables the dissemination of absolute activity quantification into clinical practice for both modalities.

12.7.1 POST-THERAPY IMAGING

In radioembolization, treatment success can be assessed with a post-therapy scan, either with bremsstrahlung SPECT/CT (bSPECT) or PET/CT (^{90}Y PET).

12.7.1.1 Bremsstrahlung SPECT/CT – The Relevance of Physics Modelling

Post-therapy assessment with ^{90}Y may be performed by bremsstrahlung imaging. This is different from mono-energetic emitters (such as ^{99m}Tc) in that ^{90}Y produces a broad and continuous energy spectrum without a photopeak. Secondly, the high flux of bremsstrahlung photons on a gamma camera will result in significant dead time, if not managed correctly (count rate linearity was estimated up-to 7.5 GBq for ^{90}Y and 1.5 GBq for ^{166}Ho [84]). Therefore, ^{90}Y image quantitation using a gamma camera was recognized early on as being non-trivial [85]. With the advent of advanced iterative reconstruction techniques that enable advanced physics modelling, several quantitative reconstruction methods have been proposed in the literature. Most of these methods utilize some kind of Monte Carlo modelling of the imaging process. Rong and colleagues achieved quantitation errors between -1.6 and 11.9 per cent for a phantom experiment by modelling all relevant energy-dependent image degrading effects [86]. Elschot and colleagues incorporated Monte Carlo simulations of photon-tissue interactions directly within the iterative reconstruction loop, increasing image contrast and activity recovery significantly (over 80% for non-small spheres), relative to a reference clinical reconstruction algorithm [87]. Minarik and colleagues performed a similar study, using the SIMIND code and achieved a quantification error around +8.5 per cent [88].

However, these methods rely on advanced Monte Carlo techniques, which are currently not easily accessible for institutions without a medical physics team that has extensive experience with these methods. Consequently, the reported accuracies will be significantly worse in normal clinical practice.

12.7.1.2 ^{90}Y PET – The Impact of Machine and Reconstruction Parameters

^{90}Y can also be imaged using PET. However, as ^{90}Y only has a minute positron branching ratio (~32 ppm) and the detectors were expected to be saturated from the bremsstrahlung photons (which was later demonstrated to be false), for a long time PET was not considered a feasible modality for post-therapy imaging. The earliest in vivo demonstration of the feasibility of ^{90}Y PET imaging was delivered by Lhommel and colleagues in 2009 [89], using a time-of-flight (TOF) PET scanner and an additional copper ring inserted in the gantry to prevent detector saturation. Later, the feasibility of ^{90}Y PET with Lutetium oxyorthosilicate (LSO) crystals in a scanner without TOF capability was demonstrated [90].

These initial proofs-of-concept were followed by studies that corroborated the quantitative reconstruction capabilities of ^{90}Y PET, using clinically available methods [91–94], which were applied to clinical data [59], [95–97]. However, the very high contribution of randoms (>90%) due to bremsstrahlung in combination with the very low coincidence count statistics was expected to impact random coincidence estimation, scatter correction and consequently, image quality. An elaborate study by Carlier and colleagues has shown that the effect of these phenomena on bias, variability, and detectability of hotspots is minor. The use of correct point spread function (PSF) modelling and TOF reconstruction kept background variability and noise at acceptable levels [98]. This was further corroborated in a fully Monte Carlo–based simulation in which ^{90}Y quantitation is compared to that of ^{18}F [99]. It was found that relative to ^{18}F, the image quality was only slightly poorer in ^{90}Y for a similar positron emission rate. Furthermore, image quality was not strongly linked to any particular physical effect or reconstruction step. This led to the conclusion that adding ^{90}Y -specific models to the PET imaging process is not needed. Furthermore, Van Elmbt and colleagues have shown that systems based on modern crystals (post-BGO) can be used for ^{90}Y dosimetry [100]. Since then, ^{90}Y image quantification has also been shown to be possible in PET/MRI [101] and solid-state digital PET/CT [94].

For clinical ^{18}FDG PET, the importance of homogenization of acquisition and reconstruction settings over centres to allow pooling and comparison of data sets is well-recognized and has resulted in the EARL guidelines and accreditation program [102]. A similar initial attempt for ^{90}Y PET has been made in the form of the QUEST study, showing that ^{90}Y PET-based dosimetry should be reproducible across scanners and centres, as long as TOF-capabilities are available [103].

Together, these studies show that PET-based ^{90}Y quantitative imaging is feasible, robust, and straightforward to implement in clinical practice when a reasonably modern PET system with TOF-capabilities is available. This is in contrast to bSPECT/CT, for which no sufficiently accurate reconstruction methods are currently available for general clinical use.

12.7.1.3 ^{90}Y PET versus bSPECT

In a direct comparison between bSPECT/CT and ^{90}Y PET/CT, the latter is found to have a higher resolution and less scatter in patient studies and several case series [89], [94], [104], [105]. In a quantitative direct comparison between a state-of-the-art clinical bSPECT/CT reconstruction algorithm and clinical PET/CT reconstruction protocols, the superior contrast, detectability, and absorbed dose estimates of PET were demonstrated [106]. However, this comes at the price of a relatively long scan duration in the case of ^{90}Y PET, which is 15 to 20 minutes per bed position. When advanced photon-tissue and photon-detector interactions were modelled with a Monte Carlo–based SPECT/CT reconstructor, image contrast improved substantially and was in some cases (in larger hot spots) higher than in PET/CT [87] (See intermezzo I).

In general, it should be noted that currently there is no standardized approach for post-therapy imaging in terms of acquisition and reconstruction settings and there may exist some systematic biases between the various approaches of different groups, even within the same modality. As a consequence, interpreting and comparing dosimetric results between different groups should be done with caution. However, in general ^{90}Y PET is currently superior to clinical bSPECT/CT in terms of resolution, accuracy and the clinical availability of accurate reconstruction methods for dosimetry.

12.7.1.4   MR & CT for ^{166}Ho

In contrast to ^{90}Y-based microspheres, ^{166}Ho does emit photons with discrete energies that are directly detectable with a gamma camera. Furthermore, it is a paramagnetic element, enabling the visualization with MRI and it has a very high x-ray attenuation, resulting in good contrast on CT [74], [107]. A quantitative SPECT/CT reconstruction using advanced Monte Carlo-based techniques has been developed [108] (achieving contrast recovery of over 80 per cent in non-small NEMA spheres), as is a hybrid method to correct for photon down-scatter from bremsstrahlung and higher energy photons [109]. In a direct comparison between SPECT- and MR-based quantification [74], both modalities are found to be suited for peri-therapy dosimetry [110].

12.8 DOSE-EFFECT RELATIONSHIPS

There is an increasing literature on dose-effect relationships in radioembolization that utilizes advanced dosimetry. An overview of recent papers that (implicitly) estimate tumour control probability (TCP) and/or non-tumour complication probability (NTCP) is given in Table 12.1. The search for the combination of tumour type, outcome measure, dosimetric model and imaging modality that yields the best predictive power is very early stage. Consequently, there is a wide variety in each of these properties amongst these studies, resulting in diffuse optimal absorbed dose limits for both liver complications (~50–97 Gy) and tumour control (~50–560 Gy). Four major factors are hypothesized to contribute to this: differences in response measures, absorbed dose calculations, microsphere type, scan modality (including acquisition and reconstruction settings), and tumour type.

12.8.1 RESPONSE MEASURES

In these studies, tumour response is assessed according to RECIST, mRECIST, vRECIST, EASL, densitometric change [111], change in total lesion glycolysis (TLG) or standardized uptake value (SUV). What is considered a complete response, partial response, stable disease, or progressive disease differs significantly between these measures [112]. For example, the RECIST criteria are sensitive to changes in tumour size, whereas TLG expresses (changes in) total glycolysis (tumour volume times mean SUV over the VOI). Consequently, minimum absorbed dose estimates that lead to tumour response are different between criteria. Although some attempts have been made to directly compare some of these methods [113], the use of such a variety of methods makes comparing these data non-trivial, if not impossible. As the most relevant clinical outcomes are overall survival and progression-free survival, it is important to establish which of the reported proxies is the most predictive of survival [114]. This may result in disease-specific outcome measures (e.g. EASL or mRECIST for hepatocellular carcinoma and RECIST or TLG for metastatic colorectal cancer).

Some studies that are reported in Table 12.1 incorporate either metabolism-based (functional) masks from a previous FDG PET [60] or, for example, the D_{70} measure [59]. It has been argued that in many cases, metabolic response has an earlier onset and is a more accurate proxy for survival than anatomical response metrics [115]. However, most studies calculate the average absorbed dose to the tumour. This may disregard the existence of necrotic volumes and, more generally, absorbed dose heterogeneity.

12.8.2 ABSORBED DOSE CALCULATIONS

Which absorbed dose calculation method best reflects the underlying radiobiological processes in the entire patient population remains an open question. Theoretically, applying EUD and/or BED-based models should be best suited to naturally incorporate differences in specific activity and absorbed-dose heterogeneity in a tissue, as described above. But, clinically, a clear advantage over average absorbed dose to the tumour is yet to be found [61], [66], [121], [125]. The authors suggest this might be linked to the outcome measure being too crudely categorized [66]. Another central finding in these studies, however, is that the apparent radio sensitivities (α and β in equation 12.7) of both the tumour and hepatic tissues in radioembolization are an order-of-magnitude lower than what is found in the EBRT setting, even when correcting for absorbed dose inhomogeneities [66]. Moreover, a significant difference between the absorbed dose needed to reach TCP(50%) for glass and for resin microspheres has been found [66], [121]. In conclusion, the values of the relevant parameters in the radiobiological models have not been well established for radioembolization. They may be specific to the type of microsphere, and it can even be expected to be different between ^{90}Y and ^{166}Ho-based microspheres. These uncertainties have a direct impact on the determination of BED and EUD.

12.8.3 MICRO-DISTRIBUTION

A possible explanation for the differences found between glass and resin microsphere dose-effect relationships is the potential difference in micro-distribution.

One of the first papers on in vivo microsphere distribution was by Fox and colleagues [126]. Using a beta-probe they showed that the activity pattern on a sub-centimetre scale was highly heterogeneous. Later Yorke and colleagues [127] used a combination of computer simulations and biopsy samples to try to find an explanation for the clinically observed lack in normal liver complications using glass microspheres at absorbed dose levels that are known to cause complications in EBRT and found that absorbed dose heterogeneity is sufficient to explain this incongruity.

TABLE 12.1

Non-exhaustive Overview of Recent Dose-response Studies Showing a Large Variety in All Relevant Parameters. This Variety in Outcome Measures and Reported Dose Thresholds Complicate Data Pooling and the Extraction of Reliable Clinical Dose Limits

Study	Tumor Type	Microsphere	Modality	Outcome	Dose Model	Tumor Dose	Liver Dose	Remarks
Chiesa [66]	HCC	Glass	^{99m}Tc-MAA SPECT	Choi 50% (CR & PR) [111]	EUD, BED, EUBED, D_{avg}	TCP(50%) 560 Gy (D_{avg})	NTCP(50%) 97 Gy (D_{avg})	No scatter correction; Dose reported here based on SPECT-based delineation; Large influence of tumour volume
Srinivas [63]	HCC	Glass	^{90}Y PET	mRECIST (CR, PR)	D_{avg}	D_{avg} Responders = 215 Gy	–	Non-significant association
Garin [116], [117]	HCC	Glass	^{99m}Tc-MAA SPECT	EASL (CR, PR & SD)	D_{avg}	Threshold for response = 205 Gy	84 Gy	Large, heterogeneous tumours probably require higher dose.
Chan [118]	HCC	Glass	^{90}Y PET	mRECIST	D_{median}, D_{70}	D_{median} Responders = 225 Gy; D_{median} Non-responders = 83 Gy; D_{70} Responders = 140 Gy; D_{70} non-responders = 24 Gy	–	
Kappadath [119]	HCC	Glass	bSPECT	mRECIST	D_{avg}, BED$_{avg}$	TCP (50%) Davg = 160 Gy (95%CI = 123 to 196 Gy) Dmedian Responders: 209 Gy; Non-Responders: 138 Gy	No complication observed for normal liver D_{avg} < 44 Gy	
Fowler [120]	HCC, NET, CRC	Resin & Glass	^{90}Y PET/MR	(v)Recist	D_{20}, D_{70}, D_{avg}	D_{avg} (29.8 Gy; sensitivity 76.9%; specificity 75.9%) and D_{70} (42.3 Gy; sensitivity 61.5%; specificity 96.6%) were predictive of response in CRC; No link found for other tumour types	–	
Strigari [121]	HCC	Resin	bSPECT	EASL / RECIST	BED	TCP(50%) 110–120 Gy	NTCP (50%) 52 Gy	
Kao [59]	HCC & Cholangio	Resin	^{90}Y PET	mRECIST + 'minor response'	D_{70}	D_{70} > 100 Gy (HCC); D_{70} > 90 Gy (Cholangio)	–	Only patients with TN>=2 on MAA SPECT were selected for this study

Study	Tumour	Sphere	Imaging	Response criteria	Dose metric	Result	Comments
Flamen [62], [122]	CRC	Resin	^{99m}Tc-MAA SPECT	TLG change >50%	D_{avg}	$D_{avg} >= 66$ Gy (c.i. 32–159 Gy) –	Chang's attenuation correction Patient-relative calibration; Assuming no LSF
Van der Hoven [123]	CRC	Resin	^{90}Y PET	TLG change > 50%	D_{avg} & LMER	D_{avg} 40–60 Gy minimally –	Higher baseline TLG leads to a higher reduction
Willowson [64]	CRC	Resin	^{90}Y PET	TLG change > 50%	D_{avg}	50 Gy –	At lower doses, heterogeneity becomes more important
Eaton [60]	Metastatic melanoma	Resin	bSPECT	TLG change & SUV_{max}	D_{max}, D_{avg}, V_{50}	Sign. associations D_{max} with decreased TLG; D_{avg} and V_{50} with an absolute decrease in SUV_{max}. Stronger effect for $D > 50$ Gy –	No scatter or attenuation correction. 12 mm post-filter; Crystal effects neglected
Chansanti [124]	NET	Resin	^{99m}Tc-MAA SPECT	mRECIST	D_{avg}	D_{avg} Responders = 285.8 Gy; D_{avg} Non-responders = 128.1 Gy	Patients with moderate to severe toxicity received $D_{avg} >$ 50 Gy on liver; Reported response at early (median 2.3 months) follow-up
Bastiaannet [28]	Various	Holmium	Quantitative SPECT	TLG change	D_{avg}	D_{avg} Responders = 210 Gy; D_{avg} Non-responders = 116 Gy	Metabolic response associated with significant increase in overall survival

HCC = hepatocellular carcinoma, NET = neuroendocrine tumour, CRC = colorectal cancer, Cholangio = cholangiocarcinoma, LMER = linear mixed-effects regression model, CR = complete response, PR = partial response, SD = stable disease.

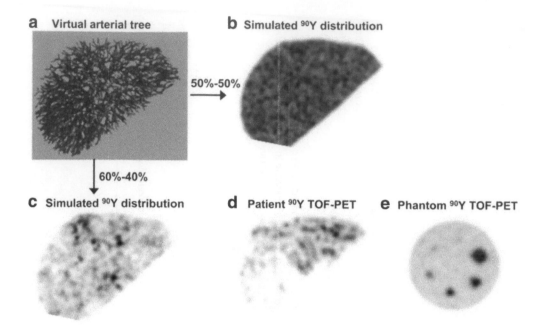

FIGURE 12.5   Simulated arterial tree (A) and subsequently simulated microsphere distribution after flow through the arterial tree (B, C), which explains PET "mottled" look often found in patients (D) but not in phantom scans (E). This research was originally published in JNM. S. Walrand, M. Hesse, C. Chiesa, R. Lhommel and F. Jamar. "The Low Hepatic Toxicity per Gray of 90Y Glass Microspheres Is Linked to Their Transport in the Arterial Tree Favoring a Nonuniform Trapping as Observed in Posttherapy PET Imaging." J Nucl Med. 2014;55: 135–40. © by the Society of Nuclear Medicine and Molecular Imaging.

More recently, Walrand and colleagues performed a simulation study of normal liver tissue, finding that the relatively low number of injected glass microspheres results in non-uniform trapping in the terminal portal artery, resulting in tissue volumes receiving sub-lethal absorbed doses. This would both explain the relatively low toxicity per Gray of glass, relative to resin microsphere and the granularity observed in post-treatment ^{90}Y PET (see Figure 12.5) [128].

This conclusion was seemingly contradicted in an elaborate histological study by Högberg and colleagues, who found that a higher concentration of microspheres (i.e. in the case of resin microspheres) leads to a higher tendency to form clusters, especially in the larger (upstream) arterioles, resulting in a more non-uniform absorbed dose distribution in the liver parenchyma [129]. According to these authors, this apparent contradiction stems from the fact that Walrand and colleagues only assumed microsphere trapping in the terminal branches of the infused artery. In a subsequent simulation study, Högberg and colleagues were able to replicate their histological findings in a mathematical model. This places further emphasis on the importance of the geometry of the arterial tree and (local) microsphere concentration as drivers for microsphere distribution inhomogeneity [130]. These models, however, predict cluster propensity as a function of arteriole generation (branch number) and lack further spatial information. Consequently, the authors conclude that the micro-scale clusterings they observed might not in themselves (fully) explain the observed macroscopic inhomogeneities, as measured by non-invasive imaging [129].

Pasciak and colleagues tried to bridge the gap between micro- and macro-scale tumour dosimetry by using Monte Carlo–based estimations of microsphere micro-distributions, given a ^{90}Y PET reconstruction of a patient [131]. These microsphere micro-distributions are simulated by drawing properties such as cluster propensity and distance from probability density functions that were constructed from histological data [132]. This resulted in realistic structures (Figure 12.6) such as clusters and strings of microspheres. Crucially, it provides a plausible link between the observations in macro- and microdosimetry.

12.9   DOSIMETRIC MODELS

With quantitative imaging, the physical quantity activity (i.e. Becquerel or Curie) of the isotope distributed in space is estimated. However, especially in the case of radionuclide therapies, the process of interest is not the activity per se, but

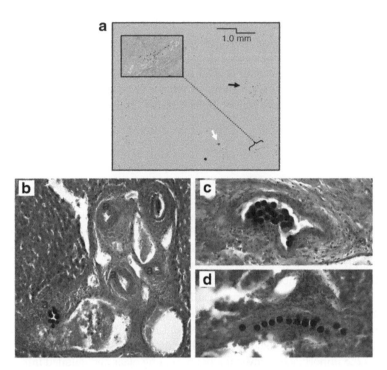

FIGURE 12.6 (a) Small clusters (white arrow) and large clusters (black arrow) are apparent in the Monte Carlo simulations by Pasciak. These simulated distributions seem to be consistent with the histological findings of (amongst others) Högberg (b–d). Panel A was originally published in JNM. A. S. Pasciak, A. C. Bourgeois, and Y. C. Bradley. "A Microdosimetric Analysis of Absorbed Dose to Tumor as a Function of Number of Microspheres per Unit Volume in 90Y Radioembolization." J Nucl Med. 2016;57:1020–26. by the Society of Nuclear Medicine and Molecular Imaging. Other panels are adapted from [130]. *This image originally published in* [38] *and reprinted according to Creative Common CC BY license (creativecommons.org).* Colour image available at www.routledge.com/9781138593299.

rather the subsequent dose absorption by the surrounding tissue (in Gray), as a result of high-energy particles (betas and photons) emitted in the process of decay. This process of dose absorption is what causes the tumour kill and constitutes a rather complex interaction that depends both on the tissue and the specific emissions from the isotope.

If the isotope distribution is known exactly, the most comprehensive and precise estimations of absorbed dose are achieved through Monte Carlo simulations of all relevant interactions between the high-energy particles and the healthy or tumour tissue. Popular codes include the EGSnrc code [133], MCNPX [134], FLUKA [135] and the GATE extension of GEANT [136].

However, these types of simulations are rather complex and time-consuming. Furthermore, the liver is a rather homogenous medium in terms of dose absorption at energies typical for radioembolization. Therefore, a frequently used method to speed up these calculations is by pre-calculating a dose point-kernel (DPK) or dose voxel-kernel (DVK), which is energy absorption in a homogeneous medium around a point source or a voxel source, respectively. Then, a convolution of the true activity distribution with the DPK/DVK will result in an accurate absorbed dose estimation for a homogeneous medium. This kernel can also be scaled to different local tissue densities [137].

The largest contribution to the total absorbed dose comes from the emitted beta particles. The maximal range for ^{90}Y betas in tissue is 1.2 cm (0.9 cm for ^{166}Ho), which is in the same order of magnitude as the resolution of both SPECT and PET. This implies that most of the energy is deposited within the voxel of origin. Consequently, a further simplification is to assume that all emitted energy is absorbed locally, which is usually called the local deposition model (LDM). In practice, this method constitutes applying an appropriate scaling factor to the voxel values of a quantitative reconstruction.

In a direct comparison of SPECT-based ^{90}Y dosimetry Monte Carlo, DVK and LDM-based dosimetry are found to be nearly identical for activity, which is not close to tissue inhomogeneities (e.g. liver-lung border) for the liver [138]. For lung tissue, it was necessary for the DVK method to be scaled to the lower local tissue density of the lung tissue to reach adequate results.

This lack of difference between LDM and the other models is likely to be explained by the fact that a SPECT-based reconstruction has a resolution that is in the same order as the average beta-range. This can be understood as a convolution of a 'blurring' kernel with a putative perfect activity distribution, obviating the need for the simulation of the beta-transport (i.e. blurring). LDM does not unnecessarily repeat this step. Indeed, Pasciak and Erwin found for ^{99m}Tc-MAA SPECT reconstructions that LDM outperformed a Monte Carlo-based absorbed dose estimation, due to this effect [139]. Later, this finding was repeated in ^{90}Y PET [140]. Although in most cases for PET, much of the theoretical benefit is obscured due to image noise, causing both techniques to have a similar absorbed-dose uncertainty. Still, the authors recommend using the LDM in post-radioembolization ^{90}Y PET dosimetry due to its accuracy and ease-of-use [140].

12.10 DISCUSSION

Recently, several phase III trials failed to show an improvement in progression-free survival and overall survival when radioembolization with SIR-Spheres was combined with first-line treatments. A reason for this might be that the methods for activity prescription used in these studies (BSA and MIRD mono-compartment) are barely personalized and are geared towards safety rather than efficacy. More personalized methods (e.g. the partition model, cDVH-based methods) are available. However, there is no consensus as to what absorbed-dose thresholds should be prescribed. In this manuscript, we have therefore reviewed the specific shortcomings of the current activity prescription methods and the current state-of-the-art of newer dosimetric methods and understanding of the underlying radiobiology.

Currently, there is a large range in the literature regarding dosimetric limits, both for the TCP and the NTCP (Table 12.1). We believe that one of the biggest drivers of these diffuse limits is the corresponding wide range in modalities, technical settings, analysis, clinical outcome measures, and relatively small sample sizes. It is therefore nearly impossible to compare data from different studies and distil a common absorbed dose limit, regardless of dosimetric method. This also highlights the importance of investigators providing clear and detailed information on the dosimetric method and analysis used in their publication. This will facilitate reproducibility and may allow for the pooling of clinical data.

With the advent of advanced iterative reconstruction techniques, image quality has improved dramatically in both PET and SPECT [80]. This is mainly due to the incorporation of models for the physics of image formation. In contrast to PET, and probably owing to the more complex (underdetermined) nature of the physics in SPECT imaging, dissemination of quantitative reconstruction algorithms started only recently for SPECT [141], [142]. For more complex isotopes (e.g. ^{90}Y bremsstrahlung SPECT), this is still in the research phase, and vendor-supported solutions are currently not available. The same holds for more complex image-degrading effects (for both SPECT and PET) such as respiratory motion and compensation for partial volume effects. These developments are beneficial to the goal of personalized dosimetry but are currently not widely available.

However, we believe that, using the currently available reconstruction techniques, reliable estimates of dosimetric limits may be established. But in order to achieve comparable results, acquisition and reconstruction settings should be standardized. An initiative similar to the EARL accreditation program for ^{18}FDG PET should lead to reconstructions that are perhaps less than optimal but are at least comparable between patients and institutions, allowing for the pooling of derived dosimetric data. To illustrate this point, it was recently shown that it is feasible to get reliable absorbed dose estimates from ^{99m}Tc-MAA, even if attenuation correction is lacking, using only a simple calibration [67]. This lowers the technical demands for more personalized dosimetry. For technical parameters in ^{90}Y PET, the QUEST initiative may be regarded as a step in the right direction [103].

Ideally, this standardization should not be limited to technical parameters of a specific imaging modality but should also include methods for the segmentation of compartments (or voxels of any VOI), the transferring of volumes (e.g. pre-therapy image delineations transferred to post-therapy images), the selection of relevant clinical outcome measures and stratification by relevant clinical factors (e.g. tumour size, tumour type, baseline liver function). We believe that this standardized acquisition and analysis pipeline may solve the biggest sources of error in current comparative studies (especially multicentre ones). Furthermore, this standardized protocol can be used for prospective studies in dosimetric limits that are relevant to clinicians.

We expect that the formulation of and adherence to such a standardized protocol would be greatly aided if it is based on guidelines formulated by a panel of experts, ideally sponsored by an authoritative entity such as the EANM, SNMMI, or similar.

In order to further refine personalized dosimetry in clinical practice, new methods need to be fast in terms of scan time, labour extensive, robust, and standardized. Some examples of developments in this direction are fully data-driven respiratory motion compensation [143], [144] and fast lung, absorbed-dose estimation [145]. These methods have in common that they are faster, often more reliable and robust and more usable in clinical practice than existing methods.

As there is a wide range of clinical parameters that have an influence on response to therapy, we believe that currently the biggest challenge for the medical physics community involved in radioembolization is not the improvement of quantitative imaging in itself, but rather the translation and dissemination of the current state-of-the-art into a usable form for the use in practical dosimetric efforts. The potential increase in clinical workload and costs associated with further refined personalized dosimetry should be weighed against the potential gains and should not, a priori, be considered a barrier for implementation.

Currently, many aspects of fundamental radiobiology in radioembolization are unknown. For example, the group of Chiesa and colleagues was unexpectedly unable to show a clear increase in predictive power for outcome when using equivalent uniform dose-based measures, as opposed to the average absorbed dose to the tumour or healthy liver tissue [66]. This illustrates that radiobiological model parameters are not well established for this modality, and that the precise relation between absorbed-dose non-homogeneity at both the macro (voxel) level and sub-millimetre level and tissue response is not well understood. We expect that a better understanding of radiobiology on this level will aid the establishment of a coherent account on the efficacy of radioembolization and enable further refinements in patient selection and/or personalized dose optimization. In that sense, the combination of statistical histological data with models that bridge between micro-distribution and clinically observable macroscopic features in reconstructed data (e.g. 'mottled look' in ^{90}Y PET) might provide additional insight into (deviations from) dose-response relationships in a wide population of patients and may result in a micro-scale equivalent uniform dose-metric.

An improved understanding of radiobiology may also facilitate other concepts from EBRT to be translated to the context of radioembolization. An example is fractionation, which uses tumour repopulation and oxygenation between fractions to increase the tumouricidal effect of subsequent irradiations. For radioembolization, this would mean improved tumour control for multiple treatments, versus the current single treatment (e.g. two times 60 Gy versus 120 Gy at once). Whether or not this effect can be exploited using radioembolization is an area of future research.

A better understanding of the dose-response relationships will lead to an improved selection of patients for which dose may be increased safely. Currently, the only available particle for treatment planning is ^{99m}Tc-MAA, which might be a suboptimal predictor of the subsequent microsphere biodistribution, both in terms of LSF [15], [16] and intrahepatic distribution [40–42]. Consequently, a particle that better matches the rheology of the therapeutic microspheres is needed, if radioembolization is to become a true theranostic modality [146]. Several efforts in this direction have been undertaken [147–149]. In this context, ^{166}Ho is a promising alternative in that exactly the same particle can be used for both planning and therapy. This was illustrated for the estimation of LSF [15].

Another approach is to apply dosimetry in an interventional setting [69]. For instance: following an AHASA (as high as safely attainable [8]) paradigm during infusion of the microspheres until thresholds for hepatic toxicity are reached. One innovation that could realize dosimetry in the interventional setting is a so-called hybrid C-arm, which combines x-ray fluoroscopy with (quantitative) nuclear imaging. The dosimetry information may allow for real-time optimization of injected dose and injection position [150][151][152], see Intermezzo II.

Furthermore, if dosimetry is found to be sufficiently reliable, EBRT could be used after radioembolization on specific target areas that might have received a sub-optimal absorbed dose from radioembolization.

Together, these developments in homogenization, accessibility and improved methods will ideally lead to the most personalized and optimal treatment, which we expect to result in improved overall survival and progression-free survival.

This chapter was originally published as: 'The physics of radioembolization.' Bastiaannet, R., Kappadath, S. C., Kunnen, B., Braat, A. J. A. T., Lam, M. G. E. H., de Jong, H. W. A. M., *EJNMMI Phys.* 2018 Nov. 2; 5(1): 22.

REFERENCES

[1] P. Gibbs, V. Gebski, M. Van Buskirk, K. Thurston, D. N. Cade, and G. a Van Hazel, "Selective Internal Radiation Therapy (SIRT) with yttrium-90 resin microspheres plus standard systemic chemotherapy regimen of FOLFOX versus FOLFOX alone as first-line treatment of non-resectable liver metastases from colorectal cancer: the SIRFLOX study," *BMC Cancer*, vol. 14, p. 897, 2014, doi: 10.1186/1471-2407-14-897.

[2] S. J. Dutton, N. Kenealy, S. B. Love, H. S. Wasan, R. A. Sharma, and FOXFIRE Protocol Development Group and the NCRI Colorectal Clinical Study Group. "FOXFIRE protocol: An open-label, randomised, phase III trial of 5-fluorouracil, oxaliplatin, and folinic acid (OxMdG) with or without interventional Selective Internal Radiation Therapy (SIRT) as first-line treatment for patients with unresectable liver-on," *BMC Cancer*, vol. 14, no. 5, p. 497, Jul. 2014, doi: 10.1186/1471-2407-14-497.

[3] G. A. Van Hazel *et al.*, "SIRFLOX: Randomized phase III trial comparing first-line mFOLFOX6 (Plus or Minus Bevacizumab) versus mFOLFOX6 (Plus or Minus Bevacizumab) plus selective internal radiation therapy in patients with metastatic colorectal cancer," *J. Clin. Oncol.*, vol. 34, no. 15, pp. 1723–31, 2016, doi: 10.1200/JCO.2015.66.1181.

[4] H. S. Wasan et al., "First-line selective internal radiotherapy plus chemotherapy versus chemotherapy alone in patients with liver metastases from colorectal cancer (FOXFIRE, SIRFLOX, and FOXFIRE-Global): A combined analysis of three multicentre, randomised, phase 3 trials," Lancet Oncol., pp. 1159–71, 2017, doi: 10.1016/S1470-2045(17)30457-6.

[5] V. Vilgrain et al., "Efficacy and safety of selective internal radiotherapy with yttrium-90 resin microspheres compared with sorafenib in locally advanced and inoperable hepatocellular carcinoma (SARAH): an open-label randomised controlled phase 3 trial," Lancet Oncol., vol. 18, no. 12, pp. 1624–36, 2017, doi: 10.1016/S1470-2045(17)30683-6.

[6] P. K. H. Chow et al., "SIRveNIB: Selective Internal Radiation Therapy Versus Sorafenib in Asia-Pacific Patients with Hepatocellular Carcinoma," J. Clin. Oncol., p. JCO.2017.76.089, 2018, doi: 10.1200/JCO.2017.76.0892.

[7] A. K. T. Tong, Y. H. Kao, C. Too, K. F. W. Chin, D. C. E. Ng, and P. K. H. Chow, "Yttrium-90 hepatic radioembolization: Clinical review and current techniques in interventional radiology and personalized dosimetry," Br. J. Radiol., vol. 89, no. 1062, 2016, doi: 10.1259/bjr.20150943.

[8] C. Chiesa et al., "The conflict between treatment optimization and registration of radiopharmaceuticals with fixed activity posology in oncological nuclear medicine therapy," European Journal of Nuclear Medicine and Molecular Imaging. 2017, doi: 10.1007/s00259-017-3707-3.

[9] A. J. A. T. Braat et al., "Adequate SIRT activity dose is as important as adequate chemotherapy dose," The Lancet Oncology. 2017, doi: 10.1016/S1470-2045(17)30811-2.

[10] K. Sjögreen Gleisner et al., "Variations in the practice of molecular radiotherapy and implementation of dosimetry: results from a European survey," EJNMMI Phys., vol. 4, no. 1, 2017, doi: 10.1186/s40658-017-0193-4.

[11] F. Giammarile, K. Muylle, R. Delgado Bolton, J. Kunikowska, U. Haberkorn, and W. Oyen, "Dosimetry in clinical radio-nuclide therapy: The devil is in the detail," Eur. J. Nucl. Med. Mol. Imaging, vol. 44, no. 12, pp. 1–3, Nov. 2017, doi: 10.1007/s00259-017-3820-3.

[12] M. L. J. Smits et al., "Radioembolization Dosimetry: The Road Ahead," Cardiovasc. Intervent. Radiol., vol. 38, no. 2, pp. 261–69, Apr. 2015, doi: 10.1007/s00270-014-1042-7.

[13] H. Ahmadzadehfar et al., "The significance of 99mTc-MAA SPECT/CT liver perfusion imaging in treatment planning for 90Y-microsphere selective internal radiation treatment.," J. Nucl. Med., vol. 51, no. 8, pp. 1206–12, 2010, doi: 10.2967/jnumed.109.074559.

[14] Sirtex Medical Limited, "Sirtex Package Insert," 2017.

[15] M. Elschot et al., "99mTc-MAA overestimates the absorbed dose to the lungs in radioembolization: a quantitative evaluation in patients treated with 166Ho-microspheres," Eur. J. Nucl. Med. Mol. Imaging, vol. 41, no. 10, pp. 1965–75, Oct. 2014, doi: 10.1007/s00259-014-2784-9.

[16] N. Yu et al., "Lung Dose Calculation With SPECT/CT for 90Yittrium Radioembolization of Liver Cancer," Int. J. Radiat. Oncol., vol. 85, no. 3, pp. 834–39, Mar. 2013, doi: 10.1016/j.ijrobp.2012.06.051.

[17] Y. H. Kao et al., "Personalized predictive lung dosimetry by technetium-99m macroaggregated albumin SPECT/CT for yttrium-90 radioembolization," EJNMMI Res., vol. 4, no. 1, p. 33, Dec. 2014, doi: 10.1186/s13550-014-0033-7.

[18] S. Ho et al., "Partition model for estimating radiation doses from yttrium-90 microspheres in treating hepatic tumours," Eur. J. Nucl. Med., vol. 23, no. 8, pp. 947–52, 1996, doi: 10.1007/BF01084369.

[19] S. A. Gulec, G. Mesoloras, and M. Stabin, "Dosimetric Techniques in 90 Y-Microsphere Therapy of Liver Cancer: The MIRD Equations for Dose Calculations," pp. 1209–12, 2016.

[20] M. L. J. Smits et al., "Holmium-166 radioembolization for the treatment of patients with liver metastases: design of the phase I HEPAR trial," J. Exp. Clin. Cancer Res., vol. 29, p. 70, 2010, doi: 10.1186/1756-9966-29-70.

[21] Biocompatibles UK Ltd, "Package Insert – TheraSphere® Yttrium-90 Glass Microspheres – Rev. 14," 2014.

[22] B. Gray et al., "Randomised trial of SIR-Spheres® plus chemotherapy vs. chemotherapy alone for treating patients with liver metastases from primary large bowel cancer," Ann. Oncol., vol. 12, no. 12, pp. 1711–20, Dec. 2001, doi: 10.1023/A:1013569329846.

[23] Sirtex Medical Limited, "SIR-Spheres Y90 Package Insert (CR1759)," 2014.

[24] J. N. Vauthey et al., "Body surface area and body weight predict total liver volume in western adults," Liver Transplant., vol. 8, no. 3, pp. 233–40, 2002, doi: 10.1053/jlts.2002.31654.

[25] M. L. J. Smits et al., "Holmium-166 radioembolisation in patients with unresectable, chemorefractory liver metastases (HEPAR trial): A phase 1, dose-escalation study," Lancet Oncol., vol. 13, no. 10, pp. 1025–34, 2012, doi: 10.1016/S1470-2045(12)70334-0.

[26] A. J. A. T. Braat, J. F. Prince, R. van Rooij, R. C. G. Bruijnen, M. A. A. J. van den Bosch, and M. G. E. H. Lam, "Safety analysis of holmium-166 microsphere scout dose imaging during radioembolisation work-up: A cohort study," Eur. Radiol., vol. 28, no. 3, pp. 920–28, 2018, doi: 10.1007/s00330-017-4998-2.

[27] M. L. J. Smits et al., "The superior predictive value of 166Ho-scout compared with 99mTc-macroaggregated albumin prior to 166Ho-microspheres radioembolization in patients with liver metastases," Eur. J. Nucl. Med. Mol. Imaging, Aug. 2019, doi: 10.1007/s00259-019-04460-y.

[28] R. Bastiaannet et al., "First evidence for a dose-response relationship in patients treated with 166 Ho-radioembolization: a prospective study," J. Nucl. Med., p. jnumed.119.232751, Oct. 2019, doi: 10.2967/jnumed.119.232751.

[29] D. Coldwell, B. Sangro, R. Salem, H. Wasan, and A. Kennedy, "Radioembolization in the treatment of unresectable liver tumors: experience across a range of primary cancers," *Am. J. Clin. Oncol.*, vol. 35, no. 2, pp. 167–77, 2012, doi: 10.1097/COC.0b013e3181f47923.

[30] A. S. Kennedy *et al.*, "Treatment Parameters and Outcome in 680 Treatments of Internal Radiation with Resin 90Y-Microspheres for Unresectable Hepatic Tumors," *Int. J. Radiat. Oncol. Biol. Phys.*, vol. 74, no. 5, pp. 1494–1500, 2009, doi: 10.1016/j.ijrobp.2008.10.005.

[31] M. N. G. J. A. Braat, K. J. van Erpecum, B. A. Zonnenberg, M. A. J. van den Bosch, and M. G. E. H. Lam, "Radioembolization-induced liver disease," *Eur. J. Gastroenterol. Hepatol.*, vol. 29, no. 2, pp. 144–52, 2017, doi: 10.1097/MEG.0000000000000772.

[32] D. Y. Sze and M. G. E. H. Lam, "Reply to 'the limitations of theoretical dose modeling for yttrium-90 radioembolization,'" *J. Vasc. Interv. Radiol.*, vol. 25, no. 7, pp. 1147–48, 2014, doi: 10.1016/j.jvir.2014.04.004.

[33] Y. H. Kao, E. H. Tan, C. E. Ng, and S. W. Goh, "Clinical implications of the body surface area method versus partition model dosimetry for yttrium-90 radioembolization using resin microspheres: a technical review," *Ann. Nucl. Med.*, vol. 25, no. 7, pp. 455–61, Aug. 2011, doi: 10.1007/s12149-011-0499-6.

[34] G. Flux *et al.*, "Clinical radionuclide therapy dosimetry: the quest for the 'Holy Gray,'" *Eur. J. Nucl. Med. Mol. Imaging*, vol. 34, no. 10, pp. 1699–1700, Sep. 2007, doi: 10.1007/s00259-007-0471-9.

[35] M. G. E. H. Lam, J. D. Louie, M. H. K. Abdelmaksoud, G. A. Fisher, C. D. Cho-Phan, and D. Y. Sze, "Limitations of body surface area-based activity calculation for radioembolization of hepatic metastases in colorectal cancer," *J. Vasc. Interv. Radiol.*, vol. 25, no. 7, pp. 1085–93, 2014, doi: 10.1016/j.jvir.2013.11.018.

[36] M. Bernardini *et al.*, "Liver Selective Internal Radiation Therapy with 90Y resin microspheres: Comparison between pretreatment activity calculation methods," *Phys. Medica*, vol. 30, no. 7, pp. 752–64, 2014, doi: 10.1016/j.ejmp.2014.05.004.

[37] M. Samim *et al.*, "Recommendations for radioembolisation after liver surgery using yttrium-90 resin microspheres based on a survey of an international expert panel," *Eur. Radiol.*, 2017, doi: 10.1007/s00330-017-4889-6.

[38] R. Bastiaannet, S. C. Kappadath, B. Kunnen, A. J. A. T. Braat, M. G. E. H. Lam, and H. W. A. M. de Jong, "The physics of radioembolization," *EJNMMI Physics*. 2018, doi: 10.1186/s40658-018-0221-z.

[39] S. Gnesin *et al.*, "Partition Model-Based 99mTc-MAA SPECT/CT Predictive Dosimetry Compared with 90Y TOF PET/CT Posttreatment Dosimetry in Radioembolization of Hepatocellular Carcinoma: A Quantitative Agreement Comparison," *J. Nucl. Med.*, vol. 57, no. 11, pp. 1672–78, 2016, doi: 10.2967/jnumed.116.173104.

[40] M. Wondergem *et al.*, "99mTc-Macroaggregated Albumin Poorly Predicts the Intrahepatic Distribution of 90Y Resin Microspheres in Hepatic Radioembolization," *J. Nucl. Med.*, vol. 54, no. 8, pp. 1294–1301, Aug. 2013, doi: 10.2967/jnumed.112.117614.

[41] H. Ilhan *et al.*, "Predictive Value of 99mTc-MAA SPECT for 90Y-Labeled Resin Microsphere Distribution in Radioembolization of Primary and Secondary Hepatic Tumors," *J. Nucl. Med.*, vol. 56, no. 11, pp. 1654–60, Nov. 2015, doi: 10.2967/jnumed.115.162685.

[42] P. Haste *et al.*, "Correlation of Technetium-99m Macroaggregated Albumin and Yttrium-90 Glass Microsphere Biodistribution in Hepatocellular Carcinoma: A Retrospective Review of Pretreatment Single Photon Emission CT and Posttreatment Positron Emission Tomography/CT," *J. Vasc. Interv. Radiol.*, pp. 1–10, 2017, doi: 10.1016/j.jvir.2016.12.1221.

[43] S. A. Gulec, G. Mesoloras, and M. Stabin, "Dosimetric techniques in 90Y-microsphere therapy of liver cancer: The MIRD equations for dose calculations," *J. Nucl. Med.*, vol. 47, pp. 1209–11, 2006, PMID: 16818957.

[44] J. K. Mikell, A. Mahvash, W. Siman, V. Baladandayuthapani, F. Mourtada, and S. C. Kappadath, "Selective Internal Radiation Therapy with Yttrium-90 Glass Microspheres: Biases and Uncertainties in Absorbed Dose Calculations Between Clinical Dosimetry Models," *Int. J. Radiat. Oncol. Biol. Phys.*, vol. 96, no. 4, pp. 888–96, 2016, doi: 10.1016/j.ijrobp.2016.07.021.

[45] Y. H. Kao *et al.*, "Image-Guided Personalized Predictive Dosimetry by Artery-Specific SPECT/CT Partition Modeling for Safe and Effective 90Y Radioembolization," *J. Nucl. Med.*, vol. 53, no. 4, pp. 559–66, Apr. 2012, doi: 10.2967/jnumed.111.097469.

[46] W. V Vogel *et al.*, "Evaluation of image registration in PET/CT of the liver and recommendations for optimized imaging," *J. Nucl. Med.*, vol. 48, no. 6, pp. 910–19, 2007, doi: 10.2967/jnumed.107.041517.

[47] J. Boda-Heggemann *et al.*, "Deep Inspiration Breath Hold – Based Radiation Therapy: A Clinical Review," *Int. J. Radiat. Oncol. Biol. Phys.*, vol. 94, no. 3, pp. 478–92, 2016, doi: 10.1016/j.ijrobp.2015.11.049.

[48] M. F. Kruis, J. B. van de Kamer, J. S. A. Belderbos, J.-J. Sonke, and M. van Herk, "4D CT amplitude binning for the generation of a time-averaged 3D mid-position CT scan," *Phys. Med. Biol.*, vol. 59, no. 18, p. 5517, 2014, doi: 10.1088/0031-9155/59/18/5517.

[49] C. Liu, L. A. Pierce II, A. M. Alessio, and P. E. Kinahan, "The impact of respiratory motion on tumor quantification and delineation in static PET/CT imaging," *Phys. Med. Biol.*, vol. 54, no. 24, pp. 7345–62, Dec. 2009, doi: 10.1088/0031-9155/54/24/007.

[50] J. R. McClelland, D. J. Hawkes, T. Schaeffter, and A. P. King, "Respiratory motion models: A review," *Med. Image Anal.*, vol. 17, no. 1, pp. 19–42, Jan. 2013, doi: 10.1016/j.media.2012.09.005.

[51] W. Siman, O. R. Mawlawi, J. K. Mikell, F. Mourtada, and S. C. Kappadath, "Effects of image noise, respiratory motion, and motion compensation on 3D activity quantification in count-limited PET images," *Phys. Med. Biol.*, vol. 62, no. 2, pp. 448–64, Jan. 2017, doi: 10.1088/1361-6560/aa5088.

[52] R. Bastiaannet, M. A. Viergever, and H. W. A. M. de Jong, "Impact of respiratory motion and acquisition settings on SPECT liver dosimetry for radioembolization," *Med. Phys.*, vol. 44, no. 10, pp. 5270–79, Oct. 2017, doi: 10.1002/mp.12483.

[53] R. M. Kessler, J. R. Ellis, and M. Eden, "Analysis of emission tomographic scan data: Limitations imposed by resolution and background," *Journal of computer assisted tomography*, vol. 8, no. 3. pp. 514–22, 1984, doi: 10.1097/00004728-198406000-00028.

[54] M. A. King, D. T. Long, and A. B. Brill, "SPECT volume quantitation: influence of spatial resolution, source size and shape, and voxel size," *Med. Phys.*, vol. 18, no. 5, pp. 1016–24, 1991, doi: 10.1118/1.596737.

[55] J. A. Lee, "Segmentation of positron emission tomography images: Some recommendations for target delineation in radiation oncology," *Radiother. Oncol.*, vol. 96, no. 3, pp. 302–07, 2010, doi: 10.1016/j.radonc.2010.07.003.

[56] E. Garin *et al.*, "Effectiveness of quantitative MAA SPECT/CT for the definition of vascularized hepatic volume and dosimetric approach: phantom validation and clinical preliminary results in patients with complex hepatic vascularization treated with yttrium-90-labeled micr," *Nucl Med Commun*, vol. 32, no. 12, pp. 1245–55, 2011, doi: 10.1097/MNM.0b013e32834a716b.

[57] E. Garin *et al.*, "Utility of Quantitative 99m Tc-MAA SPECT/CT for 90 yttrium-Labelled Microsphere Treatment Planning: Calculating Vascularized Hepatic Volume and Dosimetric Approach," *Int. J. Mol. Imaging*, vol. 2011, no. 3, pp. 1–8, 2011, doi: 10.1155/2011/398051.

[58] M. G. E. H. Lam, M. L. Goris, A. H. Iagaru, E. S. Mittra, J. D. Louie, and D. Y. Sze, "Prognostic utility of 90Y radioembolization dosimetry based on fusion 99mTc-macroaggregated albumin-99mTc-sulfur colloid SPECT," *J. Nucl. Med.*, vol. 54, no. 12, pp. 2055–61, 2013, doi: 10.2967/jnumed.113.123257.

[59] Y.-H. Kao *et al.*, "Post-radioembolization yttrium-90 PET/CT - part 2: dose-response and tumor predictive dosimetry for resin microspheres," *EJNMMI Res.*, vol. 3, no. 1, 2013, doi: 10.1186/2191-219X-3-57.

[60] B. R. Eaton *et al.*, "Quantitative dosimetry for yttrium-90 radionuclide therapy: Tumor dose predicts fluorodeoxyglucose positron emission tomography response in hepatic metastatic melanoma," *J. Vasc. Interv. Radiol.*, vol. 25, no. 2, pp. 288–95, Feb. 2014, doi: 10.1016/j.jvir.2013.08.021.

[61] M. Cremonesi *et al.*, "Radioembolization of Hepatic Lesions from a Radiobiology and Dosimetric Perspective," *Front. Oncol.*, vol. 4, no. August, pp. 1–20, 2014, doi: 10.3389/fonc.2014.00210.

[62] P. Flamen *et al.*, "Multimodality imaging can predict the metabolic response of unresectable colorectal liver metastases to radioembolization therapy with Yttrium-90 labeled resin microspheres," *Phys. Med. Biol.*, vol. 53, no. 22, pp. 6591–603, 2008, doi: 10.1088/0031-9155/53/22/019.

[63] S. M. Srinivas *et al.*, "Determination of Radiation Absorbed Dose to Primary Liver Tumors and Normal Liver Tissue Using Post-Radioembolization 90Y PET," *Front. Oncol.*, vol. 4, no. October, p. 255, 2014, doi: 10.3389/fonc.2014.00255.

[64] K. P. Willowson *et al.*, "Clinical and imaging-based prognostic factors in radioembolisation of liver metastases from colorectal cancer: a retrospective exploratory analysis," *EJNMMI Res.*, vol. 7, no. 1, p. 46, 2017, doi: 10.1186/s13550-017-0292-1.

[65] J. F. Fowler, "21 Years of biologically effective dose," *Br. J. Radiol.*, vol. 83, no. 991, pp. 554–68, 2010, doi: 10.1259/bjr/31372149.

[66] C. Chiesa *et al.*, "Radioembolization of hepatocarcinoma with 90Y glass microspheres: development of an individualized treatment planning strategy based on dosimetry and radiobiology," *Eur. J. Nucl. Med. Mol. Imaging*, vol. 42, no. 11, pp. 1718–38, 2015, doi: 10.1007/s00259-015-3068-8.

[67] F. Botta *et al.*, "Impact of missing attenuation and scatter corrections on 99mTc-MAA SPECT 3D dosimetry for liver radioembolization using the patient relative calibration methodology: a retrospective investigation on clinical images," *Med. Phys.*, doi: 10.1002/MP.12774.

[68] L. C. Jones and P. W. Hoban, "Treatment plan comparison using equivalent uniform biologically effective dose (EUBED)," *Phys. Med. Biol.*, vol. 45, no. 1, pp. 159–70, 2000, doi: 10.1088/0031-9155/45/1/311.

[69] A. C. Bourgeois, T. T. Chang, Y. C. Bradley, S. N. Acuff, and A. S. Pasciak, "Intraprocedural yttrium-90 positron emission tomography/CT for treatment optimization of yttrium-90 radioembolization," *J. Vasc. Interv. Radiol.*, vol. 25, no. 2, pp. 271–75, 2014, doi: 10.1016/j.jvir.2013.11.004.

[70] S. Walrand, M. Hesse, G. Demonceau, S. Pauwels, and F. Jamar, "Yttrium-90-labeled microsphere tracking during liver selective internal radiotherapy by bremsstrahlung pinhole SPECT: feasibility study and evaluation in an abdominal phantom," *EJNMMI Res.*, vol. 1, no. 1, p. 32, 2011, doi: 10.1186/2191-219X-1-32.

[71] C. Beijst, M. Elschot, M. A. Viergever, and H. W. A. M. de Jong, "Toward Simultaneous Real-Time Fluoroscopic and Nuclear Imaging in the Intervention Room," *Radiology*, vol. 278, no. 1, pp. 232–38, 2016, doi: 10.1148/radiol.2015142749.

[72] S. Van Der Velden, C. Beijst, M. A. Viergever, and H. W. A. M. De Jong, "Simultaneous fluoroscopic and nuclear imaging: Impact of collimator choice on nuclear image quality: Impact," *Med. Phys.*, vol. 44, no. 1, pp. 249–61, 2017, doi: 10.1002/mp.12010.

[73] S. Van Der Velden, R. Bastiaannet, A. J. A. T. Braat, M. G. E. H. Lam, M. A. Viergever, and H. W. A. M. De Jong, "Estimation of lung shunt fraction from simultaneous fluoroscopic and nuclear images," *Phys. Med. Biol.*, 2017, doi: 10.1088/1361-6560/aa8840.

[74] G. H. Van De Maat *et al.*, "MRI-based biodistribution assessment of holmium-166 poly(L-lactic acid) microspheres after radioembolisation," *Eur. Radiol.*, vol. 23, no. 3, pp. 827–35, 2013, doi: 10.1007/s00330-012-2648-2.

[75] M. L. J. Smits *et al.*, "In Vivo Dosimetry Based on SPECT and MR Imaging of 166Ho-Microspheres for Treatment of Liver Malignancies," *J. Nucl. Med.*, vol. 54, no. 12, pp. 2093–2100, 2013, doi: 10.2967/jnumed.113.119768.

[76] J. H. Seppenwoolde, L. W. Bartels, R. Van Der Weide, J. F. W. Nijsen, A. D. Van Het Schip, and C. J. G. Bakker, "Fully MR-guided hepatic artery catheterization for selective drug delivery: A feasibility study in pigs," *J. Magn. Reson. Imaging*, vol. 23, no. 2, pp. 123–29, 2006, doi: 10.1002/jmri.20479.

[77] Y. K. Dewaraja *et al.*, "MIRD Pamphlet No. 23: Quantitative SPECT for Patient-Specific 3-Dimensional Dosimetry in Internal Radionuclide Therapy," *J. Nucl. Med.*, vol. 53, no. 8, pp. 1310–25, 2012, doi: 10.2967/jnumed.111.100123.

[78] M. Pacilio *et al.*, "Impact of SPECT corrections on 3D-dosimetry for liver transarterial radioembolization using the patient relative calibration methodology," *Med. Phys.*, vol. 43, no. 7, pp. 4053–64, 2016, doi: 10.1118/1.4953203.

[79] E. C. Frey, J. L. Humm, and M. Ljungberg, "Accuracy and Precision of Radioactivity Quantification in Nuclear Medicine Images," vol. 42, no. 3, pp. 208–18, 2013, doi: 10.1053/j.semnuclmed.2011.11.003.Accuracy.

[80] D. L. Bailey and K. P. Willowson, "Quantitative SPECT/CT: SPECT joins PET as a quantitative imaging modality," *Eur. J. Nucl. Med. Mol. Imaging*, vol. 41, no. S1, pp. 17–25, May 2014, doi: 10.1007/s00259-013-2542-4.

[81] D. L. Bailey and K. P. Willowson, "An Evidence-Based Review of Quantitative SPECT Imaging and Potential Clinical Applications," *J. Nucl. Med.*, vol. 54, no. 1, pp. 83–89, 2013, doi: 10.2967/jnumed.112.111476.

[82] J. Zeintl, A. H. Vija, A. Yahil, J. Hornegger, and T. Kuwert, "Quantitative Accuracy of Clinical 99mTc SPECT/CT Using Ordered-Subset Expectation Maximization with 3-Dimensional Resolution Recovery, Attenuation, and Scatter Correction," *J. Nucl. Med.*, vol. 51, no. 6, pp. 921–28, Jun. 2010, doi: 10.2967/jnumed.109.071571.

[83] H. Vija, "Introduction to xSPECT* Technology: Evolving Multi-modal SPECT to Become Context-based and Quantitative," 2013.

[84] M. Elschot, J. F. W. Nijsen, A. J. Dam, and H. W. A. M. de Jong, "Quantitative evaluation of scintillation camera imaging characteristics of isotopes used in liver radioembolization," *PLoS One*, vol. 6, no. 11, 2011, doi: 10.1371/journal.pone.0026174.

[85] S. Shen, G. L. DeNardo, A. Yuan, D. A. DeNardo, and S. J. DeNardo, "Planar gamma camera imaging and quantitation of yttrium-90 bremsstrahlung," *J. Nucl. Med.*, vol. 35, no. 8, pp. 1381–89, 1994.

[86] X. Rong, Y. Du, M. Ljungberg, E. Rault, S. Vandenberghe, and E. C. Frey, "Development and evaluation of an improved quantitative 90Y bremsstrahlung SPECT method," *Med. Phys.*, vol. 39, no. 5, p. 2346, 2012, doi: 10.1118/1.3700174.

[87] M. Elschot, M. G. E. H. Lam, M. A. A. J. van den Bosch, M. A. Viergever, and H. W. A. M. de Jong, "Quantitative Monte Carlo-Based 90Y SPECT Reconstruction," *J. Nucl. Med.*, vol. 54, no. 9, pp. 1557–63, Sep. 2013, doi: 10.2967/jnumed.112.119131.

[88] D. Minarik, K. Sjögreen Gleisner, and M. Ljungberg, "Evaluation of quantitative (90)Y SPECT based on experimental phantom studies," *Phys. Med. Biol.*, vol. 53, no. 20, pp. 5689–703, 2008, doi: 10.1088/0031-9155/53/20/008.

[89] R. Lhommel *et al.*, "Yttrium-90 TOF PET scan demonstrates high-resolution biodistribution after liver SIRT," *Eur. J. Nucl. Med. Mol. Imaging*, vol. 36, no. 10, p. 1696, 2009, doi: 10.1007/s00259-009-1210-1.

[90] V. L. Gates, A. A. H. Esmail, K. Marshall, S. Spies, and R. Salem, "Internal Pair Production of 90Y Permits Hepatic Localization of Microspheres Using Routine PET: Proof of Concept," *J. Nucl. Med.*, vol. 52, no. 1, pp. 72–76, 2011, doi: 10.2967/jnumed.110.080986.

[91] T. Carlier *et al.*, "Assessment of acquisition protocols for routine imaging of Y-90 using PET/CT," *EJNMMI Res.*, vol. 3, no. 1, p. 11, 2013, doi: 10.1186/2191-219X-3-11.

[92] V. L. Gates, R. Salem, and R. J. Lewandowski, "Positron emission tomography/CT after yttrium-90 radioembolization: Current and future applications," *J. Vasc. Interv. Radiol.*, vol. 24, no. 8, pp. 1153–55, 2013, doi: 10.1016/j.jvir.2013.06.014.

[93] K. Willowson, N. Forwood, B. W. Jakoby, A. M. Smith, and D. L. Bailey, "Quantitative 90Y image reconstruction in PET," *Med. Phys.*, vol. 39, no. 11, pp. 7153–59, 2012, doi: 10.1118/1.4762403.

[94] C. L. Wright, K. Binzel, J. Zhang, E. J. Wuthrick, and M. V. Knopp, "Clinical feasibility of 90Y digital PET/CT for imaging microsphere biodistribution following radioembolization," *Eur. J. Nucl. Med. Mol. Imaging*, pp. 1–4, 2017, doi: 10.1007/s00259-017-3694-4.

[95] E. Fourkal *et al.*, "3D inpatient dose reconstruction from the PET-CT imaging of 90Y microspheres for metastatic cancer to the liver: feasibility study," *Med. Phys.*, vol. 40, no. 8, p. 081702, 2013, doi: 10.1118/1.4810939.

[96] Y. S. Song *et al.*, "PET/CT-Based Dosimetry in 90Y-Microsphere Selective Internal Radiation Therapy," *Medicine (Baltimore)*, vol. 94, no. 23, p. e945, Jun. 2015, doi: 10.1097/MD.0000000000000945.

[97] S. C. Ng *et al.*, "Patient dosimetry for 90Y selective internal radiation treatment based on 90Y PET imaging," *J. Appl. Clin. Med. Phys.*, vol. 14, no. 5, pp. 212–21, 2013, doi: sd.

[98] T. Carlier, K. P. Willowson, E. Fourkal, D. L. Bailey, M. Doss, and M. Conti, "90 Y -PET imaging: Exploring limitations and accuracy under conditions of low counts and high random fraction," *Med. Phys.*, vol. 42, no. 7, pp. 4295–4309, 2015, doi: 10.1118/1.4922685.

[99] J. Strydhorst, T. Carlier, A. Dieudonne, M. Conti, and I. Buvat, "A gate evaluation of the sources of error in quantitative 90Y PET," *Med Phys*, vol. 43, no. 10, pp. 5320–29, 2016, doi: 10.1118/1.4961747.

[100] L. van Elmbt, S. Vandenberghe, S. Walrand, S. Pauwels, and F. Jamar, "Comparison of yttrium-90 quantitative imaging by TOF and non-TOF PET in a phantom of liver selective internal radiotherapy," *Phys. Med. Biol.*, vol. 56, no. 21, pp. 6759–77, 2011, doi: 10.1088/0031-9155/56/21/001.

[101] M. Eldib, N. Oesingmann, D. D. Faul, L. Kostakoglu, K. Knešaurek, and Z. A. Fayad, "Optimization of yttrium-90 PET for simultaneous PET/MR imaging: A phantom study," *Med. Phys.*, vol. 43, no. 8, pp. 4768–74, 2016, doi: 10.1118/1.4958958.

[102] R. Boellaard *et al.*, "FDG PET/CT: EANM procedure guidelines for tumour imaging: version 2.0," *Eur. J. Nucl. Med. Mol. Imaging*, vol. 42, no. 2, pp. 328–54, 2014, doi: 10.1007/s00259-014-2961-x.

[103] K. P. Willowson *et al.*, "A multicentre comparison of quantitative 90Y PET/CT for dosimetric purposes after radioembolization with resin microspheres: The QUEST Phantom Study," *Eur. J. Nucl. Med. Mol. Imaging*, vol. 42, no. 8, pp. 1202–22, 2015, doi: 10.1007/s00259-015-3059-9.

[104] S. A. Padia, A. Alessio, S. W. Kwan, D. H. Lewis, S. Vaidya, and S. Minoshima, "Comparison of positron emission tomography and bremsstrahlung imaging to detect particle distribution in patients undergoing yttrium-90 radioembolization for large hepatocellular carcinomas or associated portal vein thrombosis," *J. Vasc. Interv. Radiol.*, vol. 24, no. 8, 2013, doi: 10.1016/j.jvir.2013.04.018.

[105] Y. H. Kao, E. H. Tan, C. E. Ng, and S. W. Goh, "Yttrium-90 time-of-flight PET/CT is superior to Bremsstrahlung SPECT/CT for postradioembolization imaging of microsphere biodistribution.," *Clin. Nucl. Med.*, vol. 36, no. 12, pp. e186–87, 2011, doi: 10.1097/RLU.0b013e31821c9a11.

[106] M. Elschot, B. J. Vermolen, M. G. E. H. Lam, B. de Keizer, M. A. A. J. van den Bosch, and H. W. A. M. de Jong, "Quantitative Comparison of PET and Bremsstrahlung SPECT for Imaging the In Vivo Yttrium-90 Microsphere Distribution after Liver Radioembolization," *PLoS One*, vol. 8, no. 2, 2013, doi: 10.1371/journal.pone.0055742.

[107] P. R. Seevinck *et al.*, "Factors affecting the sensitivity and detection limits of MRI, CT, and SPECT for multimodal diagnostic and therapeutic agents.," *Anticancer. Agents Med. Chem.*, vol. 7, no. 3, pp. 317–34, 2007, doi: 10.2174/187152007780618153.

[108] M. Elschot *et al.*, "Quantitative Monte Carlo-based holmium-166 SPECT reconstruction," *Med. Phys.*, vol. 40, no. 11, p. 112502, Oct. 2013, doi: 10.1118/1.4823788.

[109] T. C. de Wit *et al.*, "Hybrid scatter correction applied to quantitative holmium-166 SPECT," *Phys. Med. Biol.*, vol. 51, no. 19, pp. 4773–87, 2006, doi: 10.1088/0031-9155/51/19/004.

[110] M. L. J. Smits *et al.*, "In Vivo Dosimetry Based on SPECT and MR Imaging of 166 Ho-Microspheres for Treatment of Liver Malignancies," doi: 10.2967/jnumed.113.119768.

[111] H. Choi *et al.*, "Correlation of computed tomography and positron emission tomography in patients with metastatic gastro-intestinal stromal tumor treated at a single institution with imatinib mesylate: Proposal of new computed tomography response criteria," *J. Clin. Oncol.*, vol. 25, no. 13, pp. 1753–59, 2007, doi: 10.1200/JCO.2006.07.3049.

[112] M. N. Kim, B. K. Kim, K.-H. Han, and S. U. Kim, "Evolution from WHO to EASL and mRECIST for hepatocellular car-cinoma: Considerations for tumor response assessment," *Expert Rev. Gastroenterol. Hepatol.*, vol. 9, no. 3, pp. 335–48, 2015, doi: 10.1586/17474124.2015.959929.

[113] A. Riaz *et al.*, "Role of the EASL, RECIST, and WHO response guidelines alone or in combination for hepatocellular carcinoma: Radiologic–pathologic correlation," *J. Hepatol.*, vol. 54, no. 4, pp. 695–704, Apr. 2011, doi: 10.1016/j.jhep.2010.10.004.

[114] D. Hipps, F. Ausania, D. M. Manas, J. D. G. Rose, and J. J. French, "Selective Interarterial Radiation Therapy (SIRT) in colorectal liver metastases: How do we monitor response?" *HPB Surg.*, vol. 2013, 2013, doi: 10.1155/2013/570808.

[115] R. Bastiaannet, M. A. Lodge, H. W. A. M. de Jong, and M. G. E. H. Lam, "The Unique Role of Fluorodeoxyglucose-PET in Radioembolization," *PET Clin.*, vol. 14, no. 4, pp. 447–57, Oct. 2019, doi: 10.1016/j.cpet.2019.06.002.

[116] E. Garin *et al.*, "Boosted selective internal radiation therapy with 90Y-loaded glass microspheres (B-SIRT) for hepatocellular carcinoma patients: A new personalized promising concept," *Eur. J. Nucl. Med. Mol. Imaging*, vol. 40, no. 7, pp. 1057–68, 2013, doi: 10.1007/s00259-013-2395-x.

[117] E. Garin *et al.*, "Dosimetry Based on 99mTc-Macroaggregated Albumin SPECT/CT Accurately Predicts Tumor Response and Survival in Hepatocellular Carcinoma Patients Treated with 90Y-Loaded Glass Microspheres: Preliminary Results," *J. Nucl. Med.*, vol. 53, no. 2, pp. 255–63, 2012, doi: 10.2967/jnumed.111.094235.

[118] K. T. Chan *et al.*, "Prospective trial using internal pair-production positron emission tomography to establish the Yttrium-90 radioembolization dose required for response of hepatocellular carcinoma," *Int. J. Radiat. Oncol.*, vol. 0, no. 0, 2018, doi: 10.1016/j.ijrobp.2018.01.116.

[119] S. C. Kappadath, J. Mikell, A. Balagopal, V. Baladandayuthapani, A. Kaseb, and A. Mahvash, "Hepatocellular Carcinoma Tumor Dose Response following 90 Y-radioembolization with glass microspheres using 90 Y-SPECT/CT based Voxel Dosimetry," *Int. J. Radiat. Oncol.*, Jun. 2018, doi: 10.1016/j.ijrobp.2018.05.062.

[120] K. J. Fowler *et al.*, "PET/MRI of Hepatic 90Y Microsphere Deposition Determines Individual Tumor Response," *Cardiovasc. Intervent. Radiol.*, vol. 39, no. 6, pp. 855–64, 2016, doi: 10.1007/s00270-015-1285-y.

[121] L. Strigari *et al.*, "Efficacy and toxicity related to treatment of hepatocellular carcinoma with 90Y-SIR spheres: Radiobiologic considerations.," *J. Nucl. Med.*, vol. 51, no. 9, pp. 1377–85, 2010, doi: 10.2967/jnumed.110.075861.

[122] P. Flamen *et al.*, "Corrigendum: Multimodality imaging can predict the metabolic response of unresectable colorectal liver metastases to radioembolization therapy with Yttrium-90 labeled resin microspheres," *Phys. Med. Biol.*, vol. 59, no. 10, pp. 2549–51, May 2014, doi: 10.1088/0031-9155/59/10/2549.

[123] A. F. van den Hoven *et al.*, "Insights into the Dose-Response Relationship of Radioembolization with Resin 90Y-Microspheres: A Prospective Cohort Study in Patients with Colorectal Cancer Liver Metastases," *J. Nucl. Med.*, vol. 57, no. 7, pp. 1014–19, 2016, doi: 10.2967/jnumed.115.166942.

[124] O. Chansanti *et al.*, "Tumor Dose Response in Yttrium-90 Resin Microsphere Embolization for Neuroendocrine Liver Metastases: A Tumor-Specific Analysis with Dose Estimation Using SPECT-CT," *J. Vasc. Interv. Radiol.*, pp. 1–8, 2017, doi: 10.1016/j.jvir.2017.07.008.

[125] C. Chiesa *et al.*, "A dosimetric treatment planning strategy in radioembolization of hepatocarcinoma with 90Y glass microspheres," *Q. J. Nucl. Med. Mol. Imaging*, vol. 56, no. 6, pp. 503–9, 2012.

[126] R. A. Fox, P. F. Klemp, G. Egan, L. L. Mina, M. A. Burton, and B. N. Gray, "Dose distribution following selective internal radiation therapy," *Int. J. Radiat. Oncol. Biol. Phys.*, vol. 21, no. 2, pp. 463–67, 1991, doi: 10.1016/0360-3016(91)90797-8.

[127] E. D. Yorke, A. Jackson, R. A. Fox, B. W. Wessels, and B. N. Gray, "Can current models explain the lack of liver complications in Y-90 microsphere therapy?" *Clin. Cancer Res.*, vol. 5, no. 10 SUPPL., 1999.

[128] S. Walrand, M. Hesse, C. Chiesa, R. Lhommel, and F. Jamar, "The low hepatic toxicity per Gray of 90Y glass microspheres is linked to their transport in the arterial tree favoring a nonuniform trapping as observed in posttherapy PET imaging," *J. Nucl. Med.*, vol. 55, no. 1, pp. 135–40, 2014, doi: 10.2967/jnumed.113.126839.

[129] J. Högberg *et al.*, "Increased absorbed liver dose in Selective Internal Radiation Therapy (SIRT) correlates with increased sphere-cluster frequency and absorbed dose inhomogeneity," *EJNMMI Phys.*, vol. 2, no. 1, p. 10, Dec. 2015, doi: 10.1186/s40658-015-0113-4.

[130] J. Högberg *et al.*, "Simulation Model of Microsphere Distribution for Selective Internal Radiation Therapy Agrees with Observations," *Int. J. Radiat. Oncol.*, vol. 96, no. 2, pp. 414–21, Oct. 2016, doi: 10.1016/j.ijrobp.2016.05.007.

[131] A. S. Pasciak, A. C. Bourgeois, and Y. C. Bradley, "A Microdosimetric Analysis of Absorbed Dose to Tumor as a Function of Number of Microspheres per Unit Volume in 90Y Radioembolization," *J. Nucl. Med.*, vol. 57, no. 7, pp. 1020–26, 2016, doi: 10.2967/jnumed.115.163444.

[132] A. M. Campbell, I. H. Bailey, and M. A. Burton, "Analysis of the distribution of intra-arterial microspheres in human liver following hepatic yttrium-90 microsphere therapy," *Phys. Med. Biol.*, vol. 45, no. 4, pp. 1023–33, 2000, doi: 10.1088/0031-9155/45/4/316.

[133] I. Kawrakow, "The EGSnrc Code System: Monte Carlo Simulation of Electron and Photon Transport," *Med. Phys.*, vol. 34, pp. 4818–53, 2007, doi: 10.1118/1.598917.

[134] G. W. McKinney, J. W. Durkee, and J. S. Hendricks, "MCNPX 2.5.0 – New Features Demonstrated," *Monte Carlo Method Versatility Unbounded A Dyn. Comput. World*, no. 2005, pp. 1–14, 2005.

[135] V. Andersen *et al.*, "The application of FLUKA to dosimetry and radiation therapy," *Radiat. Prot. Dosimetry*, vol. 116, no. 1–4, pp. 113–17, 2005, doi: 10.1093/rpd/nci040.

[136] D. Sarrut *et al.*, "A review of the use and potential of the GATE Monte Carlo simulation code for radiation therapy and dosimetry applications," *Med. Phys.*, vol. 41, no. 6, p. 064301, 2014, doi: 10.1118/1.4871617.

[137] A. Dieudonne *et al.*, "Study of the Impact of Tissue Density Heterogeneities on 3-Dimensional Abdominal Dosimetry: Comparison Between Dose Kernel Convolution and Direct Monte Carlo Methods," *J. Nucl. Med.*, vol. 54, no. 2, pp. 236–43, Feb. 2013, doi: 10.2967/jnumed.112.105825.

[138] J. K. Mikell, A. Mahvash, W. Siman, F. Mourtada, and S. C. Kappadath, "Comparing voxel-based absorbed dosimetry methods in tumors, liver, lung, and at the liver-lung interface for 90Y microsphere selective internal radiation therapy," *EJNMMI Phys.*, vol. 2, no. 1, p. 16, 2015, doi: 10.1186/s40658-015-0119-y.

[139] A. S. Pasciak and W. D. Erwin, "Effect of voxel size and computation method on Tc-99m MAA SPECT/CT-based dose estimation for Y-90 microsphere therapy," *IEEE Trans. Med. Imaging*, vol. 28, no. 11, pp. 1754–58, 2009, doi: 10.1109/TMI.2009.2022753.

[140] A. S. Pasciak, A. C. Bourgeois, and Y. C. Bradley, "A Comparison of Techniques for (90)Y PET/CT Image-Based Dosimetry Following Radioembolization with Resin Microspheres," *Front. Oncol.*, vol. 4, no. May, p. 121, 2014, doi: 10.3389/fonc.2014.00121.

[141] P. Ritt, H. Vija, J. Hornegger, and T. Kuwert, "Absolute quantification in SPECT," *European Journal of Nuclear Medicine and Molecular Imaging*. 2011, doi: 10.1007/s00259-011-1770-8.

[142] I. Vija, Hans (Siemens Medical Solutions, "Introduction to xSPECT* Technology: Evolving Multi-modal SPECT to Become Context-based and Quantitative," pp. 1–28, 2013.

[143] F. Büther, T. Vehren, K. P. Schäfers, and M. Schäfers, "Impact of Data-driven Respiratory Gating in Clinical PET," *Radiology*, vol. 281, no. 1, pp. 229–38, Oct. 2016, doi: 10.1148/radiol.2016152067.

[144] A. L. Kesner *et al.*, "Validation of Software Gating: A Practical Technology for Respiratory Motion Correction in PET," *Radiology*, vol. 281, no. 1, pp. 239–48, Oct. 2016, doi: 10.1148/radiol.2016152105.

[145] R. Bastiaannet, S. Van Der Velden, M. Lam, M. Viergever, and H. de Jong, "Fast quantitative determination of lung shunt fraction using orthogonal planar projections in hepatic radioembolization," *J. Nucl. Med.*, vol. 57, no. Supplement 2, p. 537, 2016.

[146] U. Eberlein, M. Cremonesi, and M. Lassmann, "Individualized dosimetry for theranostics: Necessary, nice to have, or counterproductive?" *Journal of Nuclear Medicine*. 2017, doi: 10.2967/jnumed.116.186841.

[147] R. G. Selwyn *et al.*, "18F-labeled resin microspheres as surrogates for 90Y resin microspheres used in the treatment of hepatic tumors: a radiolabeling and PET validation study," *Phys. Med. Biol.*, vol. 52, no. 24, pp. 7397–408, 2007, doi: 10.1088/0031-9155/52/24/013.

[148] E. Schiller *et al.*, "Yttrium-86-labelled human serum albumin microspheres: relation of surface structure with in vivo stability," *Nucl. Med. Biol.*, vol. 35, no. 2, pp. 227–32, 2008, doi: 10.1016/j.nucmedbio.2007.10.008.

[149] O. S. Grosser *et al.*, "Pharmacokinetics of 99mTc-MAA- and 99mTc-HSA-Microspheres Used in Preradioembolization Dosimetry: Influence on the Liver-Lung Shunt," *J. Nucl. Med.*, vol. 57, no. 6, pp. 925–27, Jun. 2016, doi: 10.2967/jnumed.115.169987.

[150] M. M. A. Dietze *et al.*, "Performance of a dual-layer scanner for hybrid SPECT/CBCT," *Phys. Med. Biol.*, 2019, doi: 10.1088/1361-6560/ab15f6.

[151] S. van der Velden *et al.*, "A Dual-layer Detector for Simultaneous Fluoroscopic and Nuclear Imaging," *Radiology*, 2019, doi: 10.1148/radiol.2018180796.

[152] C. Beijst, M. Elschot, M. A. Viergever, and H. W. A. M. De Jong, "Toward simultaneous real-time fluoroscopic and nuclear imaging in the intervention room," *Radiology*, vol. 278, no. 1, 2016, doi: 10.1148/radiol.2015142749.

13 Thyroid Imaging and Dosimetry

Michael Lassmann and Heribert Hänscheid

CONTENTS

13.1 INTRODUCTION

The iodine isotope ^{131}I, often referred to as radioiodine, was first produced and described in 1938 [1]. The first study of iodine metabolism with ^{131}I in healthy individuals and in patients with various thyroid diseases was published only one year later [2], soon followed by radioiodine therapy (RIT) of benign [3, 4] and malignant thyroid diseases [5]. Even before the introduction of scintigraphic imaging, numerous investigations led to a detailed qualitative and quantitative understanding of the biokinetics of iodide [6]. After the invention of the rectilinear scanner [7] and the Anger camera [8], radiopharmaceuticals have mainly been used to examine the functional topography of the thyroid gland, initially exclusively with iodine isotopes, later also with ^{99m}Tc-Pertechnetate [9]. Quantitative information, for example, on the uptake of ^{99m}Tc-pertechnetate into the thyroid gland, was mainly used to consolidate a diagnosis or in the staging of the disease.

Quantitative imaging to assess the kinetics activity in the tissues under consideration is essential if a patient is to be treated with a personalized, individually optimized endoradiotherapy. Since both imaging and therapy with radiopharmaceuticals are key components of diagnosis and treatment of benign and malignant diseases of the thyroid gland with ^{131}I, this chapter provides an overview of the iodine metabolism of the thyroid gland and its clinical use for imaging, dosimetry, and therapy.

DOI: 10.1201/9780429489549-13

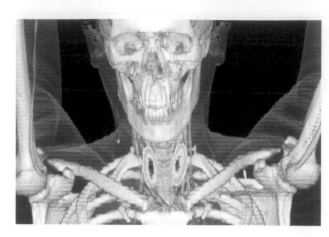

FIGURE 13.1   The thyroid, an endocrine gland adjacent to larynx and trachea, consists of two lobes connected by the thyroid isthmus, a band of thyroid tissue in front of the trachea. Colour image available at www.routledge.com/9781138593299.

13.2   IODINE METABOLISM

Stable iodine, [127]I, ingested with food is absorbed as iodide (I⁻) in the gastro-intestinal tract into the blood stream, from where it rapidly distributes into the extracellular and partly also intracellular fluid space [6]. Medically administered radioactive iodine isotopes are often also applied orally on an empty stomach. Under these conditions, absorption occurs rapidly at a rate of several per cent per minute, resulting in an almost complete transfer into the blood within about one hour. Compared to intravenous application, there is thus only a short delay, which is not relevant for imaging and dosimetry with [131]I.

Dissolved in the water contained in the blood, the iodide is circulated throughout the body, where it distributes into the easily exchangeable parts of the body water. While the distribution into the extracellular fluid space is rapid, the rate of diffusion into the intracellular fluid depends on the tissue, so that the final distribution is reached with some delay. In the blood, the concentration of iodide in the intracellular water of the erythrocytes equals that in the plasma because the iodide ion I⁻ can move readily through the membrane of the red blood cells. A few hours after radioactive iodide enters the blood pool, its distribution volume, defined as the ratio of plasma concentration to total iodide in the blood pool, is about 35 per cent of the total body volume in a normal person [6]. As the water in the blood accounts for some 5.5-6 per cent of the body volume, the whole blood theoretically accounts for about 16 per cent of the iodide in the blood pool.

Scintigraphically, active accumulation is observed in the thyroid and in the salivary and gastric glands (Figure 13.2). In females, during late pregnancy and lactation, the breasts also concentrate iodide, which is necessary to supply the breastfed child with iodine. The salivary glands and the stomach accumulate iodide, but do not store it. Instead, they return secreted iodine to the system via the gastrointestinal tract. Activity in the esophagus visible in scintigraphic imaging with iodine isotopes is often due to contamination by saliva. Only thyroid tissue is able to accumulate iodine and store it. When absorbing the iodide out of the blood, the thyroid competes with the kidneys, in which iodide is filtered in the glomeruli and only partially reabsorbed in the tubules.

13.2.1   THE THYROID

The thyroid is a well-perfused endocrine gland located under the front surface of the neck adjacent to larynx and trachea. Shaped like a butterfly, it consists of two lobes connected by the thyroid isthmus, a band of thyroid tissue in front of the trachea. The main function of the thyroid gland is the regulated production and secretion of thyroid hormones, which are essential for a variety of metabolic processes throughout the body. Iodine, which is present in normal food as a trace element in the form of the stable isotope [127]I, is necessary for the production of thyroid hormones. In healthy persons, a certain fraction of iodine that enters the body is absorbed by the thyroid gland, depending on the average iodine supply.

Microscopically, the thyroid is composed of colloid-filled iodine storing follicles whose surface consists of a layer of thyrocytes, follicular cells with functionally asymmetric membrane domains. In the basolateral cell membrane, that is, the cell membrane facing away from the colloid-filled follicular lumen, thyrocytes are able to absorb the anion iodide I⁻ from the blood by active transport through an ion channel. This ion channel, which is formed by a transmembrane protein, the sodium iodide symporter (NIS), simultaneously transports one iodide ion I⁻ and two positively charged

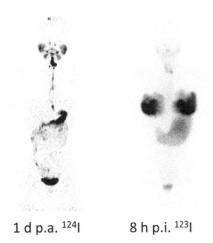

1 d p.a. ^{124}I   8 h p.i. ^{123}I

FIGURE 13.2 Scintigraphic images of two patients with differentiated thyroid carcinoma, left: one day after 20 MBq ^{124}I, right: breast-feeding woman 8 hours after 180 MBq ^{123}I. Imaging was performed after thyroidectomy to exclude lymph node metastases. Besides increased activity concentrations in the salivary glands, stomachs, and the postoperative thyroid remnants, contamination by saliva (left) and strong accumulation in the lactating breasts (right) are visible.

sodium ions Na^+ into the cell [10, 11], even at very low iodide concentrations in the blood and against a considerable electrochemical gradient. While some of the imported iodide diffuses back into the blood following the concentration gradient, most of it is rapidly transported through the apical membrane into the follicular lumen, where it is oxidized and bound to the hormone precursor thyroglobulin (Tg) in a process called iodide organification. A healthy thyroid can store several milligrams of iodine organically bound to Tg, thus ensuring the hormone supply even during periods without external iodine supply.

In response to demand for thyroid hormones, iodinated Tg is released from the follicular lumen back into the thyrocytes, where it is converted into thyroid hormones, which are then secreted into the blood. The concentrations in the blood of the most important thyroid hormones, triiodothyronine (T3) and thyroxine (T4), are kept constant within their normal ranges by the pituitary gland adjusting the rate of the thyroid metabolism via the thyroid-stimulating hormone (TSH). When thyroid hormone levels in the blood are low, TSH is upregulated and, by activating TSH receptors in the basolateral membrane, stimulates the production and release of T3 and T4 as well as the expression of NIS and thus iodide uptake [12–14].

Since the NIS identifies I⁻ by its ionic volume, it also carries other anions of the same size, such as perchlorate and pertechnetate. These, however, are not transferred to the follicle and organified, but diffuse back into the blood following the concentration gradient.

13.3 IMAGING

13.3.1 ^{99m}Tc PERTECHNETATE

^{99m}Tc pertechnetate (^{99m}TcO$_4^-$), the most commonly used tracer for thyroid scintigraphy, is accumulated via the NIS in the first step of the concentration process but, as it is not organified, leaves the thyroid relatively quickly. A balance of supply and back diffusion is established about a quarter of an hour after an i.v. injection of ^{99m}TcO$_4^-$, resulting in a fixed ratio of concentrations in thyroid and blood. The activity concentration in the thyroid remains more or less constant at its maximum value between 10 and 25 min after the injection. The joint EANM/SNMMI guideline [15] recommends gamma camera imaging with measurement of the maximum fractional thyroid uptake (TcU) by count-rate evaluation in the region of interest (ROI) at 15–20 min after 74–111 MBq ^{99m}TcO$_4^-$. The TcU is sufficiently closely correlated with the iodide clearance for clinical purposes as clearance equivalent.

The field of view of the gamma camera and the computer matrix used must match each other, so that a pixel size of < 3 mm is guaranteed. While 128 × 128 matrix size can be adequate for a dedicated small field camera, 256 × 256 and zoom factors of 1.5 to 2 should be used for neck imaging with standard large field cameras. The use of a special thyroid collimator or a collimator with high resolution for low energies and a 15–20 per cent energy window centred on the photopeak are recommended to achieve the best resolution possible with the 140 keV photons of ^{99m}Tc.

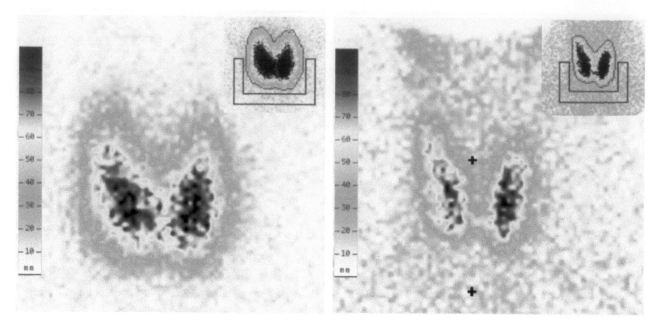

FIGURE 13.3 Scintigraphic images of the thyroid gland of a patient with Graves's disease, left: 4.5 h after 4 MBq ^{131}I (64% retention) for pretherapeutic dosimetry; right: 20 min after 50 MBq ^{99m}TcO$_4^-$ (0.9% TcU) half a year after RIT. While the thyroid gland was significantly enlarged before RIT, size and kinetics returned to normal after treatment. ROI positions are shown in the overexposed images at the top right. Sizes and relative count rates are indicated by the rulers to the left. Colour image available at www.routledge.com/9781138593299.

The investigation proceeds as follows:

- Camera acquisition and count-rate assessment of the syringe with the activity to be administered in a neck phantom or, if the sensitivity of the camera in counts per seconds per MBq ^{99m}TcO$_4^-$ is known from calibration, input of the activity measured with the activimeter.
- Measurement and correction for the residual activity in the syringe.
- Neck imaging and evaluation of the net count rate in the thyroid by ROI-technique.
- Calculation of the TcU as thyroid to administered activity count- rate ratio.

Scintigraphic images should contain at least a hundred thousand counts registered from decays in the thyroid gland. This usually means a recording time of 5 to 10 minutes. The measuring geometry must not be altered during this time. The thyroid ROI should be as small as possible without excluding organ activity. This is usually best achieved by an irregular ROI. Focal uptake in a thyroid nodule may need to be quantified with a separate ROI. The net count rate is obtained by correcting the measured count rate by the count rate per area measured in a background ROI caudally or laterally of the thyroid gland, which apparently contains only blood pool activity (Figure 13.3).

13.3.2 ^{131}I SODIUM IODIDE

Imaging with ^{131}I today is generally performed in conjunction with RIT, always for diagnostic purposes and often as part of dosimetry. Dosimetries for benign diseases of the thyroid gland are often carried out using probe measurements. The use of a gamma camera (planar or SPECT/CT) instead of a probe to perform retention measurements increases the expense for dosimetry but is advantageous in individual patients because it adds information on the distribution of the activity enabling more adequate background correction. A single head acquisition of anterior views is sufficient in many cases, especially for benign diseases. The camera must be suited for radioiodine scintigraphy featuring a high-energy collimator with low septal penetration and good imaging characteristics with a full width at tenth maximum of the point spread function not exceeding 3 times the full width at half maximum.

The ^{131}I activity required for imaging depends on the objective of the scan. For benign thyroid diseases, scintigraphy and dosimetry is possible with 1–3 MBq; for malignant lesions, retentions of 0.001 per cent are detectable after 7 GBq and 0.01 per cent after 100 MBq [16]. 10 MBq are sufficient to detect lesions with 0.05 per cent retention, and to determine the specific blood-absorbed dose. If available, a camera with a thick crystal (1/2" or 5/8" equivalent to 1.27 cm or 1.59 cm, respectively) should be selected to increase the count rate. Such cameras can be expected to register about 50 counts per second per MBq [131]I (free air) in a 15 per cent window centred on the peak at 364.5 keV [17].

Two aspects in particular are disadvantageous for the accuracy of quantitative imaging, the relatively poor spatial resolution and the higher-energy photons of [131]I. The spatial resolution for ^{131}I imaging with high-energy collimators is much worse than that for ^{99m}Tc with low-energy high-resolution collimators. Even more disadvantageous is the high proportion of photons emitted in about 9 per cent of decays with energies above 600 keV. These photons are likely to penetrate even high-energy collimators or are detectable after tissue scattering in the patient. If the energy loss in the detector of the camera falls into the photopeak window at 364.5 keV, such a high-energy gamma is registered as a valid event with incorrect position information, resulting in a considerable background in the camera image [18]. As a consequence, the count rate per activity measured with a point source increases strongly with the size of the ROI (Figure 13.4). In order to achieve the highest possible accuracy in quantifying the count rate of a structure in the image, the size of the ROI must be selected based on test measurements on a phantom and suitable calibration, depending on the size of the structure.

The use of a phantom, for example, a thyroid uptake neck phantom according to specifications by IAEA or ANSI (Figure 13.5), is also recommended for retention measurements in benign thyroid disease. The phantom shall mimic

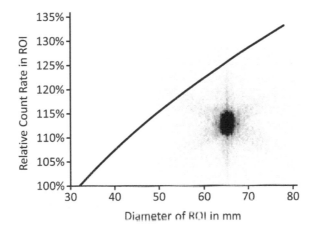

FIGURE 13.4 Zoomed scintigraphic image of a ^{131}I capsule. The star-like background indicates penetration of the collimator septa. The count rate increases with the diameter of the ROI used for quantification.

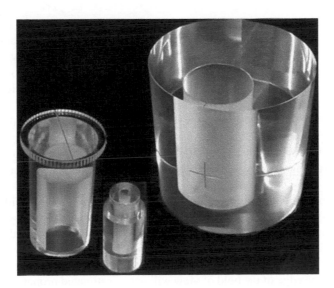

FIGURE 13.5 Anthropomorphic neck phantom.

a thyroid gland in a neck to determine the sensitivity, that is, the count rate per activity in a typical target tissue, of the measuring device during in-vivo assessments. For a realistic representation, the phantom material should have similar radiation absorption and scatter characteristics as human soft tissue and the calibration depth that is, the mean depth of the activity distribution under the surface should be about 2 to 2.5 cm.

If a dedicated phantom is not available and cannot be purchased, the calibration of the device should be performed by measuring the activity standard through a 2 cm plastic plate, for example, Lucite. The surface of the plate must have the same distance to the detector as the neck surface in patient assessments, and the activity standard must be as close as possible to the opposite side of the plate to adequately mimic both attenuation depth and distance of a typical target tissue.

The tracer activity to be used for the pre-therapy dosimetry should be measured in the phantom prior to the administration. The resulting count-rate value represents 100 per cent uptake and can be used as a constancy check for the sensitivity of the device if it is related to the actual activity. Alternatively, the tracer activity can be initially measured at a fixed distance in air. In this case, the count rate must be corrected by a calibration factor accounting for the differences in the sensitivities in activity measurements in the phantom and in free air to represent 100 per cent uptake in typical target tissue.

13.3.3 ^{123}I Sodium Iodide

Like all isotopes of iodine, ^{123}I is organified in the thyroid gland. With a physical half-life of 13 h, quantitative measurements of the activity in thyroid tissue with a gamma camera are still possible one day after administration. This can be diagnostically valuable in certain cases, but is too short to pretherapeutically evaluate the kinetics of ^{131}I. Compared to the pure gamma emitter ^{99m}Tc with its 6 hours half-life, the radiation exposure, in particular of the accumulating tissues, is significantly higher in an examination with ^{123}I. Since ^{123}I is usually not available daily, is considerably more expensive, and also the imaging properties are inferior to those of the ^{99m}Tc, it is usually only used in the scintigraphy of thyroid tissue for certain questions in selected individuals.

Early imaging is recommended at 2–6 hours, late imaging one day after ^{123}I administration [15]. Imaging and data evaluation are similar to that with ^{99m}TcO$_4^-$ but with an energy window on the photopeak at 159 keV. In some low-energy collimators, the higher energy leads to high septum penetration, which makes it necessary to use a medium-energy collimator, even if its spatial resolution is inferior.

13.3.4 ^{124}I Sodium Iodide

PET with the iodine isotope ^{124}I is a superior method for measuring the uptake and biokinetics of iodide in the patient. ^{124}I has a half-life of 4.2 days and emits positrons usable for PET with a probability of about 23 per cent during decay. An activity of about 25 MBq ^{124}I is sufficient for diagnostically adequate image quality and kinetics measurements. Since the nuclide is not commercially available at reasonable prices and with the necessary marketing authorization, the ^{124}I PET is reserved for a few specialized centres with the necessary expertise and the possibility of producing it themselves.

The decay scheme of ^{124}I is complex as it contains positron emission, electron capture, and emission of x-rays and γ-rays. Due to the positron emission, PET-imaging is possible; however, the branching ratio of positron emission with 22.8 per cent is much lower than that for ^{18}F (96.7%). Longer measurements or higher activity concentrations are therefore necessary to get a similar image quality as compared to ^{18}F. Furthermore, the emitted positrons have higher emission energies and, thus, a 2–3 mm higher mean range, which leads to a reduced spatial resolution of the PET images.

A major problem of PET with ^{124}I is the emission of a prompt gamma photon with energy 602.7 keV (emission probability: 62.9%) that lies within the standard energy window of LSO detectors (typically 425–650 keV). Most PET scanners will recognize these photons as valid coincidences if concurrently monitored with 511 keV photons. The 602.7 keV photons are emitted in cascade with nearly 50 per cent of the positron emissions, so the probability of such coincidences is high, thus increasing the dead time of the system and impairing the count-rate performance significantly [19].

To avoid biased quantification and degradation of the image quality the prompt coincidences have to be accounted for and corrected by a prompt-gamma compensation algorithm. This can be achieved by calculating the distribution of the prompt coincidences from a convolution of a prompt-gamma correction kernel with acquired data corrected for attenuation and random coincidences [20, 21]. After compensation, the ^{124}I image quality and quantification accuracy become comparable to that of ^{18}F and ^{68}Ga images after a 5-fold longer acquisition time [22]. Without compensation, the prompt coincidence level at the edge of the field of view will not be estimated properly while in the centre too many coincidences are subtracted because of an overestimation of the scatter contribution.

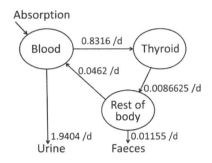

FIGURE 13.6 Simple model of iodine kinetics [6, 25].

13.4 ABSORBED DOSE FROM ^{131}I

Very precise mathematical models of the biokinetics of iodine in the organism exist [23], which take into account a large number of compartments and iodine flows. For routine clinical dosimetry, the use of overly detailed models, which by their nature require the individual adaptation of a large number of free parameters, is not possible, or not statistically justified due to the limited number and accuracy of the available information [24]. A simple model of the thyroid gland, proposed in [6] (Figure 13.6), was adopted by the International Commission on Radiological Protection (ICRP) as a useful model for radiation protection calculations [25]. The rate constants of iodine transfer in the model, which apply to a healthy standard adult individual with normal iodine supply, can be quite different in patients with thyroid diseases.

In RIT, dosimetry is performed to determine the average absorbed dose per administered activity for diseased thyroid tissue or in critical organs, such as the red bone marrow or the lungs, in the case of disseminated pulmonary metastasis. This can be useful both for treatment planning to determine the activity required achieving a targeted absorbed dose, and during therapy to determine the doses actually administered. According to the generally accepted formalism of the MIRD, the total mean absorbed dose $D(r_T)$ to a target tissue r_T is [26]:

$$D(r_T) = \sum_{r_S} \int_0^\infty A(r_S,t) \cdot S(r_T \leftarrow r_S,t)dt \qquad (13.1)$$

where $A(r_S,t)$ is the time-dependent activity in any source tissue r_S contributing to the dose absorbed in r_T, and the 'S-value' $S(r_T \leftarrow r_S,t)$ is the mean absorbed dose to r_T per decay in r_S at time t after the activity administration. The time dependence of the S-value is usually neglected in dosimetry in the context of thyroid diseases.

13.4.1 DOSIMETRY OF THYROID TISSUE

RIT is reasonable only if the ^{131}I concentration in the diseased target tissue r_T is much higher than in other tissues r_S. The dose rate in r_T is mainly due to self-irradiation by short-range ß-radiation and contributions from source tissues other than the target tissue itself can be neglected. Eqn. 13.1 can be simplified:

$$D(r_T) = S(r_T \leftarrow r_T) \cdot A_0 \cdot \int_0^\infty a(r_T,t)dt \qquad (13.2)$$

where r_T is the considered tissue of thyroidal origin, for example, the entire thyroid in Graves's disease, a toxic nodule within the thyroid, or a tumourous lesion. A_0 is the administered activity and $a(r_T,t)$ the fractional uptake in r_T at time t: $a(r_T,t) = A(r_T,t) / A_0$.

The S-value of a macroscopic tissue r_T with several millimeters diameter or larger can be calculated from the contributions by particle and photon radiation and its volume V_T. The mean energy per decay released from ^{131}I by ß-radiation is 192 keV/(Bq·s) = 2.654 Gy·g/(MBq·d) [27], which is almost completely absorbed within r_T. For thyroid tissue of density $\rho=1.04$ g/ml this leads to a dose per decay in r_T of $2.55/V_T$ Gy·ml/(MBq·d). The energy deposition by photons in a thyroid gland approximated by two spheres with a mass of 10 g each is 0.154

Gy·g/(MBq·d) [28]. As the energy deposition is proportional to $V_T^{1/3}$ [29], the absorbed dose per decay is $0.148/V_T$ Gy·ml/(MBq·d) · $(V_T/9.6ml)^{1/3}$ = 0.07 Gy/(MBq·d) · $(V_T/ml)^{2/3}$:

$$S(r_T \leftarrow r_T) = \left(\frac{2.55}{V_T / ml} + \frac{0.07}{(V_T / ml)^{\frac{2}{3}}} \right) \frac{Gy}{MBq \cdot d} \tag{13.3}$$

In addition to the administered activity A_0 and the volume V_T of the target tissue, the time function of the activity retention in r_T, which must be determined by measurements, must be known in order to calculate the dose according to Eqn. 13.2.

In order to keep the number of necessary activity measurements in clinical routine as small as possible, it is necessary to further simplify the model in Figure 13.6 to reduce the number of unknown parameters. The iodine released into the remainder of the body is bound to thyroid hormones, which are metabolized, whereby most of the iodine is reduced, becoming available again as I⁻. This should be taken into account in compartment models as it theoretically modifies the kinetics in the gland. It is, however, not the correct determination of the individual transfer rates that are important for dosimetry, but a sufficiently precise representation of the retention function in the target tissue. With radioiodine therapy, an effective half-life can be measured soon after administration of the activity, which is relevant for dosimetry and remains unchanged later [30]. A sufficiently accurate description of the retention function in thyroid tissue r_T can be derived assuming first order kinetics in a model with two compartments, blood pool, and thyroid [31–33] (Figure 13.7).

With the total activity present at the time of administration ($t=0$), the retention in the blood pool changes according to:

$$\frac{da(r_B,t)}{dt} = k_B \cdot a(r_B,t) \tag{13.4}$$

where $k_B = k_p + k_r + k_t$ is the total rate of activity elimination from the blood pool by physical decay, k_p=0.0864/d for ^{131}I, renal clearance, k_r, and target tissue uptake, k_t. The blood activity is expected to decrease mono-exponentially. Retention in the thyroid increases by uptake from the blood, k_t, and decreases with rate $k_T = k_p + k_h$ by physical decay, k_p, and release of organically bound ^{131}I, k_h:

$$\frac{da(r_T,t)}{dt} = k_t \cdot a(r_B,t) - k_T \cdot a(r_T,t) \tag{13.5}$$

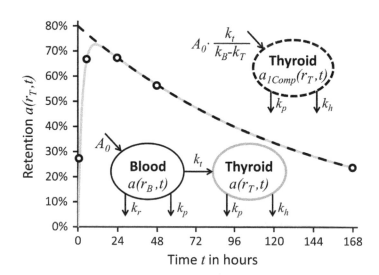

FIGURE 13.7 Hypothetical example of ^{131}I retention measurements in a thyroid of a patient with Graves's disease (circles) and fit of the retention function a(r_T,t) in Eqn. 13.6 (solid grey line). The retention function a$_{1Comp}$(r_T,t) expected after direct activity injection into a single compartment (Eqn. 13.8) is shown by the dashed black line.

The solution of the differential Eqn. 13.5 is:

$$a(r_T,t) = \frac{k_t}{k_B - k_T} \cdot \left(e^{-k_T \cdot t} - e^{-k_B \cdot t} \right)$$

(13.6)

The decay rate k_T is related to the effective half-life T_{eff} of the activity in r_T by $T_{eff} = ln(2)/k_T$. $a(r_T,t)$ in Eqn. 13.6 rises from zero at the time of administration ($t=0$) to a maximum at time

$$t_{max} = \frac{\ln(k_B) - \ln(k_T)}{k_B - k_T}$$

(13.7)

and afterwards decreases again approaching the mono-exponential decay function

$$a_{1Comp}(r_T,t) = \frac{k_t}{k_B - k_T} \cdot e^{-k_T \cdot t}$$

(13.8)

when the ^{131}I iodide concentration in the blood becomes negligible. $a_{1Comp}(r_T,t)$ in Eqn. 13.8 represents the retention function after bolus injection of the activity $A_0 \cdot k/(k_B - k_T)$ into the target tissue as expected according to a one-compartment model (Figure 13.7). In euthyroid adults with adequate iodine supply, the time t_{max} of maximum uptake is most often observed between 24 h and 48 h after the activity administration. The time t_{max} can be earlier in hyperthyroid patients who often show a higher transfer rate k_t into the thyroid and a shorter half-life T_{eff} of the activity in the thyroid due to stimulation and iodine depletion of the target tissue. By definition, the rate k_T must not be less than the rate of physical decay k_p, therefore k_T must always be set to k_p if a fit to measured values results in a smaller value.

At least three measurements of $a(r_T,t)$ are necessary to fix the unknown transfer rates k_t, k_B, and k_T in Eqn. 13.6, which should best be carried out a few hours after the administration in the main phase of accumulation, at or just after t_{max}, and after some days when the activity retention in r_T has already decreased significantly. Measurements at about 4 to 6 hours, 1 to 2 days, and 5 to 8 days after the activity administration are recommended for dosimetry of target tissues in benign thyroid disease [31]. With known transfer rates, the absorbed dose can be determined from Eqs. 13.2 and 13.3 and from the time integral of Eqn. 13.6 to be

$$D(r_T) = S(r_T \leftarrow r_T) \cdot A_0 \cdot \frac{k_T}{k_B \cdot k_T}$$

(13.9)

Often, an estimate of the absorbed dose based on the one-compartment model with a retention function according to Eqn. 13.8 is sufficiently accurate. It requires at least two measurements to fix the parameters k_T and $k_t/(k_B-k_T)$ in Eqn. 13.8, which must be performed not too early and with a sufficiently long time interval. The first measurement after time t_1 should be performed after the accumulation phase is largely finished, the second after t_2 when the retention has already decreased significantly. The rate k_T is then calculated from the measured retentions $a(r_T,t_1)$ and $a(r_T,t_2)$ by

$$k_T = \frac{\ln\left(a(r_{T,t_1}) \right) - \ln\left(a(r_T,t_2) \right)}{t_2 - t_1}$$

(13.10)

and the factor $k_t/(k_B-k_T)$ in Eqn. 13.8 by back-extrapolation according to

$$\frac{k_t}{k_B - k_T} = a(r_T,t_2) \cdot e^{k_T \cdot t_2}$$

(13.11)

The absorbed dose in the target tissue is overestimated with the one-compartment model kinetics because the second addend in brackets in Eqn. 13.6 is neglected. In dosimetry of benign thyroid disease, where effective half-lives are a few hours in the blood and several days in the target tissue, the resulting error is usually only a few per cent [33]. The EANM guideline for dosimetry in benign disease recommends using a factor of 0.97 to compensate for the initial increase in retention [31]. Integration of $a_{1Comp}(r_T,t)$ in Eqn. 13.8 over time leads to:

$$D_{1Comp}(r_T) = 0.97 \cdot S(r_T \leftarrow r_T) \cdot A_0 \cdot \frac{a(r_T,t_2) \cdot e^{k_T \cdot t_2}}{k_T} \tag{13.12}$$

The aim of dosimetric measurements is to determine the time integral over $a(r_T,t)$ as accurately as possible. Individual kinetic parameters like k_T are used for calculation but are of minor diagnostic interest. It is a characteristic of the decay function that its values are with good accuracy representative of its time integral within a certain time range [33]. The factor $e^{k_T t_2}/k_T$ in Eqn. 13.12, representing the dependence of the dose estimate on k_T, can be approximated with less than 6 per cent error by the factor $2 \cdot t/ln(2)$ if the factor $k_T \cdot t_2$ is between 0.58 and 1.58 or, related to the effective half-life, the time of measurement t_2 is between $0.84 \cdot T_{eff}$ and $2.28 \cdot T_{eff}$. A dose estimate based on only one measurement is possible by:

$$D_{1Meas}(r_T) = \frac{2 \cdot 0.97}{ln(2)} \cdot S(r_T \leftarrow r_T) \cdot A_0 \cdot a(r_T,t_2) \cdot t_2 \tag{13.13}$$

The measurement should preferably be performed after 6 or 7 days for dosimetry of target tissues in benign thyroid disease [31, 33].

13.4.2   RIT OF BENIGN THYROID DISEASES

In benign thyroid diseases, RIT is usually performed to treat hyperthyroidism in Graves's disease or toxic adenoma aiming at euthyroidism or, in an ablative concept for Graves's disease, hypothyroidism compensated by thyroxine medication [34, 35]. The tissue to be treated usually is highly stimulated by the disease and has a high iodide uptake, in toxic adenoma, much in contrast to the down-regulated healthy tissue. Patients with a large, non-toxic goiter, most commonly diagnosed in regions with nutritional iodine deficiency, can be treated to reduce thyroid volume while maintaining thyroid function. In goiters with areas with insufficient iodide uptake, metabolism can be stimulated by externally administered artificial TSH (recombinant human TSH, rhTSH). While fixed standard activities are still often administered, personalized treatment requires pre-therapeutic dosimetry to determine the therapeutic activity necessary to administer a predefined dose to the diseased tissue. Empirically determined values for the absorbed dose are targeted, for example 150 Gy for Graves's disease if euthyroidism is targeted, or 200–300 Gy for ablation, and 300–400 Gy for ablation of autonomous nodules [34].

Dosimetry for planning an RIT is valid only if it is based on a reliable mass estimate from current imaging, and if the kinetics during the therapy is more or less unchanged. Aspects like a long delay, change of medication with anti-thyroid drugs or thyroid hormones, change of supply or contamination with stable iodine, intake of food prior to oral activity administration, or change of fluid intake can modify the iodine kinetics between dosimetry and therapy and thus should be avoided [34].

The pre-therapy dosimetry should include the following tasks:

- Target mass delineation by sonography or other adequate procedures.
- Quantification of the tracer activity with a dose calibrator.
- Measurement of the tracer activity with the test device, probe or gamma camera, with the activity located in the phantom or in free air with according count-rate correction.
- Verification that the observed count rate per activity matches the expected sensitivity value of the device.
- Administration of the tracer activity with accurate documentation.
- Patient measurements.
- Calculation of the absorbed dose and the activity required to administer a specified target dose.

13.4.3 CALCULATION EXAMPLE

As a numerical example, a thyroid gland with $V_T = 43$ ml (Eqn 13.3: $S(r_T \leftarrow r_T) = 0.065$ Gy/MBq/d) and the ^{131}I kinetics in Figure 13.7 is assumed, which is to be treated with 200 Gy target dose. Fit of Eqn. 13.6 to the data yields the red curve in Figure 13.7 with $k_t = 7.06$/d, $k_B = 9$/d, and $k_T = 0.1729$/d corresponding to 4 d effective half-life in the gland. The specific absorbed dose according to Eqn. 13.9 is $D(r_T)/A_0 = 0.2949$ Gy/MBq. With unchanged kinetics, the target dose is achieved with $A_0 = 678$ MBq.

Evaluation from the last two measurements $a(r_T, t_1 = 48h) = 0.566$ and $a(r_T, t_2 = 168h) = 0.238$ results: $k_T = 0.1729$/d (Eqn. 13.10), $k_t/(k_B - k_T) = 0.80$ (Eqn. 13.11), and $D_{1Comp}(r_T)/A_0 = 0.2917$ Gy/MBq (Eqn. 13.12). The calculated therapy activity is $A_0 = 686$ MBq. An estimate based on the late measurement $a(r_T, t_2 = 168h) = 0.238$ alone yields $D_{1Meas}(r_T)/A_0 = 0.3036$ Gy/MBq (Eqn. 13.13) and $A_0 = 659$ MBq.

13.4.4 RIT FOR THYROID CANCER

Differentiated thyroid carcinoma is cancer that develops from the tissues of the thyroid gland, most often with preserved iodide uptake and metabolism. The disease is initially treated by thyroidectomy, that is, surgical removal of the thyroid gland. The athyreotic patients must then externally supply the essential thyroid hormones for the rest of their lives, usually by oral application of thyroxine. Thyroidectomy is usually followed by an RIT to eliminate residual thyroid tissue or metastatic lesions. Since, in contrast to the therapy of benign diseases, the iodide uptake into the tissue to be treated is not already stimulated by the disease, treatment is generally performed at elevated TSH levels to optimize tumour uptake and dose. High TSH levels are reached after 3–4 weeks of thyroid hormone withdrawal leading to deep hypothyroidism, or in euthyroidism by intramuscular injection of rhTSH. Compared to external stimulation with rhTSH, hypothyroidism has the disadvantage of very unpleasant side effects and a more or less pronounced deterioration of renal function, resulting in slower excretion of radioiodine and increased exposure per administered activity. However, since, as can be seen from Eqn. 13.9, the dose in the target tissue is also inversely proportional to the rate of loss k_B and thus approximately the blood-absorbed dose, the ratio of doses in target tissue and residual body is virtually unaffected.

Standard activities are generally applied in RIT for thyroid cancer in accordance with current guidelines and recommendations for action [36, 37], which leads to very different treatment conditions and radiation exposures for individual patients due to individual differences in radioiodine kinetics [38, 39]. Nevertheless, treatment based on individual dosimetry remains the exception.

If a diagnostic activity of ^{131}I is administered before the first RIT for remnant ablation in order to measure the remaining retention or assess the need for further surgery, the activity must not exceed a few MBq. The earlier customary administration of higher diagnostic radioiodine activities for pretherapeutic imaging in the context of a more precise determination of the tumour stage and the kinetics in the target tissue is contraindicated, at least before the first radioiodine therapy, as this can have a considerable influence on the biokinetics and reduce the tumour dose administered by the therapy [40]. Nevertheless, individualized, dosimetry-optimized therapies are possible in patients with thyroid carcinoma, whereby two different approaches exist: tumour dosimetry based on measurements of iodine kinetics in the malignoma (Figure 13.8) and the determination of the blood dose representative of dosimetry of the dose-limiting organ, the bone marrow.

For the application of tumour dosimetry, the kinetics in the target volume must be measured prior to therapy; similar to the procedure for the treatment of benign thyroid diseases, and from this the activity must be calculated which at the lowest radiation exposure is still therapeutically effective with a high probability. Ideally, ^{124}I PET should be used for this purpose, which allows superior measurements with low radiation exposure in the target volume, that is, little influence on the kinetics by pre-damage of the target tissue.

The first studies using ^{131}I for tumour dosimetry in a larger patient population with the aim of determining the doses required for a high probability of successful target tissue elimination found that in ablation therapy the dose in the thyroid remnant should reach 300 Gy and should exceed 80 Gy in the treatment of cervical lymph node metastases [41, 42]. A study on ablation therapy and treatment of metastases after pretherapeutic dosimetry with ^{124}I PET confirmed these values [43]. A dose dependence of therapeutic success has further been reported in [44–46].

Tumour doses determined from ^{131}I retention after RIT under stimulation with rhTSH and estimates of tumour volumes from radiological images showed a high variability with dose ranging from 1.3–368 Gy after therapy with standard activities; only 5 of 25 lesions examined received doses of more than 80 Gy [47]. Similar results were found in another study, where 17 of 20 lesions evaluated received less than 80 Gy [45], and in pretherapeutic dosimetry at

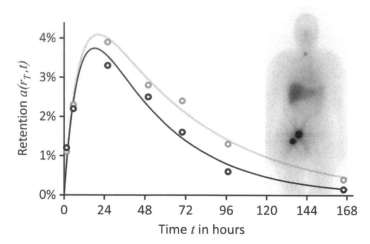

FIGURE 13.8 Retention in pelvic metastases of a patient with differentiated thyroid carcinoma measured in successive scans after therapy with 3.7 GBq ^{131}I. The scintigraphic image shows the scan after 72 hours.

voxel level with ^{124}I PET [48]. These data suggest that at least patients in advanced tumour stage are not adequately treated by the administration of standard activities, that is, with too-low tumour doses. In particular, repeated treatment of inadequately treated lesions has shown that the absorbed dose per administered activity can decrease drastically from therapy to therapy, which leads to a further loss of therapeutic efficacy of ^{131}I [45, 47]. For patients with lymph node metastases and distant metastases, a retrospective mono-institutional study showed an improved response rate using tumour dosimetry before RIT [49].

13.4.5 BLOOD-BASED DOSIMETRY

Prior to ablation therapy after thyroidectomy, reliable dosimetry with ^{131}I for the thyroid gland is difficult because the target mass must be known, a requirement that is almost never met. In the case of voxel-based dosimetry of the thyroid remnant, as performed by some groups [50], errors caused by imaging artefacts cannot be excluded [51]. Even the therapy of metastases of known mass after tumour dosimetry is not uncontroversial, as different metastases in the same patient can have quite different kinetics and extremely different doses have been measured even within individual tumours [45, 48]. The dosage of therapeutic activity based on the mean kinetics in dosimetrically recorded lesions carries the risk that unconsidered manifestations or areas within the measured tumours receive too low radiation doses. To increase the probability of therapy success, it may therefore be appropriate to administer more radioiodine than is potentially sufficient and to accept a higher radiation exposure.

The tolerable radiation exposure during radioiodine therapy is limited by the toxicity in the critical organ, most often the red bone marrow, for which a reliable direct determination of the dose is not feasible. A recognized method to optimize the tumour dose while avoiding threatening myelotoxic effects is to limit the blood dose. Since the free iodide is distributed uniformly in the organism in the easily exchangeable fraction of body water, it can be safely assumed that the absorbed dose in the blood represents an upper estimate of the dose in well-perfused organs, including the bone marrow.

An upper limit for the blood dose from RIT of 2 Gy proposed in an early study, below which no significant hematological problems occurred [52], is now considered very conservative. A significant proportion of patients reach this dose already with the application of the fixed activity of 7 GBq ^{131}I [53, 54], which is typically used in tumour therapies, without any side effects. Even when significantly higher fixed activities are administered, the rate of side effects remains low [55] and even in a study in which a bone marrow dose of maximum 3 Gy was targeted [44], only transient myelotoxic effects were observed. A therapy with 2 Gy absorbed dose to the blood can therefore be considered safe. Since the median specific blood dose observed in carcinoma patients is about 0.1 Gy/GBq ^{131}I or less, therapy activities can be increased on average by 2–3 times after blood dosimetry, compared to the application of standard activities. In patients for whom standard activities are not sufficient, blood dosimetry allows the increase of the administered activity and thus the achievable doses in the target tissue. Patients in whom even the maximum administrable activity does not lead to a promising dose can be spared further ineffective treatments [56].

Measurement of the blood-absorbed dose according to Eqn. 13.1 requires the determination of retention functions in blood and whole body as source tissues:

$$D\left(r_{blood}\right) = A_0 \cdot \left(S\left(r_{blood} \leftarrow r_{blood}\right) \cdot \int_0^\infty a\left(r_{blood}, t\right) dt + S\left(r_{blood} \leftarrow r_{body}\right) \int_0^\infty a\left(r_{body}, t\right) dt \right) \qquad (13.14)$$

The S-value of the contribution of photon radiation from the blood and the residual body, that is the whole body to the blood can be approximated by the S-value determined by Monte Carlo simulation for total body self-irradiation by photons, $0.0188 \ /(wt/\text{kg})^{2/3}$ Gy/(GBq·h) [57], where wt is the body mass. With regard to the S-factor of the self-irradiation of the blood by ß-radiation, it must be considered that about 65 per cent of the total blood volume resides in blood vessels with diameters less than 5 mm [58]. Especially in thin vessels, the released energy is not completely absorbed within the vessel but diffuses into vessel walls and surrounding tissues. On the other hand, since these tissues also contain iodide in lower concentrations, the loss is partially compensated for by irradiation of the blood by ß-radiation from the residual body. The EANM dosimetry guideline [17] recommends neglecting the ß component from the body and instead assume complete ß-absorption in the blood with an S-value of 108 Gy·ml/(GBq·h), which is about a factor of 1.5 higher than determined for blood self-irradiation [58]. This leads to the following conservative estimate of the specific blood-absorbed dose:

$$\frac{D\left(r_{blood}\right)}{A_0} = 108 \frac{Gy \cdot ml}{GBq \cdot h} \cdot \int_0^\infty a\left(r_{ml\ of\ blood}, t\right) dt + \frac{0.0188}{\left(wt/kg\right)^{2/3}} \frac{Gy}{GBq \cdot h} \cdot \int_0^\infty a\left(r_{body}, t\right) dt \qquad (13.15)$$

where $a(r_{ml\ of\ blood}, t)$ is the retention in one millilitre of blood.

Pretherapeutic evaluation of the blood-absorbed dose per administered activity is reliably feasible with low activities of about 10 MBq ^{131}I by measuring body retention with a gamma camera and activity concentrations in whole blood samples in a well counter (Figure 13.9). The EANM guideline [17] recommends a first measurement up to two hours after the administration after complete activity retention in the blood pool without interim excretion. Further whole-body scans and whole blood sampling should follow at 6 hours, 1 day, and 4 days after the administration with an additional measurement after 6 days in case of a retarded decline in blood activity. Mono- or bi-exponential retention functions should be fit to the measured values, whatever is more adequate.

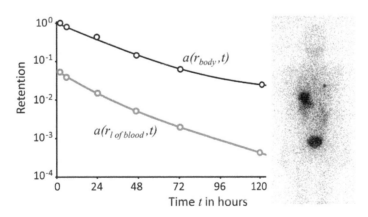

FIGURE 13.9 Retention in total body and per liter of whole blood and the 24 hours posterior image of a 14-year-old female (43 kg, 160 cm) measured after 9.5 MBq ^{131}I for treatment planning. After diagnosis of differentiated thyroid carcinoma and total thyroidectomy, a post-therapeutic scan after a first RIT performed with 2.2 GBq ^{131}I for thyroid remnant ablation revealed distant metastasis in the form of small lung lesions. A second therapy with increased activity was scheduled four months later, before which a dosimetry was performed to determine the specific blood absorbed dose. Time integrated retention was 0.00109 h per ml of blood and 30.5 h in the body. Specific blood-absorbed dose (Eqn. 13.15) was 0.164 Gy/GBq ^{131}I and tolerable activity for 2 Gy blood dose 12.2 GBq [131]I.

During therapy, too, blood-dose measurement is useful for estimating the radiation exposure caused by therapy, since exposure cannot be meaningfully derived from the activity administered alone due to the wide range of doses caused [59]. The absorbed dose to the blood, however, is a good surrogate measure of radiation exposure. As explained above, the iodide is dissolved in exchangeable water. In the dose-relevant organs the water content and thus theoretically the absorbed dose is 10-20 per cent lower than in the blood, which was confirmed in measurements with ^{124}I PET [60].

Accurate blood dosimetry is time consuming, too costly for routine use, and burdensome for the patient because of the additional blood samples. For simplification, the blood dose can be estimated from a single measured value of the whole-body retention [61]. The accuracy of dosimetry is then slightly reduced, but sufficient for post-therapeutic dose evaluation.

13.5   SUMMARY AND CONCLUSION

Scintigraphic imaging is an important aspect in diagnosis and therapy of benign and malignant thyroid diseases. In addition to the qualitative evaluation of the functional status of the examined tissue, the quantitative analysis of iodine kinetics, which is necessary for an individualized treatment, is becoming increasingly important in therapy. Nevertheless, radioiodine therapy remains largely empirical, especially in the treatment of differentiated thyroid carcinoma. The reasons for omitting dosimetry are the additional burden on the patient, a lack of trained personnel and expertise available, and that there are hardly any prospective, randomized studies on therapy optimization that demonstrate a superiority of individual therapy over the administration of standard activities and, thus, a compelling medical necessity to perform individual dosimetry.

However, evidence increases that treatment optimized by dosimetry improves outcome especially in high-risk patients for whom standard activities are not sufficient. Dosimetry allows the administration of the highest possible doses in the target tissue and potentially prevents ineffective treatments.

REFERENCES

[1] J. J. Livingood and G. T. Seaborg, "Radioactive isotopes of iodine," *The Physical Review,* vol. 54, no. 10, pp. 775–83, 1938.

[2] J. G. Hamilton and M. H. Soley, "Studies in iodine metabolism by the use of a new radioactive isotope of iodine," *American Journal of Physiology,* vol. 127, pp. 557–72, 1939.

[3] J. G. Hamilton and J. H. Lawrence, "Recent clinical developments in the therapeutic application of radiophosphorus and radioiodine," *J Clin Invest,* vol. 21, p. 624, 1942.

[4] S. Hertz and A. Roberts, "Application of radioactive iodine in Graves disease," *J Clin Invest,* vol. 21, 1942.

[5] S. M. Seidlin, L. D. Marinelli, and E. Oshry, "Radioactive iodine therapy: Effect on functioning metastases of adenocarcinoma of the thyroid," *JAMA,* vol. 132, pp. 838–47, 1946.

[6] D. S. Riggs, "Quantitative aspects of iodine metabolism in man," *Pharmacol Rev,* vol. 4, no. 3, pp. 284–370, 1952.

[7] B. Cassen, L. Curtis, C. Reed, and R. Libby, "Instrumentation for 131I use in medical studies," *Nucleonics,* vol. 9, pp. 46–50, 1951.

[8] H. O. Anger, "Use of a gamma-ray pinhole camera for in vivo studies," *Nature,* vol. 170, no. 4318, pp. 200–201, 1952.

[9] P. V. Harper, K. A. Lathrop, R. J. McCardle, and G. Andros, *The Use of Technetium-99m as a Clinical Scanning Agent for Thyroid, Liver and Brain.* International Atomic Energy Agency: IAEA, 1964.

[10] N. Carrasco, "Iodide transport in the thyroid-gland," *Biochim Biophys Acta,* vol. 1154, no. 1, pp. 65–82, 1993.

[11] S. Eskandari, D. D. Loo, G. Dai, O. Levy, E. M. Wright, and N. Carrasco, "Thyroid Na+/I- symporter. Mechanism, stoichiometry, and specificity," *J Biol Chem,* vol. 272, no. 43, pp. 27230–8, 1997.

[12] T. Saito *et al.*, "Increased expression of the Na+/I- symporter in cultured human thyroid cells exposed to thyrotropin and in Graves' thyroid tissue," *J Clin Endocrinol Metab,* vol. 82, no. 10, pp. 3331–6, 1997.

[13] V. Lazar *et al.*, "Expression of the Na+/I- symporter gene in human thyroid tumours: A comparison study with other thyroid-specific genes," *J Clin Endocrinol Metab,* vol. 84, no. 9, pp. 3228–34, 1999.

[14] D. P. Carvalho and C. Dupuy, "Thyroid hormone biosynthesis and release," *Mol Cell Endocrinol,* vol. 458, pp. 6–15, 2017.

[15] L. Giovanella *et al.*, "EANM practice guideline/SNMMI procedure standard for RAIU and thyroid scintigraphy," *European Journal of Nuclear Medicine and Molecular Imaging,* vol. 46, no. 12, pp. 2514–25, 2019.

[16] H. Hanscheid, M. Lassmann, A. K. Buck, C. Reiners, and F. A. Verburg, "The limit of detection in scintigraphic imaging with I-131 in patients with differentiated thyroid carcinoma," *Phys Med Biol,* vol. 59, no. 10, pp. 2353–68, 2014.

[17] M. Lassmann, H. Hanscheid, C. Chiesa, C. Hindorf, G. Flux, and M. Luster, "EANM Dosimetry Committee series on standard operational procedures for pre-therapeutic dosimetry I: Blood and bone marrow dosimetry in differentiated thyroid cancer therapy," *Eur J Nucl Med Mol Imaging,* vol. 35, no. 7, pp. 1405–12, 2008, doi: 10.1007/s00259 008 0761 x.

[18] Y. K. Dewaraja, M. Ljungberg, A. J. Green, P. B. Zanconico, and E. C. Frey, "MIRD Pamphlet No. 24: Guidelines for Quantitative 131I- SPECT in Dosimetry Applications," *J Nucl Med,* vol. 54, pp. 2182–8, 2013.

[19] B. J. Beattie, R. D. Finn, D. J. Rowland, and K. S. Pentlow, "Quantitative imaging of bromine-76 and yttrium-86 with PET: A method for the removal of spurious activity introduced by cascade gamma rays," *Med Phys,* vol. 30, pp. 2410–23, 2003.

[20] P. Hetkamp, V. Stebner, I. Binse, and W. Jentzen, "Quantitative PET imaging for dosimetry as exemplified by ^{124}I, ^{86}Y, ^{68}Ga, and ^{44}Sc," *Der Nuklearmediziner,* vol. 41, no. 01, pp. 37–51, 2018, doi: 10.1055/s-0043-120726.

[21] C. C. Watson, "New, faster, image-based scatter correction for 3D PET," *Ieee T Nucl Sci,* vol. 47, no. 4, pp. 1587–94, 2000.

[22] V. Preylowski *et al.*, "Is the image quality of I-124-PET impaired by an automatic correction of prompt gammas?" *PLoS One,* vol. 8, no. 8, p. e71729, 2013, doi: 10.1371/journal.pone.0071729.

[23] F. Paquet *et al.*, "ICRP Publication 137: Occupational intakes of radionuclides: Part 3," *Annals of the ICRP,* vol. 46, no. 3–4, pp. 1–486, 2017.

[24] G. Glatting, P. Kletting, S. N. Reske, K. Hohl, and C. Ring, "Choosing the optimal fit function: Comparison of the Akaike information criterion and the F-test," *Med Phys,* Research Support, Non-U.S. Gov't vol. 34, no. 11, pp. 4285–92, 2007.

[25] ICRP78, "Individual monitoring for internal exposure of workers replacement of ICRP publication 54," *Ann ICRP,* vol. 27, no. 3–4, pp. i-x, 1–161, 1997.

[26] W. E. Bolch, K. F. Eckerman, G. Sgouros, and S. R. Thomas, "MIRD Pamphlet No. 21: A generalized schema for radiopharmaceutical dosimetry—standardization of nomenclature," *J Nucl Med,* vol. 50, no. 3, pp. 477–84, 2009, doi: 10.2967/jnumed.108.056036.

[27] K. F. Eckerman and A. Endo, S. o. N. Medicine, Ed. *MIRD: Radionuclide Data and Decay Schemes.* Reston, VA: Society of Nuclear Medicine, 2008.

[28] W. S. Snyder, *"S," Absorbed Dose Per Unit Cumulated Activity for Selected Radionuclides and Organs* (NM/MIRD pamphlet no 11). New York: Society of Nuclear Medicine, 1975.

[29] W. S. Snyder, H. L. Fisher, M. R. Ford, and G. G. Warner, "Estimates of absorbed fractions for monoenergetic photon sources uniformly distributed in various organs of a heterogeneous phantom," *Journal of Nuclear Medicine,* vol. 10, no. 3S, p. 7, 1969.

[30] W. Eschner, C. Kobe, and H. Schicha, "Follow-up on thyroidal uptake after radioiodine therapy: How robust is the peri-therapeutic dosimetry?" *Z Med Phys,* vol. 21, no. 4, pp. 258–65, 2011.

[31] H. Hanscheid *et al.*, "EANM Dosimetry Committee series on standard operational procedures for pre-therapeutic dosimetry II. Dosimetry prior to radioiodine therapy of benign thyroid diseases," *Eur J Nucl Med Mol Imaging,* vol. 40, no. 7, pp. 1126–34, 2013, doi: 10.1007/s00259-013-2387-x.

[32] T. Rink, F. J. Bormuth, S. Braun, M. Zimny, and H. J. Schroth, "Concept and validation of a simple model of the intrathyroidal iodine kinetics," *Nuklearmedizin,* vol. 43, no. 1, pp. 21–5, 2004.

[33] H. Hänscheid, M. Lassmann, and C. Reiners, "Dosimetry prior to ^{131}I-therapy of benign thyroid disease," *Z Med Phys,* vol. 21, no. 4, pp. 250–57, 2011.

[34] M. P. Stokkel, D. Handkiewicz Junak, M. Lassmann, M. Dietlein, and M. Luster, "EANM procedure guidelines for therapy of benign thyroid disease," *Eur J Nucl Med Mol Imaging,* vol. 37, no. 11, pp. 2218–28, 2010, doi: 10.1007/s00259-010-1536-8.

[35] D. S. Ross *et al.*, "2016 American Thyroid Association Guidelines for Diagnosis and Management of Hyperthyroidism and Other Causes of Thyrotoxicosis," *Thyroid,* vol. 26, no. 10, pp. 1343–1421, 2016.

[36] B. R. Haugen *et al.*, "2015 American Thyroid Association Management Guidelines for Adult Patients with Thyroid Nodules and Differentiated Thyroid Cancer: The American Thyroid Association Guidelines Task Force on Thyroid Nodules and Differentiated Thyroid Cancer," *Thyroid,* vol. 26, no. 1, pp. 1–133, 2016.

[37] M. Luster *et al.*, "Guidelines for radioiodine therapy of differentiated thyroid cancer," *Eur J Nucl Med Mol Imaging,* vol. 35, no. 10, pp. 1941–59, 2008, doi: 10.1007/s00259-008-0883-1.

[38] H. Hänscheid *et al.*, "Iodine biokinetics and dosimetry in radioiodine therapy of thyroid cancer: procedures and results of a prospective international controlled study of ablation after rhTSH or hormone withdrawal," *J Nucl Med,* vol. 47, no. 4, pp. 648–54, 2006, PMID: 16595499.

[39] F. A. Verburg *et al.*, "I-131 activities as high as safely administrable (AHASA) for the treatment of children and adolescents with advanced differentiated thyroid cancer," *J Clin Endocrinol Metab,* vol. 96, no. 8, pp. E1268–71, 2011, doi: 10.1210/jc.2011-0520.

[40] M. Lassmann, M. Luster, H. Hänscheid, and C. Reiners, "Impact of ^{131}I diagnostic activities on the biokinetics of thyroid remnants," *J Nucl Med,* vol. 45, no. 4, pp. 619–25, 2004.

[41] H. R. Maxon *et al.*, "Relation between effective radiation dose and outcome of radioiodine therapy for thyroid cancer," *N Engl J Med,* vol. 309, no. 16, pp. 937–41, 1983.

[42] H. R. Maxon, 3rd, and H. S. Smith, "Radioiodine-131 in the diagnosis and treatment of metastatic well differentiated thyroid cancer," *Endocrinol Metab Clin North Am,* vol. 19, no. 3, pp. 685–718, 1990.

[43] W. Jentzen *et al.*, "Assessment of lesion response in the initial radioiodine treatment of differentiated thyroid cancer using ^{124}I PET imaging," *J Nucl Med,* vol. 55, no. 11, pp. 1759–65, 2014, doi: 10.2967/jnumed.114.144089.

[44] R. Dorn, J. Kopp, H. Vogt, P. Heidenreich, R. G. Carroll, and S. A. Gulec, "Dosimetry-guided radioactive iodine treatment in patients with metastatic differentiated thyroid cancer: Largest safe dose using a risk-adapted approach," *J Nucl Med,* vol. 44, no. 3, pp. 451–6, 2003.

[45] C. Chiesa et al., "Individualized dosimetry in the management of metastatic differentiated thyroid cancer," *Q J Nucl Med Mol Imaging,* vol. 53, no. 5, pp. 546–61, 2009, PMID: 19910908.

[46] G. D. Flux et al., "A dose-effect correlation for radioiodine ablation in differentiated thyroid cancer," *Eur J Nucl Med Mol Imaging,* vol. 37, no. 2, pp. 270–75, 2010, doi: 10.1007/s00259-009-1261-3.

[47] B. de Keizer et al., "Tumour dosimetry and response in patients with metastatic differentiated thyroid cancer using recombinant human thyrotropin before radioiodine therapy," *Eur J Nucl Med Mol Imaging,* vol. 30, no. 3, pp. 367–73, 2003, doi: 10.1007/s00259-002-1076-y.

[48] G. Sgouros et al., "Patient-specific dosimetry for 131I thyroid cancer therapy using 124I PET and 3-dimensional-internal dosimetry (3D-ID) software," *J Nucl Med,* vol. 45, pp. 1366–72, 2004, PMID: 15299063.

[49] J. Klubo-Gwiezdzinska et al., "Efficacy of dosimetric versus empiric prescribed activity of ^{131}I for therapy of differentiated thyroid cancer," *J Clin Endocrinol Metab,* vol. 96, no. 10, pp. 3217–25, 2011, doi: 10.1210/jc.2011-0494.

[50] P. Minguez, G. Flux, J. Genolla, A. Delgado, E. Rodeno, and K. Sjogreen Gleisner, "Whole-remnant and maximum-voxel SPECT/CT dosimetry in ^{131}I-NaI treatments of differentiated thyroid cancer," *Med Phys,* vol. 43, no. 10, pp. 5279–87, 2016, doi: 10.1118/1.4961742.

[51] J. Tran-Gia, M. Salas-Ramirez, and M. Lassmann, "What you see is not what you get – On the accuracy of voxel-based dosimetry in molecular radiotherapy," *J Nucl Med,* 2019, doi: 10.2967/jnumed.119.231480.

[52] R. S. Benua, N. R. Cicale, M. Sonenberg, and R. W. Rawson, "The relation of radioiodine dosimetry to results and complications in the treatment of metastatic thyroid cancer," *Am J Roentgenol Radium Ther Nucl Med,* vol. 87, pp. 171–82, 1962.

[53] R. M. Tuttle et al., "Empiric radioactive iodine dosing regimens frequently exceed maximum tolerated activity levels in elderly patients with thyroid cancer," *J Nucl Med,* vol. 47, no. 10, pp. 1587–91, 2006.

[54] K. Kulkarni, D. Van Nostrand, F. Atkins, M. Aiken, K. Burman, and L. Wartofsky, "The relative frequency in which empiric dosages of radioiodine would potentially overtreat or undertreat patients who have metastatic well-differentiated thyroid cancer," *Thyroid,* vol. 16, no. 10, pp. 1019–23, 2006.

[55] C. Menzel et al., "'High-dose' radioiodine therapy in advanced differentiated thyroid carcinoma," *J Nucl Med,* vol. 37, no. 9, pp. 1496–503, 1996.

[56] W. Jentzen et al., "Assessment of lesion response in the initial radioiodine treatment of differentiated thyroid cancer using I-124 PET imaging," *Journal of Nuclear Medicine,* vol. 55, no. 11, pp. 1759–65, 2014.

[57] M. G. Stabin, R. B. Sparks, and E. Crowe, "OLINDA/EXM: The second-generation personal computer software for internal dose assessment in nuclear medicine," *J Nucl Med,* vol. 46, no. 6, pp. 1023–7, 2005, PMID: 15937315.

[58] H. Hänscheid, M. Fernandez, and M. Lassmann, "The absorbed dose to blood from blood-borne activity," *Phys Med Biol,* vol. 60, no. 2, pp. 741–53, 2015.

[59] F. A. Verburg, M. Lassmann, U. Mader, M. Luster, C. Reiners, and H. Hanscheid, "The absorbed dose to the blood is a better predictor of ablation success than the administered ^{131}I activity in thyroid cancer patients," *Eur J Nucl Med Mol Imaging,* vol. 38, no. 4, pp. 673–80, 2011, doi: 10.1007/s00259-010-1689-5.

[60] K. S. Kolbert et al., "Prediction of absorbed dose to normal organs in thyroid cancer patients treated with ^{131}I by use of [124]I PET and 3-dimensional internal dosimetry software," *J Nucl Med,* vol. 48, no. 1, pp. 143–9, 2007.

[61] H. Hänscheid, M. Lassmann, M. Luster, R. T. Kloos, and C. Reiners, "Blood dosimetry from a single measurement of the whole-body radioiodine retention in patients with differentiated thyroid carcinoma," *Endocr Relat Cancer,* vol. 16, no. 4, pp. 1283–9, 2009, doi: 10.1677/ERC-09-0076.

14 Bone Marrow Dosimetry

Cecilia Hindorf

CONTENTS

The calculation of absorbed dose to bone marrow is performed to avoid and/or understand haematological toxicity caused by radionuclide therapy. However, bone marrow dosimetry is less utilized nowadays when radionuclide therapies commonly are administered in fractions several weeks apart, compared to earlier when radionuclide therapies commonly were administered as a single injection. The time period between each fraction administered allows the physician to follow the decrease in blood counts and recovery. The administered activity per fraction is also generally smaller than if the radionuclide therapy is administered as a single injection. Bone marrow dosimetry has a role to play in the development of new radiopharmaceuticals for therapeutic nuclear medicine. Bone marrow dosimetry is performed in diagnostic nuclear medicine, although with the aim to optimize imaging procedures, that is, to receive an image quality sufficiently good for the physician to diagnose the patient with the smallest possible dose to the patient, develop new radiopharmaceuticals, or to compare different imaging modalities to diagnose the patient.

This chapter begins with an overview of anatomy, physiology, and haematologic toxicity expected to be received from irradiation of the bone marrow during radionuclide therapy. The development of anatomical models for calculation of S values (absorbed dose per decay) is reviewed, a guide on how to perform clinical bone marrow dosimetry is presented, and at the end is a review of absorbed dose and toxicity presented for common radiopharmaceuticals.

14.1 ANATOMY, PHYSIOLOGY AND TOXICITY

The bone marrow is a dispersed organ, present within all bones of the body. The weight of the bone marrow is approximately 5 per cent of the total-body weight. The reference value for weight of total marrow for a 35-year-old male is 3650 g and 2700 g for a 35-year-old female [1].

The role of the bone marrow is to produce mature blood cells, the haemopoiesis. Bone marrow is often divided into red and yellow marrow. Red marrow is haemopoietically active and gets its colour from red blood cells (erythrocytes), whilst yellow marrow mainly consists of fat cells. The red marrow produces almost all blood cells, that is, red blood cells, white

DOI: 10.1201/9780429489549-14

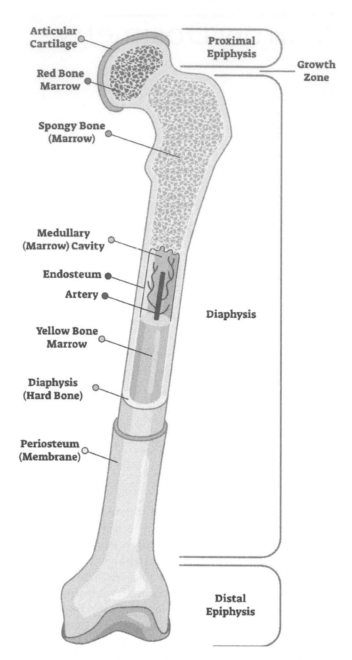

FIGURE 14.1   The anatomy of a long bone and the sites for red and yellow bone marrow. Colour image available at www.routledge.com/9781138593299.

blood cells (all granulocytes and monocytes and the main part of the lymphocytes), and the platelets. Yellow marrow does not produce blood cells, although it can be converted into red marrow if an unusual demand for blood cells should occur. The anatomy of a long bone, and the sites for red and yellow bone marrow within the bone, can be seen in Figure 14.1.

The proportions of red and yellow marrow within the body change with the age of the person. For an infant, all of the bone marrow is red. However, the red marrow is transformed into yellow with age. The transformation occurs at different paces in different bones. The red marrow within a given bone, expressed as per cent of total red marrow within the body at different ages can be seen in Table 14.1.

The bone marrow is a complex organ as it is distributed in the body to produce blood cells, which in their turn supply the organism with oxygen, defend it from disease and protect it from blood loss. Both macroscopic and microscopic perspectives are needed. Three aspects are of special importance for haemopoiesis: the dynamics of blood cell renewal, the sub-structure of the bone marrow, and the regulation of the bone marrow as one organ [3].

TABLE 14.1
Red, Active, Marrow in a Given Bone Expressed as a Percentage of Total Active Marrow in the Body [1, 2]

Bone	Percentage of active (red) marrow at different ages		
	1 year	10 years	40 years
Cranium	25.1	11.6	7.6
Sternum	0.8	2.1	3.1
Ribs	8.9	10.9	16.1
Lumbar vertebrae	4.3	8.4	12.3
Sacrum	2.4	6.7	9.9
Femur, upper half	4.1	9.4	6.7
Humerus, upper half	2.4	2.5	2.3

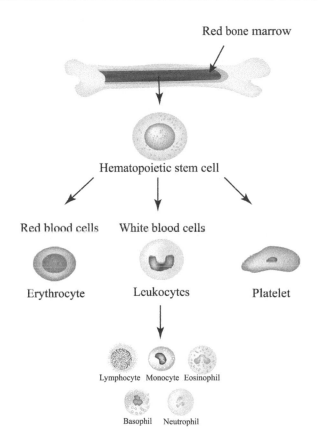

FIGURE 14.2 A simplified model of haematopoiesis, from stem cells present in red bone marrow to differentiated blood cells. Colour image available at www.routledge.com/9781138593299.

14.1.1 Blood Cells, Their Function and Renewal

Haemopoietic stem cells, present in bone marrow, have the ability of self-duplication and differentiation and to produce most blood cells, although maturation, activation, and proliferation of some cells occur at other sites, as in the spleen, thymus, and/or lymph nodes. An overview of the hemopoiesis, the production and development of differentiated blood cells (red, white and platelets), from stem cells within the bone marrow can be seen in Figure 14.2.

The function of the red blood cells (also named erythrocytes) is to deliver oxygen to the tissues. The red blood cells take up oxygen in the lungs, transport it via blood flow through the circulatory system, and release the oxygen in the capillaries. The production/maturation time from stem cell to mature red blood cell is about 7 days. A red blood cell has a lifetime of about 100–120 days. Women have 4–5 million red blood cells per microlitre of blood, and men have 5–6 million red blood cells per microlitre of blood, and it is the most common blood cell.

White blood cells (also named leukocytes) are part of the immune system and help to protect the body against infectious diseases and foreign invaders. There are three main types of white blood cells: granulocutes (eosinophils, basofils, and neutrophils), lymphocytes, and monocytes. The process from stem cell to mature granulocyte takes 10–14 days. Each day $1.6 \cdot 10^4$ granulocytes per kg body weight may be produced within the human body. Normal white blood cell counts usually is between $4 \cdot 10^9 – 1.1 \cdot 10^{10}$ per litre of blood.

Platelets (also named thrombocytes) protect against blood loss by promoting clotting at sites of injury. The platelets are produced by the megacaryocytes, which have an estimated maturation time from stem cell to platelet-producing megacaryocyte of 10 days. The average life span of a circulating platelet is 8–9 days, and there are about 150,000–400,000 platelets per microlitre of peripheral blood. However, the number of platelets can increase by 150–200 per cent of its initial level in case of excessive bleeding.

14.1.2 THE SUBSTRUCTURE OF THE BONE MARROW

Each bone marrow unit within the trabecular bone is surrounded by a bone capsule. Within the capsule is a vascular system, nerves, and parenchyma (the essential/functional part of the tissue) present. The stem cells are inhomogeneously distributed in the parenchyma, localized close to the endosteum of the bone. The rigid structure of the bone capsule makes the volume constant, which must make the production of cells inside the sub-unit to result in an increase of the pressure. To maintain equilibrium, the production of one cell must result in one cell lost, either by senescence or migration, from the prenchyma, via the sinusoids and out to the venous side of the blood circulation. Proliferation and blood flow in the sub-unit makes the pressure to increase or decrease. The nerves are thought to give signals of the local pressure within the unit and regulates the blood flow to the sub-unit. A high cell production within the sub-unit increases the pressure, and the blood flow decreases the pressure. It has been shown that the specific microstructure within the sub-unit is important for regeneration of blood cell production after irradiation.

14.1.3 REGULATION AS ONE ORGAN

The result from a bone marrow biopsy in the sternum gives essentially the same composition of the marrow tissue as a biopsy in the iliac crest in a normal person. It is also known that biopsies at different sites from a person diagnosed with leukaemia give very similar results. Thus, regulation of the individual bone marrow sub-units to act as one organ have to take place even though they act as individuals and are dispersed throughout the body. The regulation is thought to be performed both from factors relating to the circulation and from factors relating to nerve impulses. Experimental data suggest that the circulating stem cells have a function to assure a sufficient concentration of stem cells in the individual bone marrow sub-units, and the migration of stem cells is important for the function of the haematopoietic bone marrow organ system. Extramedullary haematopoiesis can be found in spleen, liver, and lymph nodes in a diseased patient. This and the local effect caused by bone marrow irradiation can be seen in PET images after injection of ^{18}F-FLT, a thymidine analog and a radiopharmaceutical to image cell proliferation [4].

All types of toxicity are defined by the Common Terminology Criteria for Adverse Events (CTCAE) developed to give a standardized nomenclature [5]. Many clinical trials use CTCAE to describe toxicity. The severity of the toxicity

TABLE 14.2

The Most Common Types of Haematological Toxicity due to Bone Marrow Toxicity During Radionuclide Therapy and Their Definitions According to CTCAE v5.0. LLN = Lower Limits of Normal

Type of toxicity	Grade 1	Grade 2	Grade 3	Grade 4
Platelet count decreased	<LLN - 75,000 /mm³	<75,000–50,000 /mm³	<50,000–25,000 /mm³	<25,000 /mm³
Neutrophil count decreased	<LLN – 1500 /mm³	<1500–1000 /mm³	<1000–500 /mm³	<500 /mm³
White blood cell decreased	<LLN – 3000 /mm³	<3000–2000 /mm³	<2000–1000 /mm³	<1000 /mm³
Anaemia (hemoglobin)	<LLN – 100 g/L	<100 0 g/L	<80 g/L	Life-threatening consequences

is scaled into five levels in which Grade 1 is considered as mild, Grade 2 moderate, Grade 3 severe, Grade 4 life-threatening, and Grade 5 death related to the adverse event. Myelotoxicity (damage to the bone marrow) is generally determined indirectly as a haematological toxicity, that is, as a drop in blood counts in peripheral blood. The CTCAE has defined levels of number of blood cells for which a certain grade of toxicity is defined. The response of the bone marrow after irradiation depends on whether the irradiation is acute or prolonged, and whether the total body or parts of it are irradiated [6]. The most common major group of toxicity related to treatment with radiopharmaceuticals is haematological, and Table 14.2 shows the most common types and their definitions according to CTCAE v5.0. [7].

14.2 ANATOMICAL MODELS AND S VALUES FOR BONE MARROW

Bone marrow and the trabecular bone have been investigated with an aim for internal dosimetry by several researchers. Spiers and co-workers at the University of Leeds investigated the trabecular bone structure and determined mean cavity pathlengths for persons at different ages and in different types of bones. Spiers and co-workers [8, 9] also calculated dose factors for both volume-seeking and surface-deposited beta emitters based on the previously determined bone structure. These dose factors were calculated from particle track-lengths, determined by the continuous slowing down approximation (CSDA). The typical structure of trabecular bone, in which the red marrow is found, can be seen in Figure 14.3.

The dosimetry due to Spiers and co-workers [10–12] was used for calculation of limits of intake of radionuclides by workers [13] and for S values (dose factors representing the absorbed dose in a target volume per decay in the source volume) presented in MIRD Pamphlet 11 [14]. The absorbed doses based in Spiers's work were conservative, especially for photons below 300 keV, as the original aim was radiation protection, not dosimetry for radionuclide therapy [15], and improvements were made [16]. Bolch and his research group at the University of Florida have continued the work that Spiers began, by investigating the anatomy of the trabecular bone and the cellularity of the bone marrow [17–19]. The increase in knowledge of the anatomy and technical improvements in the form of computer power has led to new absorbed fractions (or S values) having been calculated and published over the last twenty years [20–24].

The distribution of stem cells within the trabecular bone plays an essential role for the absorbed dose when particles with a short range are utilized for radionuclide therapy. Therefore, Watchman and colleagues published absorbed fractions that depended on the cellularity of the bone marrow [25] and Hobbs and colleagues developed a toxicity model for ^{223}Ra, an alpha particle emitter commonly used for radionuclide therapy [26].

14.3 CLINICAL BONE MARROW DOSIMETRY

The mean absorbed dose to a target region, which in this case is the bone marrow (BM), $\bar{D}_{BM}$, is calculated as the cumulated activity, $\tilde{A}_{source}$, (the number of decays in a source region) multiplied by the S value, $S_{BM \leftarrow source}$, (absorbed

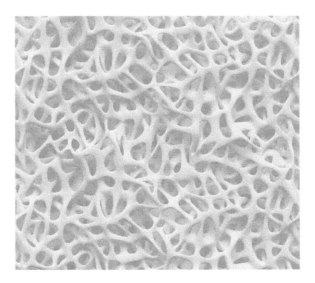

FIGURE 14.3 Structure of trabecular bone, in which the bone marrow is present.

dose to bone marrow per decay in a source region) as described by the MIRD formalism (Medical Internal Radiation Dose) [27–29].

The total mean absorbed dose to the bone marrow ($\bar{D}_{BM}$) is the sum of the self- and the cross-absorbed dose. The self-absorbed dose is the absorbed dose from activity present in the bone marrow itself ($\bar{D}_{BM\leftarrow BM}$), whilst the cross-absorbed dose originates from activity present in tissues other than bone marrow – for example, bone ($\bar{D}_{BM\leftarrow bone}$), major organs or tissues ($\bar{D}_{BM\leftarrow h}$), or the remainder of the body ($\bar{D}_{BM\leftarrow RoB}$) (Eqn. 14.1).

$$\bar{D}_{BM} = \bar{D}_{BM\leftarrow BM} + \bar{D}_{BM\leftarrow bone} + \sum_h \bar{D}_{BM\leftarrow h} + \bar{D}_{BM\leftarrow RoB} \tag{14.1}$$

The relative proportions of the self- and the cross-absorbed dose, which source regions to include, and how they are calculated, depends on the biodistribution of the radiopharmaceutical. The data necessary to acquire to perform bone marrow dosimetry therefore depends on the radiopharmaceutical applied. However, the activity in the total body should always be determined, as it can be used to calculate the activity in the remainder of the body (Eqn. 14.2).

$$A_{RoB} = A_{WB} - \sum_h A_h \tag{14.2}$$

where h indicates an organ with an activity of A_h.

In a clinical setting, the contributions from the four source regions in Eqn. 14.1 can be determined as [30]:

- If the activity does not accumulate in bone, bone marrow, or components of the blood, the activity in plasma should be determined. However, if there is an activity uptake in any components of the blood, the activity concentration in blood should be determined via blood sampling (section 14.3.1).
- If there is an activity uptake in bone or bone marrow, quantitative imaging should be applied (section 14.3.2).
- The contribution from major organs or tissues is generally small, but if there is a suspicion that this could be of importance, then the activity in relevant organs/tissues should be determined via quantitative imaging (Chapters 25 and 26 in Volume I).
- For some radiopharmaceuticals, for example ^{131}I-MIBG, a correlation between the absorbed dose to whole body and haematological toxicity has been found, which indicates that whole-body dosimetry would suffice to be able to predict or avoid haematologic toxicity (section 3.3).

14.3.1 Dosimetry Based on Blood Samples

Blood samples should be drawn from a vessel in the arm opposite to where the administration of the radiopharmaceutical was performed. The blood should be put in tubes that are individually weighed before and after the blood sampling is performed to be able to determine the exact mass and activity concentration of the blood. The activity in the tube can be measured in an automatic sample exchanger equipped with a well-type scintillation detector. The sample exchanger must be rigorously calibrated for the radionuclide, the type of tubes, and for the volume of the blood within the tubes. If the tubes are centrifuged, it will be possible to separate plasma from the blood cells. The plasma is put in another pre-weighted tube with a pipette. The tube is weighted again after the plasma is put in the tube, and the activity is determined within an automatic sample exchanger. Serial blood sampling must be performed at different points in time after the administration of the radiopharmaceutical to be able to calculate the cumulated activity. The points in time after administration, and the number of time points should be chosen so that the area under the time-activity curve gives an accurate representation of the number of decays.

The activity concentration in red marrow can be calculated from the activity concentration in blood or plasma by the blood method, which has been described by Sgouros [31]. The method assumes that the radiopharmaceutical is rapidly distributed in plasma and the extracellular space of the bone marrow, and that the radiopharmaceutical does not bind to any blood, bone marrow, or bone components.

$$\frac{[A]_{RM}}{[A]_{BL}} = \frac{RMECFF}{1-HCT} = RMBLR \tag{14.3}$$

If the activity concentration in a blood sample, $[A]_{BL}$, from the patient is determined, the activity concentration in the red marrow, $[A]_{RM}$, can be calculated via the red marrow-to-blood activity concentration ratio (RMBLR). The value for the red marrow-to-blood activity concentration ratio (RMBLR) equals 0.36, when a red marrow extra cellular fluid fraction (RMECFF) of 0.19 and a haematocrit value (HCT) of 0.47 is assumed. A RMBLR equal to 0.36 is commonly used and could be considered as a baseline value. Alternatively, if the patient's haematocrit value is known, the RMBLR can be calculated as 0.19/(1-HCT).

To calculate the cumulated activity, the activity concentration must be multiplied by the total amount of red marrow in the body of each patient. However, the total amount of red marrow cancels out in the equations when the S value is scaled to the patient-specific amount of red marrow (Eqn. 14.4).

$$\bar{D}_{BM} = \tilde{A}_{BM} \cdot S_{BM \leftarrow BM} =$$
$$= \int [A](t)_{BL} \, dt \cdot RMBLR \cdot m_{BM,patient} \cdot S_{BM \leftarrow BM} \cdot m_{BM,phantom} / m_{BM,patient} \qquad (14.4)$$
$$= \int [A](t)_{BL} \, dt \cdot RMBLR \cdot S_{BM \leftarrow BM} \cdot m_{BM,phantom}$$

14.3.2 IMAGE-BASED DOSIMETRY

The activity in bone marrow can be quantified from nuclear medicine images, commonly SPECT images, but PET images can also be used. The images must be quantitative, that is, they must be corrected for attenuation, scatter, septum penetration, and scaled by a camera calibration factor, as appropriate. Also, the recovery of activity for the segmented volume has to be assessed. The recovery depends on the spatial resolution, and the activity present in the surrounding areas has to be taken into account. A comprehensive description of activity quantification from patient images can be found elsewhere in this book (for example, Chapters 25 and 26 in Volume I).

Nuclear medicine images (SPECT and PET) have a spatial resolution in the order of magnitude of mm to cm that makes it impossible to determine if the quantified activity is present in bone marrow, cortical bone, or trabecular bone, and whether it is distributed on the bone surface or within the whole bone volume. Values on the amount of trabecular and cortical bone present in different bones in the body for a reference can be found in *ICRP Report 70* [1] together with the size of the surface of cortical and trabecular bone in different bones.

Since it is exceedingly difficult to segment the whole bone marrow to determine the total activity in bone marrow for each patient, it is important to choose a region that is representative for the red marrow within the whole body. The chosen region should be reasonably large to avoid partial-volume effect, be relatively easy to segment, contain a large part of the red marrow, and be placed at a distance from regions in the body with a high activity uptake to avoid spill-in of counts into the target volume. The most appropriate region to use for bone marrow dosimetry therefore must be assessed for each radiopharmaceutical and sometimes for each individual patient. Commonly, the activity in the sacrum and/or the lumbar vertebrae are regions chosen to represent the red marrow [32]. The quantified activity within the chosen region has to be divided by the fraction of red marrow present within the region, that is, if the sacrum is chosen, the activity present in the red marrow in the sacrum has to be divided by 0.099 to represent the activity in red marrow in the whole of the body ($A_{BM} = A_{sacrum}/0.099$). The percentage of the total red marrow that is present in a specific skeletal region can be found in Table 14.1.

Voxel-based dosimetry is another option that can be applied for bone marrow dosimetry based on activity quantification from images. The activity within each voxel of the image is convolved with a dose point kernel or by a full Monte Carlo–based calculation to receive an image that displays the absorbed dose within each voxel. Voxel-based dosimetry is described in more detail in Chapter 10.

14.3.3 TOTAL BODY ACTIVITY BASED ON PROBE MEASUREMENTS

The absorbed dose to total body has been used as a surrogate for the absorbed dose to bone marrow. The method is relatively simple and has been found useful for some radiopharmaceuticals – for example, ^{131}I-MIBG, for which the total body absorbed dose has been found to correlate to haematological toxicity [33].

The total body content of the radiopharmaceutical is measured at different time points after administration of the radiopharmaceutical. Commonly, a single probe for measurement of dose rate or a scintillation detector is used [34]. All measurements for a given patient must be performed in a fixed geometry to be able to estimate the activity of the radiopharmaceutical. The measurement should be performed with the detector held at the mid-gut level of the patient,

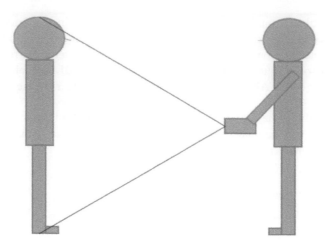

FIGURE 14.4   The distance between the patient and the detector is a compromise between uniform exposition of the detector and the level of the detected signal. The distance is recommended to be at least 1 metre.

and the distance between the patient and the detector should be at least 1 m. Ideally, activity in all parts of the patient should expose the detector equally. The longer the distance the better, as all parts of the patient should expose the detector equally. However, the detected signal will decrease with distance and thereby increase the uncertainty of the measurement. If the patient has a height of 2 m and the measurement is performed at the height and distance of 1 m, then the distance from the head or feet to the detector will be $(1^2+1^2)^{1/2} = 1.4$ m, according to Figure 14.4 and the Pythagorean Theorem. If the measurement is performed at the height 1 m and the distance 2 m, then the distance from the head or feet to the detector will be $(1^2+2^2)^{1/2} = 2.2$ m.

The first measurement should be performed immediately after the administration so that the detected counts or the measured dose rate can be normalized to a given activity. Both prone and supine measurements should be performed to take into account effects of redistribution of the radiopharmaceutical within the body.

The activity in whole body, A_{WB}, at the time of the measurement $t=T$ is calculated according to Eqn. 14.5, where c_{prone} and c_{supine} are the detected number of counts (or the measured dose rate) in the prone and supine positions, respectively, at a given time point, t=T. The time point t=0 equals the time for administration of the radiopharmaceutical.

$$A_{WB,t=T} = A_{WB,t=0} \cdot \frac{\sqrt{c_{prone,t=T} \cdot c_{supine,t=T}}}{\sqrt{c_{prone,t=0} \cdot c_{supine,t=0}}} \tag{14.5}$$

The absorbed dose to the patient is calculated via the MIRD formalism [28, 29]. Briefly, the cumulated activity is calculated either via the time integral of the activity in whole body obtained by fitting measured data to an exponential as function of time or via the trapezoidal method. The cumulated activity is multiplied by a factor that gives the absorbed dose to whole body per activity in total body, that is, the S value.

14.4   DOSIMETRY AND TOXICITY FOR SOME RADIOPHARMACEUTICALS

Several pharmaceuticals for radionuclide therapy have hitherto been approved by EMA (European Medicines Agency www.ema.europa.eu) and/or by the FDA (Federal Drug Agency www.fda.gov). In the summary of product characteristics for these radiopharmaceuticals, the absorbed dose, together with the toxicity, is reported. During treatment with these, thrombocytopenia, neutropenia, leukocytopenia, and anaemia are the most common types of haematological toxicities.

Iodine-131, in the form of sodium iodide (^{131}I-NaI), is the radiopharmaceutical most used for therapy. It is used to treat both benign (thyrotoxicosis) and malignant (thyroid cancer) diseases. The biodistribution is highly dependent on the disease to treat, that is, whether the patient has undergone a thyroidectomy or not, and whether the patient has received pre-treatment with Thyrogen or not. The absorbed dose to red marrow [35, 36] is reported to be 0.035 mGy/MBq when no uptake of iodine is present in the thyroid, which is the case for a patient who receives treatment for thyroid cancer as he/she has undergone a thyroidectomy. This corresponds to 0.26 Gy to red marrow for a treatment with

7400 MBq of ^{131}I-NaI. However, treatment with ^{131}I for thyroid cancer is commonly preceded by injections of Thyrogen to stimulate TSH (Thyroid Stimulating Hormone). As Thyrogen increases the elimination of iodine from normal tissues, this will affect the absorbed dose. Myelodepression and haematological toxicity (thrombocytopenia, erythrocytopenia and/or leukocytopenia) may appear after treatment with ^{131}I-NaI, but the frequencies are not reported in the summary of product characteristics.

It is recommended to administer 3700–4700 MBq of **^{131}I-MIBG**. The absorbed dose to red marrow is reported to be 0.067 mGy/MBq, which corresponds to 0.5 Gy for one treatment of 7400 MBq ^{131}I-MIBG [35]. The radiopharmaceutical is reported to cause myelosuppression, anaemia, thrombocytopenia and neutropenia, but no frequency is reported.

Samarium-153-EDTMP (Quadramet, approved by FDA in 1997 and by EMA in 1998) is used for treatment of bone pain caused by multiple osteoblastic skeletal metastases and is recommended to be administered as a single injection of 37 MBq per kg of body weight. The absorbed dose to red marrow is 1.54 mGy/MBq, which corresponds to 4 Gy for one treatment (2590 MBq for a 70 kg person) [37]. White blood cell and platelet counts have in clinical trials been reported to decrease to a nadir of approximately 40 to 50 per cent of baseline 3 to 5 weeks after treatment, and generally returned to baseline levels by 8 weeks after treatment.

Yttrium-90-ibritumomab tiuxetan (Zevalin, approved by FDA in 2002 and by EMA in 2009) is recommended to be administered once, with an injected activity of 15 MBq/kg of body weight of the patient or 1200 MBq at maximum, to patients diagnosed with a non-Hodgkin lymphoma. The median absorbed dose to red marrow is 1.3 mGy/MBq (range 0.6–1.8 mGy/MBq), which corresponds to 1.4 Gy for one treatment (1050 MBq for a 70 kg patient). Thrombocytopenia, leukocytopenia, neutropenia, and anaemia are reported as very common (>10% of the patients) adverse effects for patients treated with ^{90}Y-ibritumomab tiuxetan.

The recommended activity to administer of **^{131}I-tositumomab** (Bexxar, approved by FDA in 2003) is the activity to deliver 0.75 Gy in total body absorbed dose, based on a pre-therapeutic infusion of 185 MBq ^{131}I-tositumomab for assessment of biodistribution and dosimetry, for patients diagnosed with a lymphoma. The median absorbed dose to total body is reported to be 0.24 mGy/MBq (range 0.2–0.3 mGy/MBq), which would correspond to an administered activity of 3125 MBq for a total body absorbed dose of 0.75 Gy. The median absorbed dose to the marrow space is reported to be 0.65 mGy/MBq (range 0.5–1.1 mGy/MBq), which would correspond to 2 Gy for one treatment of 3125 MBq. Treatment with ^{131}I-tositumomab results in a decrease in number of platelets and neutrophils, which reach a nadir within 3–6 weeks for over 70 per cent of patients [38, 39].

Radium-223-dichloride, ^{223}Ra-Cl$_2$, (Xofigo, approved by both FDA and EMA in 2013) is indicated for treatment of symptomatic bone metastases from metastatic castration-resistant prostate cancer without known visceral metastases. Radium-223-dichloride should be administered as six injections, four weeks apart, of 55 kBq/kg of body weight of the patient. The reported absorbed dose to red marrow is 0.13879 Gy/MBq (with a coefficient of variation of 41%) which corresponds to 0.53 Gy per treatment (3.85 MBq for a 70 kg patient) and a total of 3.2 Gy over a period of 20 weeks (six treatments, four weeks apart). Grade 3–4 thrombocytopenia was observed in 6.3 per cent of the patients who received ^{223}Ra-dichloride and grade 3–4 neutropenia were seen in 2.2 per cent of the patients. Platelet and neutrophil count nadirs were reached 2–3 weeks after administration.

Lutetium-177-DOTATATE (^{177}Lu-oxodotreotid) is a radiolabelled peptide used for treatment of patients diagnosed with a neuroendocrine tumour. The recommended administration schedule for ^{177}Lu-DOTATATE (Lutathera, approved by EMA in 2017 and by FDA in 2018) is four infusions of 7400 MBq, eight weeks apart. The summary of product characteristics reports that bone marrow is the critical organ and that the absorbed dose to bone marrow is 0.03 mGy/MBq (standard deviation 0.03 mGy/MBq), which corresponds to 0.2 Gy per infusion of 7400 MBq of ^{177}Lu-DOTATATE and a total absorbed dose of 0.9 Gy over a period of 24 weeks (four treatments, 8 weeks apart). The dosimetry is based on data from 20 patients. In summary of product characteristics, it is reported that the most expected haematological adverse reactions due to bone marrow toxicity were thrombocytopenia (25%), lymphopenia (22.3%) and anaemia (13.4%) [40]. About 5–10 per cent of the patients who receive treatment with ^{177}Lu-DOTATATE display haematological toxicity grade 3–4 [41–45]. Nadir in blood counts is reached within 4–6 weeks after which recovery starts.

Models to understand or predict bone marrow toxicity from absorbed dose have been developed by several researchers. Fliedner and colleagues developed a biomathematical model to describe the number of granulocytes in peripheral blood after continuous and acute external total body irradiation. The model was tested and found to correlate for humans who received autologus stem cell transfusion [6]. Sas and colleagues developed a compartmental model of mouse thrombopoiesis and erythropoiesis to predict toxicity after internal irradiation [46]. However, in a clinical setting, a correlation between absorbed dose to bone marrow (or red marrow) and myelotoxicity has been difficult to find.

TABLE 14.3

Absorbed Dose to Bone Marrow per Administered Activity for Some Radiopharmaceuticals. The Absorbed Dose to Bone Marrow for One Treatment and the Reported Toxicity. One Treatment Has Been Specified as How the Radiopharmaceutical Commonly Is Prescribed

Radiopharmaceutical	Absorbed dose per administered activity	"One treatment"	Absorbed dose[Gy]	Reported toxicity
^{131}I, NaI	0.035 mGy/MBq	One administration of 7400 MBq	0.26	Myelosuppression and haematological toxicity (thrombocytopenia, erythrocytopenia and/or leukocytopenia).
^{131}I-MIBG	0.067 mGy/MBq	One administration of 7400 MBq	0.5	Myelodepression, anemia, thrombocytopenia and neutropenia.
^{153}Sm-EDTMP	1.54 mGy/MBq	One injection of 37 MBq/kg	4	Decrease in white blood cell and platelet counts.
^{90}Y-ibritumomab tiuxetan	1.3 mGy/MBq	One injection of 15 MBq/kg	1.4	Thrombocytopenia, leukocytopenia, neutropenia and anaemia (>10%)
^{131}I-tositumomab	0.65 mGy/MBq	One injection of activity to give 0.75 Gy absorbed dose to total body	2	Decrease in platelets and neutrophils (70%)
^{223}Ra-Cl$_2$	0.14 Gy/MBq	Six injections of 55 kBq/kg	3.2	Grade 3–4 thrombocytopenia (6.3%), grade 3–4 neutropenia (2.2%)
^{177}Lu-DOTATATE	0.03 mGy/MBq	Four infusions of 7400 MBq	0.9	Thrombocytopenia (25%), lymphopenia (22.3%) and anaemia (13.4%)

Absorbed doses between approximately 0.3 Gy and 4 Gy have been reported (Table 14.3), but the assumptions made, and the methods to determine the absorbed dose to bone marrow, are generally not reported. Also, alpha and beta particles are known to introduce different biological effects, based on their pattern to interact with media. Furthermore, the biodistribution of the radiopharmaceutical on a microscopic scale, together with the short range of particles will make the absorbed dose to be non-uniform over the bone marrow. All the above factors have been shown to influence the correlation between the absorbed dose and toxicity. Furthermore, as can be seen in Table 14.3, the reported toxicities are described differently for different radiopharmaceuticals. Another factor that might affect the biological response is whether the patient has received myelotoxic treatments prior to treatment with the radiopharmaceutical. Furthermore, genomic instability and bystander effects, and their impact on radiobiology in radiotherapy for treatment of cancer still need to be clarified [47]. Despite all these difficulties, one can conclude that an improved method for dosimetry improves the correlation to toxicity [48–51].

REFERENCES

[1] ICRP, 1995. *Basic Anatomical & Physiological Data for Use in Radiological Protection – The Skeleton.* ICRP Publication 70, Ann. ICRP 25 (2).

[2] M. Cristy, "Active bone marrow distribution as a function of age in humans," *Phys Med Biol,* vol. 26, no. 3, pp. 389–400, 1981, doi: 10.1088/0031-9155/26/3/003.

[3] T. M. Fliedner, D. Graessle, C. Paulsen, and K. Reimers, "Structure and function of bone marrow hemopoiesis: Mechanisms of response to ionizing radiation exposure," *Cancer Biother Radiopharm,* vol. 17, no. 4, pp. 405–26, 2002, doi: 10.1089/108497802760363204.

[4] A. Agool, A. W. Glaudemans, H. H. Boersma, R. A. Dierckx, E. Vellenga, and R. H. Slart, "Radionuclide imaging of bone marrow disorders," *Eur J Nucl Med Mol Imaging,* vol. 38, no. 1, pp. 166–78, 2011, doi: 10.1007/s00259-010-1531-0.

[5] "Common terminology criteria for adverse events v5.0 (CTCAE)," U.S. Department of Health and Human Services,

[6] T. M. Fliedner, B. Tibken, E. P. Hofer, and W. Paul, "Stem cell responses after radiation exposure: A key to the evaluation and prediction of its effects," *Health Phys,* vol. 70, no. 6, pp. 787–97, 1996, doi: 10.1097/00004032-199606000-00002.

[7]   D. Murray and A. J. McEwan, "Radiobiology of systemic radiation therapy," *Cancer Biother Radiopharm*, vol. 22, no. 1, pp. 1–23, 2007, doi: 10.1089/cbr.2006.531.

[8]   A. H. Beddoe, P. J. Darley, and F. W. Spiers, "Measurements of trabecular bone structure in man," *Phys Med Biol*, vol. 21, no. 4, pp. 589–607, 1976, doi: 10.1088/0031-9155/21/4/010.

[9]   F. W. Spiers and A. H. Beddoe, " 'Radial' scanning of trabecular bone: consideration of the probability distributions of path lengths through cavities and trabeculae," *Phys Med Biol*, vol. 22, no. 4, pp. 670–80, 1977, doi: 10.1088/0031-9155/22/4/002.

[10] F. W. Spiers, A. H. Beddoe, and J. R. Whitwell, "Mean skeletal dose factors for beta-particle emitters in human bone. Part I: Volume-seeking radionuclides," *Br J Radiol*, vol. 51, no. 608, pp. 622–27, 1978, doi: 10.1259/0007-1285-51-608-622.

[11] F. W. Spiers, J. R. Whitwell, and A. H. Beddoe, "Calculated dose factors for the radiosensitive tissues in bone irradiated by surface-deposited radionuclides," *Phys Med Biol*, vol. 23, no. 3, pp. 481–94, 1978, doi: 10.1088/0031-9155/23/3/011.

[12] F. W. Spiers, A. H. Beddoe, and J. R. Whitwell, "Mean skeletal dose factors for beta-particle emitters in human bone. Part II: Surface-seeking radionuclides," *Br J Radiol*, vol. 54, no. 642, pp. 500–4, 1981, doi: 10.1259/0007-1285-54-642-500.

[13] ICRP, 1979. *Limits for Intakes of Radionuclides by Workers*. ICRP Publication 30 (Part 1), Ann. ICRP 2 (2–4).

[14] W. Snyder, M. Ford, G. Warner, and S. Watson. *MIRD Pamphlet No 11: "S," absorbed dose per unit cumulated activity for selected radionuclides and organs*. (1975). Society of Nuclear Medicine. New York.

[15] M. G. Stabin, K. F. Eckerman, W. E. Bolch, L. G. Bouchet, and P. W. Patton, "Evolution and status of bone and marrow dose models," *Cancer Biother Radiopharm*, vol. 17, no. 4, pp. 427–33, 2002, doi: 10.1089/108497802760363213.

[16] M. Cristy and K. F. Eckerman, *Specific Absorbed Fractions of Energy at Various Ages from Internal Photon Sources. Report ORNL/TM-8381/V1-V7*. Oak Ridge National Laboratory, Oak Ridge, TN, 1987.

[17] J. M. Brindle *et al.*, "Linear regression model for predicting patient-specific total skeletal spongiosa volume for use in molecular radiotherapy dosimetry," *J Nucl Med*, vol. 47, no. 11, pp. 1875–83, 2006.

[18] J. C. Pichardo, R. J. Milner, and W. E. Bolch, "MRI measurement of bone marrow cellularity for radiation dosimetry," *J Nucl Med*, vol. 52, no. 9, pp. 1482–89, 2011, doi: 10.2967/jnumed.111.087957.

[19] A. P. Shah, P. W. Patton, D. A. Rajon, and W. E. Bolch, "Adipocyte spatial distributions in bone marrow: Implications for skeletal dosimetry models," *J Nucl Med*, vol. 44, no. 5, pp. 774–83, 2003.

[20] K. F. Eckerman and M. G. Stabin, "Electron absorbed fractions and dose conversion factors for marrow and bone by skeletal regions," *Health Phys*, vol. 78, no. 2, pp. 199–214, 2000, doi: 10.1097/00004032-200002000-00009.

[21] L. G. Bouchet, W. E. Bolch, R. W. Howell, and D. V. Rao, "S values for radionuclides localized within the skeleton," *J Nucl Med*, vol. 41, no. 1, pp. 189–212, 2000.

[22] A. P. Shah, W. E. Bolch, D. A. Rajon, P. W. Patton, and D. W. Jokisch, "A paired-image radiation transport model for skeletal dosimetry," *J Nucl Med*, vol. 46, no. 2, pp. 344–53, 2005.

[23] M. Zankl, K. F. Eckerman, and W. E. Bolch, "Voxel-based models representing the male and female ICRP reference adult: The skeleton," *Radiat Prot Dosimetry*, vol. 127, no. 1–4, pp. 174–86, 2007, doi: 10.1093/rpd/ncm269.

[24] M. Hough, P. Johnson, D. Rajon, D. Jokisch, C. Lee, and W. Bolch, "An image-based skeletal dosimetry model for the ICRP reference adult male: Internal electron sources," *Phys Med Biol*, vol. 56, no. 8, pp. 2309–46, 2011, doi: 10.1088/0031-9155/56/8/001.

[25] C. J. Watchman, D. W. Jokisch, P. W. Patton, D. A. Rajon, G. Sgouros, and W. E. Bolch, "Absorbed fractions for alpha-particles in tissues of trabecular bone: Considerations of marrow cellularity within the ICRP reference male," *J Nucl Med*, vol. 46, no. 7, pp. 1171–85, 2005.

[26] R. F. Hobbs *et al.*, "A bone marrow toxicity model for ^{223}Ra alpha-emitter radiopharmaceutical therapy," *Phys Med Biol*, vol. 57, no. 10, pp. 3207–22, 2012, doi: 10.1088/0031-9155/57/10/3207.

[27] R. Loevinger, T. F. Budinger, and E. E. Watson, "MIRD primer for absorbed dose calculations," 1988.

[28] W. E. Bolch, K. F. Eckerman, G. Sgouros, and S. R. Thomas, "MIRD pamphlet 21: A generalized schema for radiopharmaceutical dosimetry – standardization of nomenclature," *J Nucl Med*, vol. 50, pp. 477–84, 2009, doi: 10.2967/jnumed.108.056036.

[29] C. Hindorf, "Internal dosimetry," in *Nuclear Medicine Physics: A Handbook for Teachers and Students*, D. L. Bailey, A. van Aswegen, A. Todd-Pokropek, and J. H. Humm Eds. Vienna: International Atomic Energy Agency (IAEA), 2014.

[30] C. Hindorf, G. Glatting, C. Chiesa, O. Lindén, and G. Flux, "EANM Dosimetry Committee guidelines for bone marrow and whole-body dosimetry," *Eur J Nucl Med Mol Imaging*, vol. 37, no. 6, pp. 1238–50, 2010, doi: 10.1007/s00259-010-1422-4.

[31] G. Sgouros, "Bone marrow dosimetry for radioimmunotherapy: Theoretical considerations," *J Nucl Med*, vol. 34, pp. 689–95, 1993.

[32] J. A. Siegel, R. E. Lee, D. A. Pawlyk, J. A. Horowitz, R. M. Sharkey, and D. M. Goldenberg, "Sacral scintigraphy for bone marrow dosimetry in radioimmunotherapy," *Int J Rad Appl Instrum B*, vol. 16, no. 6, pp. 553–59, 1989, doi: 10.1016/0883-2897(89)90070-6.

[33] S. E. Buckley, S. J. Chittenden, F. H. Saran, S. T. Meller, and G. D. Flux, "Whole-body dosimetry for individualized treatment planning of 131I-MIBG radionuclide therapy for neuroblastoma," *J Nucl Med*, vol. 50, no. 9, pp. 1518–24, 2009, doi: 10.2967/jnumed.109.064469.

[34] S. J. Chittenden *et al.*, "Optimization of equipment and methodology for whole body activity retention measurements in children undergoing targeted radionuclide therapy," *Cancer Biother Radiopharm,* vol. 22, no. 2, pp. 243–49, 2007, doi: 10.1089/cbr.2006.315.

[35] ICRP, 1988. *Radiation Dose to Patients from Radiopharmaceuticals.* ICRP Publication 53, Ann. ICRP 18 (1–4)

[36] ICRP, 1991. *1990 Recommendations of the International Commission on Radiological Protection.* ICRP Publication Ann. ICRP 60 (Users Edition)

[37] "Quadramet." www.ema.europa.eu/en/documents/product-information/quadramet-epar-productinformation_en.pdf.

[38] R. L. Wahl, "Tositumomab and (131)I therapy in non-Hodgkin's lymphoma," *J Nucl Med,* vol. 46 Suppl 1, pp. 128s–40s, 2005.

[39] "Bexxar." www.accessdata.fda.gov/drugsatfda_docs/label/2012/125011s0126lbl.pdf.

[40] "Summary of product characteristics (EMA)." www.ema.europa.eu/en/documents/productinformation/lutathera-epar-product-information_en.pdf.

[41] D. J. Kwekkeboom *et al.*, "Treatment with the radiolabeled somatostatin analog [177 Lu-DOTA 0,Tyr3]octreotate: toxicity, efficacy, and survival," *Journal of Clinical Oncology: Official journal of the American Society of Clinical Oncology,* vol. 26, no. 13, pp. 2124–30, 2008, doi: 10.1200/jco.2007.15.2553.

[42] S. K. Gupta, S. Singla, and C. Bal, "Renal and hematological toxicity in patients of neuroendocrine tumors after peptide receptor radionuclide therapy with 177Lu-DOTATATE," *Cancer Biother Radiopharm,* vol. 27, no. 9, pp. 593–99, 2012, doi: 10.1089/cbr.2012.1195.

[43] A. Sabet *et al.*, "Long-term hematotoxicity after peptide receptor radionuclide therapy with 177Lu-octreotate," *J Nucl Med,* vol. 54, no. 11, pp. 1857–61, 2013, doi: 10.2967/jnumed.112.119347.

[44] L. Bodei *et al.*, "Long-term tolerability of PRRT in 807 patients with neuroendocrine tumours: The value and limitations of clinical factors," *Eur J Nucl Med Mol Imaging,* vol. 42, no. 1, pp. 5–19, 2015, doi: 10.1007/s00259-014-2893-5.

[45] H. Bergsma *et al.*, "Subacute haematotoxicity after PRRT with (177)Lu-DOTA-octreotate: Prognostic factors, incidence and course," *Eur J Nucl Med Mol Imaging,* vol. 43, no. 3, pp. 453–63, 2016, doi: 10.1007/s00259-015-3193-4.

[46] N. Sas *et al.*, "A compartmental model of mouse thrombopoiesis and erythropoiesis to predict bone marrow toxicity after internal irradiation," *J Nucl Med,* vol. 55, no. 8, pp. 1355–60, 2014, doi: 10.2967/jnumed.113.133330.

[47] C. Mothersill and C. Seymour, "Low-dose radiation effects: experimental hematology and the changing paradigm," *Exp Hematol,* vol. 31, no. 6, pp. 437–45, 2003, doi: 10.1016/s0301-472x(03)00078-x.

[48] M. E. Juweid, C. H. Zhang, R. D. Blumenthal, G. Hajjar, R. M. Sharkey, and D. M. Goldenberg, "Prediction of hematologic toxicity after radioimmunotherapy with (131)I-labeled anticarcinoembryonic antigen monoclonal antibodies," *J Nucl Med,* vol. 40, no. 10, pp. 1609–16, 1999.

[49] J. A. Siegel *et al.*, "Red marrow radiation dose adjustment using plasma FLT3-L cytokine levels: improved correlations between hematologic toxicity and bone marrow dose for radioimmunotherapy patients," *J Nucl Med,* vol. 44, no. 1, pp. 67–76, 2003.

[50] L. Ferrer *et al.*, "Three methods assessing red marrow dosimetry in lymphoma patients treated with radioimmunotherapy," *Cancer,* vol. 116, no. 4 Suppl, pp. 1093–100, 2010, doi: 10.1002/cncr.24797.

[51] L. Hagmarker *et al.*, "Bone marrow absorbed doses and correlations with hematologic response during (177)Lu-DOTATATE treatments are influenced by image-based dosimetry method and presence of skeletal metastases," *J Nucl Med,* vol. 60, no. 10, pp. 1406–13, 2019, doi: 10.2967/jnumed.118.225235.

15 Cellular and Multicellular Dosimetry

Roger W. Howell

CONTENTS

15.1 INTRODUCTION

The regulatory approvals of the α-particle emitting radiopharmaceutical (RP) radium-223 dichloride (Xofigo®) and the β-particle emitting lutetium-177 Dotatate (LUTATHERA®), and implementation in the clinic, has contributed to reinvigorated interest in radiopharmaceutical therapy (RPT) of cancer. RPT entails the delivery of radioactive drugs to the primary tumour, metastases, and disseminated tumour cells (DTC). Different classes of radionuclides have been advocated for therapy, including α, β, and Auger emitters. The different ranges of these radiations in tissue, and their differences in relative biological effectiveness (RBE), contribute to the complexity of predicting therapeutic efficacy. However, like external beam radiation therapy, the future of RPT will depend in part on our capacity to plan treatments that maximize therapeutic effect while minimizing adverse effects in normal tissues. Key to the long-term success of RPT is to overcome limitations of the intrinsic nonuniform uptake of the radiopharmaceutical by cancer cells that can impact our capacity to sterilize tumours, metastases, and DTC. While primary tumours can often be addressed with external beams of radiation, micrometastases and DTC cannot. While there are commercial tools to assist with calculating absorbed dose to macroscopic disease based on external imaging and using it to predict response, there is a dearth of readily available tools that can be used to optimize and plan RPT of microscopic disease. This chapter describes the rationale and some of the approaches that have been used for modelling the dosimetry and biological response of disseminated tumour cells and micrometastases. It then goes on to present examples of multicellular dose response modelling with the open-source software MIRDcell [1].

DOI: 10.1201/9780429489549-15

15.2 DEFINITION OF CELLULAR AND MULTICELLULAR DOSIMETRY

In this chapter we define cellular dosimetry as the calculation of absorbed dose to a cell from radionuclide decays that occur within the cell of interest. This is also known as the self-dose to a cell. The cell is often modelled as two concentric spheres (Figure 15.1).

As specified in the MIRD schema [3, 4], the cell compartment that contains radioactivity is referred to as the *source region*. This can be the nucleus, cytoplasm, or cell surface. Subcellular organelles could also be considered if modelled suitably [5]. The cell compartment for which the absorbed dose is calculated is known as the *target region*. This is most often taken as the cell nucleus because it houses the nuclear DNA, which is the primary radiosensitive target; however, other compartments may be considered because there are targets in the cytoplasm and on the cell surface, albeit less sensitive [6, 7]. While the concentric sphere model has been used commonly for cellular dosimetry, some models have shifted the centre of the cell nucleus from the centre of the cell [8]. Concentric ellipsoids have also been used [2, 9] (Figure 15.2). Depending on the range of the particles emitted by the radionuclides of interest, these geometries can result in significant changes in the calculated self-dose.

In this chapter we define multicellular dosimetry as the calculation of absorbed doses to cells from radionuclide decays that occur within the target cell(s) of interest as well as the absorbed dose from decays in surrounding cells.

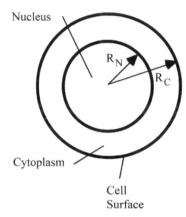

FIGURE 15.1 Model of cell consisting of two concentric spheres making up the nuclear, cytoplasmic, and cell surface compartments. This figure was originally published in MIRD Cellular S values: self-absorbed dose per unit cumulated activity for selected radionuclides and monoenergetic electron and alpha particle emitters incorporated into different cell compartments. S. M. Goddu, R. W. Howell, L. G. Bouchet, W. E. Bolch, and D. V. Rao, Society of Nuclear Medicine, 1997, © SNMMI [2].

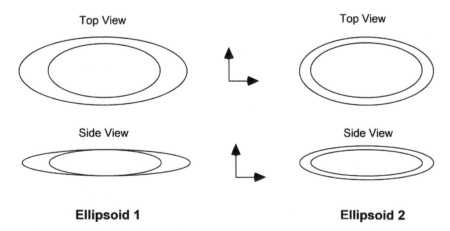

FIGURE 15.2 Ellipsoidal geometry for cellular dosimetry. This figure was originally published in MIRD Cellular S values: self-absorbed dose per unit cumulated activity for selected radionuclides and monoenergetic electron and alpha particle emitters incorporated into different cell compartments. S. M. Goddu, R. W. Howell, L. G. Bouchet, W. E. Bolch, and D. V. Rao, Society of Nuclear Medicine, 1997, © SNMMI [2].

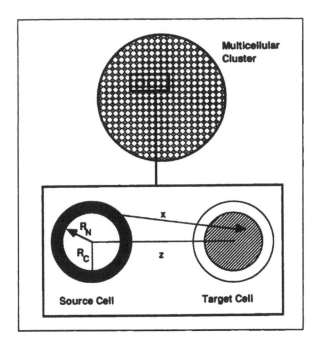

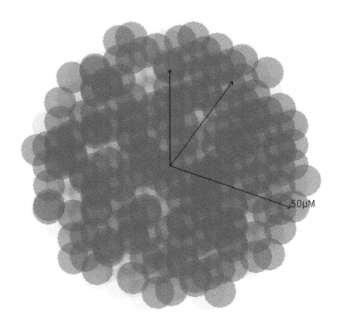

FIGURE 15.3 Spherical multicellular cluster consisting of spherical cells in close packed arrays [1, 10]. The left figure was originally published in *JNM*. S. M. Goddu, D. V. Rao, and R. W. Howell, Multicellular dosimetry for micrometastases: Dependence of self-dose versus cross-dose to cell nuclei on type and energy of radiation and subcellular distribution of radionuclide. J Nucl Med, vol. 35, pp. 521–530, 1994. © SNMMI [10].

The latter is also known as the cross-dose to a cell(s). Multicellular structures are modelled frequently as cubic close-packed or hexagonal close-packed lattices of spherical cells (Figure 15.3); however, more intricate multicellular geometries have also been modelled. These models are often used to represent spheroids used in cell culture experiments or micrometastases in vivo.

Often cells and multicellular structures are located within complex anatomical structures of organs such as the testes, kidneys, liver, bone marrow, and so forth. Such models, often referred to as small-scale dosimetry, provide a greater degree of realism and enable calculating the absorbed dose contributions from distant tissues in the organ. Furthermore, radiopharmaceutical therapies can deliver significant absorbed doses to specific cells within normal tissues. Estimation of risks to these cells can require multicellular dosimetry approaches. For example, a multicellular liver dosimetry model is shown below (Figure 15.4).

15.3 RATIONALE FOR CELLULAR AND MULTICELLULAR DOSIMETRY

It long been recognized that the mean absorbed dose to an organ or tumour is often of limited use in predicting biological response to RPT because of the nonuniform distributions of radioactivity that arise in tissue. The importance of cell-level dosimetry for RPT arose at least as early as the 1950s with the advent of therapeutic use of ^{131}I and [32]P [12, 13]. Multicellular dosimetry was explored by Sinclair in his study on cellular self-dose versus cross-dose (from other cells) when cells labelled with beta particle emitting radionuclides are suspended in the presence of other labelled cells [14]. The imperative of cellular and multicellular dosimetry for predicting the effects of radionuclides was recognized particularly for emitters of low-energy beta particles and alpha particles due to the short range of these radiations in tissue [15]. However, it was not recognized until some years later that cellular dosimetry was most important in the context of radionuclides that emit Auger electrons such as [125]I [16–19]. These Auger-electron emitting radionuclides can be as radiotoxic as alpha-particle emitters when the radionuclide is incorporated into DNA in the cell nucleus [20, 21]. Their radiotoxicity is largely due to the shower of low-energy electrons that are emitted and which produce highly localized energy deposition in the immediate vicinity of the decay site (Figure 15.5) [22–25]. The relative biological effectiveness (RBE) of Auger electron emitters has been shown to depend linearly on the fraction of cellular activity incorporated into nuclear DNA [26].

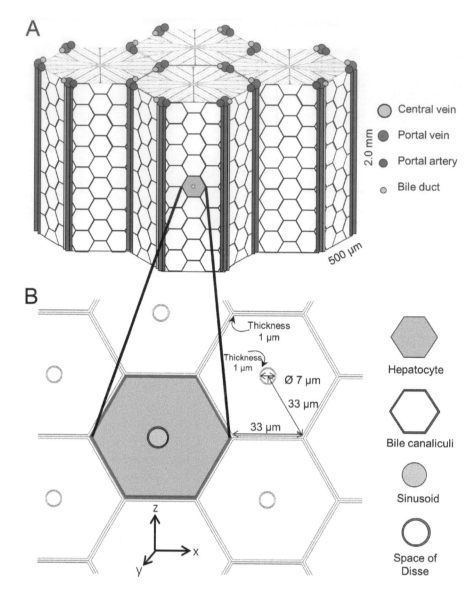

FIGURE 15.4 The small-scale dosimetry model of the liver [11]. Image courtesy Anna Stenvall, Medical Radiation Physics, Lund University, Lund, Sweden. Colour image available at www.routledge.com/9781138593299.

Radionuclides that emit Auger electrons typically emit other radiations as well. For example, ^{111}In also emits internal conversion electrons, the most prominent being 0.145 and 0.219 keV. Electrons of these energies have ranges of many cell diameters and therefore contribute significantly to cross-dose. Therefore, when an ^{111}In-labeled radiopharmaceutical is localized in the cell nucleus, the RBE of the self-dose may be higher than the RBE of the cross-dose. This can also impact DNA-incorporated beta particle emitters. There is evidence that the RBE for self-dose from DNA-incorporated ^{131}I-iododeoxyuridine is substantially higher than that for the cross-dose [28]. The impact that this has on the response of the cell population depends on the self-dose to cross-dose ratios and the activity distribution among the cell population [10, 29].

There is a multitude of published theoretical and experimental studies that support the need for cellular and multicellular dosimetry to predict the effects of the inherent nonuniform distribution of radiopharmaceuticals. Models to calculate absorbed doses to cells from radiopharmaceuticals and predict their responses have been developed over the years to address this problem [2, 10, 28–61]. Many of these models are not interactive, and they are only accessible to the few individuals who have created them, yet each one makes important points regarding the importance of cellular and multicellular dosimetry when predicting effects of radiopharmaceuticals. Their importance for optimization of therapy has been echoed by experts in the field [62–65].

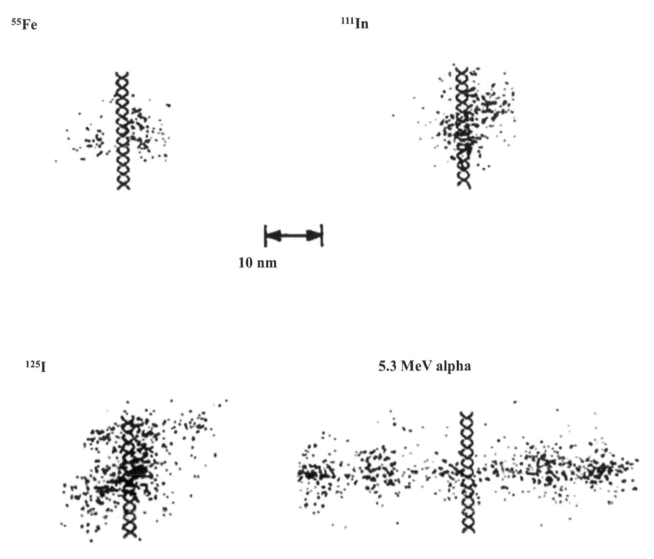

^{55}Fe

^{111}In

10 nm

^{125}I

5.3 MeV alpha

FIGURE 15.5 Initial positions of reactive chemical species produced by Auger cascades from several radionuclides compared to those along the track of a 5.3-MeV α-particle. The two helical strands of simulated DNA are depicted (reproduced from [27]). An average of 5, 15, and 25 Auger electrons per decay are emitted by ^{55}Fe, ^{111}In, and ^{125}I, respectively [23].

The multitude of models precludes the description and significance of each one in this chapter. Accordingly, this author apologizes to all those whose important citations have been omitted.

15.4 MIRD SCHEMA FOR CELLULAR AND MULTICELLULAR DOSIMETRY

The MIRD Schema, developed in the 1960s, has been applied to organ dosimetry for decades [66, 67]. Later, it was emphasized by the MIRD Committee that the MIRD Schema is equally relevant to cellular and multicellular dosimetry [3, 4]. In this application of the MIRD Schema, calculation of absorbed doses, specifically the self-dose D_k^{self} and cross-dose D_k^{cross}, to each cell in a population is required where the subscript denotes the kth cell of the population. These quantities are mean absorbed doses as defined by ICRU [65, 68]. As defined in the MIRD Schema [69], the time-integrated activity $\tilde{A}(r_S, \tau)$ is the total number of nuclear transformations in source region r_S that occur over the dose-integration period τ such that $\tilde{A}(r_S, \tau) = \int_0^\tau A(r_S, t)dt$. The absorbed dose to a given target region r_T is given by

$$D(r_T, \tau) = \sum_{r_S} \tilde{A}(r_S, \tau)\, S\,(r_T \leftarrow r_S) \qquad (15.1)$$

where $S(r_T \leftarrow r_S)$ is the mean absorbed dose to r_T per decay in r_S. Dropping the dose integration period for brevity and rewriting this equation for calculating the self-dose D_k^{self} to the nucleus (N) of the kth cell from radioactivity in the nucleus (N), cytoplasm (Cy), and cell surface (CS) of the kth cell:

$$D_k^{self}(N_k) = \tilde{A}(N_k)\, S(N_k \leftarrow N_k) + \tilde{A}(Cy_k)\, S(N_k \leftarrow Cy_k) + \tilde{A}(CS_k)\, S(N_k \leftarrow CS_k) \qquad (15.2)$$

The cross-dose to the nucleus of the kth cell comprises contributions from each of the i surrounding cells.

$$D_k^{cross}(N_k) = \sum_i \tilde{A}(N_i)\, S(N_k \leftarrow N_i) + \tilde{A}(Cy_i)\, S(N_k \leftarrow Cy_i) + \tilde{A}(CS_i)\, S(N_k \leftarrow CS_i) \qquad (15.3)$$

If the cellular activity is confined to a single subcellular compartment and the cell nucleus is taken as the target region, these equations reduce to:

Activity restricted to cell nucleus

$$D_k^{self}(N_k) = \tilde{A}(N_k)\, S(N_k \leftarrow N_k) \qquad (15.4)$$

$$D_k^{cross}(N_k) = \sum_i \tilde{A}(N_i)\, S(N_k \leftarrow N_i) \qquad (15.5)$$

Activity restricted to cytoplasm

$$D_k^{self}(N_k) = \tilde{A}(Cy_k)\, S(N_k \leftarrow Cy_k) \qquad (15.6)$$

$$D_k^{cross}(N_k) = \sum_i \tilde{A}(Cy_i)\, S(N_k \leftarrow Cy_i) \qquad (15.7)$$

Activity restricted to cell surface

$$D_k^{self}(N_k) = \tilde{A}(CS_k)\, S(N_k \leftarrow CS_k) \qquad (15.8)$$

$$D_k^{cross}(N_k) = \sum_i \tilde{A}(CS_i)\, S(N_k \leftarrow CS_i) \qquad (15.9)$$

Similar equations can be written for other targets in the cell or for the entire cell.

15.5   CELLULAR MODELS (SELF-DOSE)

As mentioned above, cell-level dosimetry for predicting effects in radiopharmaceutical therapies began at least as early as 1950 with the advent of the therapeutic use of ^{131}I and ^{32}P [12, 13]. Numerous cellular dosimetry calculations were conducted in the years that ensued. However, the tools to conveniently calculate cellular absorbed doses were not available until Goddu and colleagues tabulated cellular S values for determination of self-doses for about 20 radionuclides [70]. The MIRD Committee published an expanded list of S values for hundreds of radionuclides in the MIRD Cellular S Values monograph [2]. These tabulations were based on the cell model illustrated in Figure 15.1, and mean absorbed doses to the cell or cell nucleus were calculated for radioactivity uniformly distributed in the nucleus, cytoplasm, or on the cell surface. The computational approach used point-kernels and geometric factors. The geometric factors for the various source target configurations are published [10, 70].

The MIRD cellular S values did not fold in microdosimetric considerations that can play a role in resulting distribution of absorbed doses received by cells, particularly for alpha particle emitters where only several disintegrations are often required to sterilize a cell. Microdosimetric cellular dosimetry was studied extensively by Charlton [71, 72], Fisher [73, 74], Humm [75, 76], Stinchcomb [77, 78], and Roeske [79]. The conditions that require microdosimetry to assess the radiobiological effects of radiopharmaceuticals was discussed extensively in a review by Roeske and colleagues [80]. Due to the limited scope of this chapter, readers interested in microdosimetric applications in cellular and multicellular dosimetry are encouraged to read this review.

Several computer codes for calculating self-dose S values have been distributed. For example, an Excel spreadsheet application for single-cell alpha particle dosimetry was published with offer to send personal copies as per requests [81]. The downloadable program MIRDcell V2.1 provides the capacity to calculate self-dose S values for hundreds of radionuclides with user selectable dimensions for spherical cells [1]. The COOLER code for single-cell dosimetry for select beta particle emitters can be downloaded from the Danish Technical University website [55]. Although it appears to require considerable user expertise to implement, it does facilitate dose calculations for flattened cell geometries. Figure 15.6 shows comparisons of cellular dosimetry calculations performed with COOLER, MIRDcell V2 and the Monte Carlo radiation transport codes PARTRAC and GEANT4-DNA. Considerable differences are seen, particularly in the 20–30 keV electron energy range where the range of the electron is of the order of the cell dimensions. Some differences have also been observed by others that used the MCNP Monte Carlo radiation transport code [82]. Work is under way to understand the source of these differences.

15.6 MULTICELLULAR DOSIMETRY MODELS (SELF-DOSE AND CROSS-DOSE)

15.6.1 EVOLUTION OF MULTICELLULAR DOSIMETRY

Among the earliest multicellular models for radiopharmaceutical dosimetry was a report prepared by Haydock and Sastry for New England Nuclear (NEN) Corporation and published concurrently in the *Journal of Nuclear Medicine* [30, 59]. The model consisted of spherical cells hexagonally close-packed in spherical clusters of 53–5000 μm diameter. All the cells were labelled with activity uniformly distributed within the cell or on the cell surface. The NEN report provided multicellular dosimetry calculations for [111]Ag and ^{90}Y in the context of comparing a low- and high-energy beta emitters for radioimmunotherapy of small tumours and micrometastases. The calculated results favoured [111]Ag for treating micrometastases and alluded to [119]Sn as another possible candidate. The concurrent publication by Kassis and colleagues pointed out the importance of cellular dosimetry for low energy Auger electron emitters [59]. This story was elaborated further in a subsequent publication [83]. There, Sastry and colleagues calculated the fraction of electron energy absorbed in the cluster as a function of energy and cluster diameter (Figure 15.7). These data suggested that small micrometastasis could be treated most efficiently with low-energy electrons whereas high-energy electrons were more suitable for larger ones. Due to its low emission of low-energy electrons [119]Sb was considered optimal for therapy of small micrometastases (diameter ~ 100 μm). Interestingly, this radionuclide has resurfaced as a candidate for Auger therapy [84].

The Haydock and Sastry model that was used to calculate the absorbed fractions in Figure 15.7 was built upon by Howell and colleagues to obtain absorbed dose rate profiles for several radionuclides of interest for therapeutic nuclear medicine [31]. When the radioactivity was distributed uniformly among the cells, it was shown that the optimal electron energy for irradiating micrometastases corresponds to that which has a range that is about the same as the cluster radius (Figure 15.8).

However, while low-energy electron emitters can offer substantial therapeutic advantages when the radiopharmaceutical is distributed uniformly among the cells in small micrometastases, this advantage can be enhanced even further when the radionuclide is localized in the cell nucleus to leverage the high RBE that arises when Auger electron emitters are incorporated into DNA [31]. However, this advantage is mitigated when penetration into the micrometastasis is poor, as represented by an exponentially decreasing activity concentration as one moves from the surface of the cluster to the centre of the cluster (Figure 15.9) [31]. Poor penetration into the micrometastasis can be problematic for alpha particle emitters as well as demonstrated in experimental spheroid models [85]. However, recent work has demonstrated that penetration can be improved markedly using liposomes [86].

Goddu and colleagues expanded this model by considering nonuniform activity distributions that entailed labelling only 1, 10, or 100 per cent of the cells in the cluster [10]. Cells in multicellular clusters were labelled with ^{90}Y, ^{125}I, or [210]Po, which emit energetic beta particles, low-energy Auger electrons, and 5.3 MeV alpha particles, respectively. As

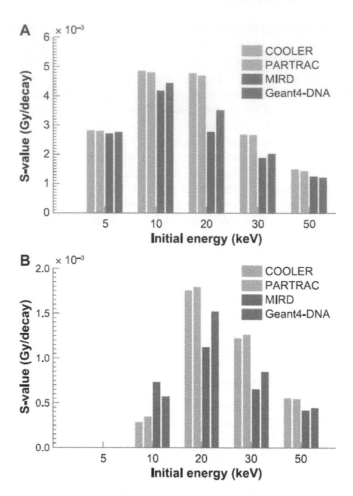

FIGURE 15.6 Results with Geant4-DNA were obtained from (53) for the N←N (panel A) and N←CS (panel B) cases, with a spherical cell geometry (cell radius = 5 μm; nucleus radius = 4 μm). COOLER/PARTRAC results were obtained from dedicated calculations with the same cell model. Reprinted from Siragusa M, Baiocco G, Fredericia PM, Friedland W, Groesser T, Ottolenghi A, Jensen M. The COOLER Code: A Novel Analytical Approach to Calculate Subcellular Energy Deposition by Internal Electron Emitters. Radiat Res. 2017;188(2):204–20 with permission from Radiation Research. © 2021 Radiation Research Society [55]. Colour image available at www.routledge.com/9781138593299.

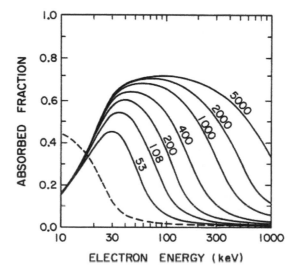

FIGURE 15.7 Absorbed fractions for monoenergetic electrons as a function of electron energy [83]. The dashed curve represents the self-absorbed fraction for a labelled cell. The solid curves are the contribution from other labelled cells to the target cell. Each curve is designated by the cell cluster diameter in μm. Reproduced from [83].

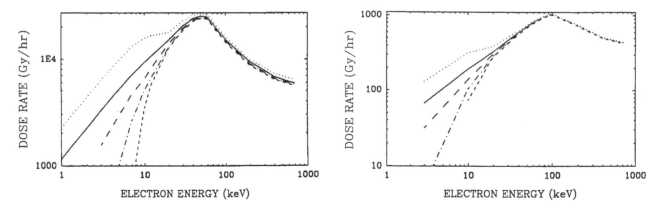

FIGURE 15.8 Average dose rate to cell or cell nucleus for 1 MBq of hypothetical monoenergetic electron emitters distributed equally between cells in a 108 μm (left) and 400 μm (right) diameter multicellular cluster [31]. A cell and cell nucleus are represented by concentric spheres with the radii of 5 μm and 4 μm, respectively. The fives curves represent different combinations of target and subcellular distribution (target < source): dotted (nucleus < nucleus), solid (cell < cell), long dash (nucleus < cell surface), dot dash (nucleus < cytoplasm), and short dash (nucleus < cell surface). Maximum dose rate occurs at energy for which the pathlength is of the order of the cluster radius.

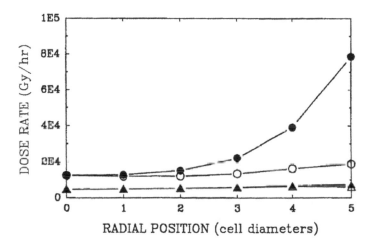

FIGURE 15.9 Radial dose rate profiles in a spherical multicellular cluster (diameter 108 μm) containing 1 MBq of either ^{193m}Pt (circles) or ^{90}Y (triangles) distributed exponentially at the macroscopic level. The solid and open circles represent the dose rates to cell nuclei when the radioactivity is localized in the cell nucleus and cell surface, respectively.

shown in Figure 15.10, the absorbed doses received by individual cells within the cluster can vary drastically depending on the radionuclide, subcellular distribution of the radionuclide, and percentage of cells labelled. This enabled consideration of responses to targeted cells (labelled) and non-targeted cells (unlabelled).

A dosimetric and radiobiological analysis by O'Donoghue and colleagues, on the basis of tumour-control probability (TCP) for multicellular clusters, demonstrated a linear relationship between tumour diameter and optimal electron energy (Figure 15.11) [87]. Given that patients generally have several or more metastasis of varying sizes, they concluded that a mixture of low- and high-energy electron emitters was suggested for targeted radionuclide therapy.

Charlton published a program for multicellular dosimetry that used analytical approaches to predict cell survival in micrometastases consisting of two cell types (Figure 15.12) [32]. This model featured overlapping cells, each with a distribution of cell sizes. Computational results showed that for an average of 1 decay of ^{211}At or ^{213}Bi per cell, cell survival decreased somewhat (57% to 37%) as the spheroid diameter increased (75 μm to 225 μm). A similar reduction in survival was achieved by increasing the packing of the cells from 40 per cent to 70 per cent. As anticipated based on the data in Figure 15.10, the presence of small regions of unlabelled cells (79% labelled and 21% unlabelled) within the spheroids did not significantly change cell survival even at this very low cellular time-integrated activity (1 decay per

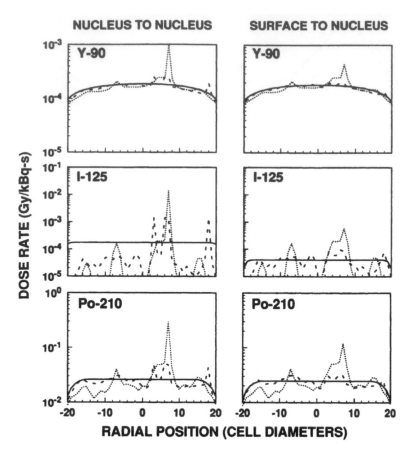

FIGURE 15.10 Dose-rate profiles in 400-μm diameter multicellular dusters containing 1 kBq of either ^{90}Y, ^{125}I, or [210]Po. The radioactivity is uniformly distributed either in the cell nucleus (left) or on the cell surface (right) and the radioactivity is confined to 1 per cent (dotted line), 10 per cent (dashed line) or 100 per cent (solid line) of the cells in the duster at random. The spikes observed for the 1 per cent and 10 per cent labelling cases correspond to cells that are labelled. The increasing importance of the subcellular distribution and the self-dose Is apparent as the percentage of cells that are labelled decreases, particularly for the Auger emitter [125]I. This figure was originally published in *JNM*. S. M. Goddu, D. V. Rao, and R. W. Howell, Multicellular dosimetry for micrometastases: Dependence of self-dose versus cross-dose to cell nuclei on type and energy of radiation and subcellular distribution of radionuclide. J Nucl Med, vol. 35, pp. 521–530, 1994. © SNMMI [10].

cell). However, restricting the decays to the outer layers of the spheroid increased cell survival as observed by Kennel and colleagues [85]. As stated in his publication, Charlton offered to provide the code upon request.

A number of other codes for multicellular dosimetry have also been published over the years. Malaroda and colleagues created a voxel-based code for small-scale dosimetry [35, 36]. Hobbs and colleagues created a GEANT4-based program for multicellular dosimetry with features to calculate tumour control probability [48]. Howell and colleagues expanded on their earlier work mentioned above by studying the impact of lognormal distributions of activity among the cell population in multicellular clusters [88]. This concept arose out of experimental studies that demonstrated lognormal activity distributions of among targeted cells can have a profound impact on biological response of the population [39]. The importance of lognormal distributions of radioactivity were highlighted by leading scientists in three different invited contributions [62–64]. Marcatili and colleagues developed general-purpose software tools to generate randomized 3D cell culture geometries based on experimentally determined parameters (cell size, cell density, cluster density, average cluster size, cell cumulated activity). These models were used in conjunction with analytical and Monte Carlo dosimetry calculations to predict the fraction of surviving cells following uptake of ^{177}Lu radiopharmaceuticals [52]. Cai and colleagues developed a multicellular model that used MCNP radiation transport [82]. Sizeable differences up to about 30 per cent in the cross-dose S values produced by their code versus MIRDcell V2 were noted. The most detailed model was published recently by Raghavan and colleagues [51]. This multicellular cluster model has the capacity to account for the time-dependent nature of diffusion of short-lived radiopharmaceuticals into the cluster (Figure 15.13). The diffusion rate constants can have a profound effect on the resulting absorbed dose profile.

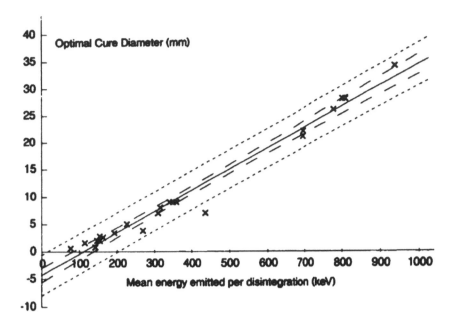

FIGURE 15.11 Relationship between optimal cure diameter and mean beta-particle energy emitted per disintegration. Linear regression yielded the equation of $D_{optimal} = 0.039\ E_{total} - 4$, where E_{total} is the mean beta particle energy emitted per disintegration which may be used to predict optimal cure size. This research was originally published in JNM. O'Donoghue JA, Bardiès M, Wheldon TE. Relationships between tumor size and curability for uniformly targeted therapy with beta-emitting radionuclides. J Nucl Med. 1995;36:1902–1909. Figure 6. © SNMMI.

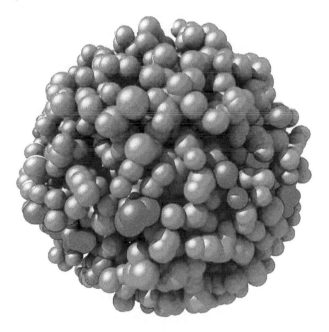

FIGURE 15.12 Mosaic multicellular cluster model created by Charlton [32]. Two distinct cell populations are distinguished by red (labelled) and blue (unlabelled). Cell survival was calculated for alpha particle emitters distributed among the labelled cells. Colour image available at www.routledge.com/9781138593299.

15.6.2 MIRDcell V2

Although many multicellular dosimetry programs have been developed, they are largely in the hands of their creators and not available widely for general use. This is likely due to the effort required to create a graphic user interface (GUI) with a variety of options that can be used by both novice and expert users. MIRDcell V2 is perhaps the only freely available application that launches easily and provides a user-friendly interface [1].

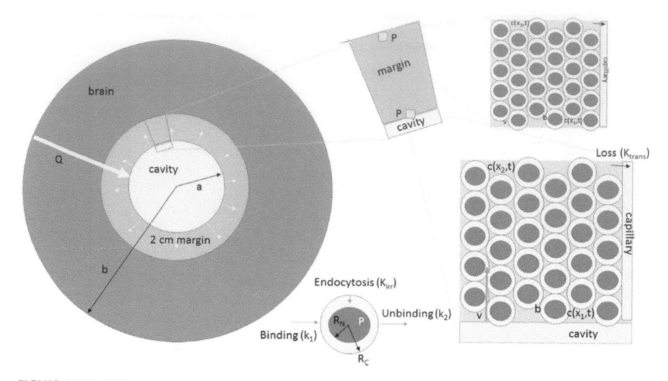

FIGURE 15.13 Basic components and assumptions of the multicellular dosimetry model that accounts for time-dependent diffusion of a radiopharmaceutical into the wall of a resection cavity in the brain [51]. Top left: the brain is considered a sphere with a concentric spherical cavity created after resection of visible tumour (SCRC). The entire spherical wall of the cavity is the source of an infusion of a macromolecule (for example, an MNT labelled with radionuclide) in fluid suspension. The target for the therapy is a shell or margin of tissue between the SCRC wall and an outer sphere: to simulate the region where cancer is most likely to recur first. Two places in this margin are of particular interest, both denoted P (magnified view, top centre). One is the inner wall of the margin and the other is the outer sphere defining the extent of the margin. All cells are considered identical spheres arranged in closed-packed arrangement (see text for further details). The macromolecule has an association or binding rate, and dissociation or unbinding rate at the cell membrane surface. It can also internalize (endocytosis) and ultimately reside in the cell nucleus; no escape from there is allowed in the current model. The concentrations of interstitial MNT, bound MNT, and internalized MNT are denoted c, b, and X, all functions of spatial location x in and time t.

Figure 15.14 shows one tab (3-D Cluster) of the interface that enables users to pick a radionuclide, location of radioactivity within the cell, target within the cell, radii of the cell and cell nucleus, distance between cells, geometry of the cell population, and distribution of activity among the cells (uniform, normal, and lognormal). Three models were created including 1D, 2D, and 3D. The 1D interface has two cells. 2D has a monolayer cell population that lies on a plane – this can be used to represent a colony in a cell culture assay or cells attached to the wall of a vessel [33]. The 3D model is for multicellular clusters of different selectable shapes. The distance between cells can be varied to eliminate cross-dose as in the case of isolated tumour cells. These user interfaces provide multicellular dosimetry and cell survival analysis. Developed in collaboration with the MIRD Committee, this tool can be accessed at http://mirdcell.njms.rutgers.edu; a description of MIRDcell is published in *J Nucl Med* [1]. The *J Nucl Med* article is accompanied by a supplement to describe its implementation. New users will note that the software has moved from a Web-based Java applet (MIRDcell V2.0) to a downloadable Java program (MIRDcell V2.1) due to the disallowance of Java applets on all web browsers due to security concerns with the applet platform. This has not affected the functionality of MIRDcell V2.1 in any way. This ease of use and ready availability of MIRDcell V2.1 has led to its widespread use around the world with over 200 users and over 8,900 logged uses (Figure 15.15).

MIRDcell V3 was launched in September 2021 and will serve as an indispensable educational tool for dosimetry and radiobiology of radiopharmaceuticals. Students will be able to operate MIRDcell V3 and learn about how the selection of different radionuclides and other parameters are expected to affect cell killing. The influence of particle range, RBE, activity distribution and other parameters can be explored. This educational element is perhaps one of the most

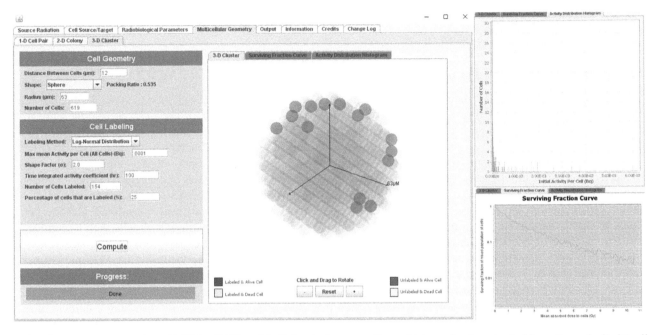

FIGURE 15.14 Screen shot of MIRDcell V2 multicellular dosimetry toolbox which can be downloaded from the web site http://mirdcell.njms.rutgers.edu. Arrows point to Activity Distribution Histogram tab (top right) and Surviving Fraction Curve tab (lower right) that correspond to selected parameters (left). MIRDcell V2 is patented under USPTO 9,623,262 [89]. Colour image available at www.routledge.com/9781138593299.

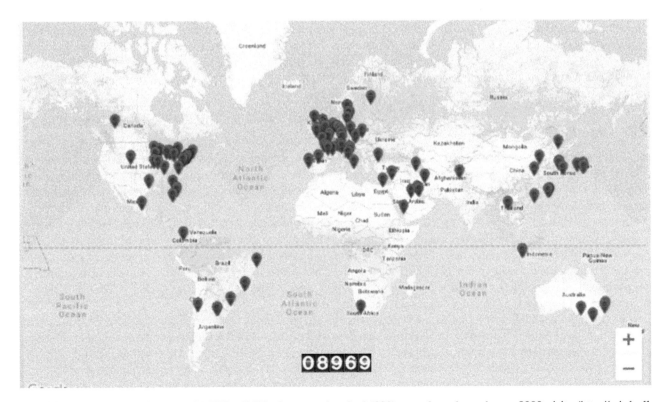

FIGURE 15.15 Worldwide use of MIRDcell V2. Over two hundred (200) users have logged over 8900 visits (http://mirdcell.njms.rutgers.edu/map) to run the code.

important aspects of MIRDcell V3. The teaching and learning made possible by its predecessor, MIRDcell V2, has spurred other studies [50–55].

15.7 LIMITATIONS OF CELLULAR AND MULTICELLULAR DOSIMETRY MODELS

It is often said that dosimetry calculations must account for the stochastic nature of the radiation field required to kill cell populations, especially with alpha particle emitters [80, 90]. The lower the number of decays, and, correspondingly, the tumour-control probability, the more important become the stochastic processes of radionuclide uptake, decay, direction of alpha particle emission, track segment lengths through cells, and cell death itself having received a given absorbed dose [61, 91]. MIRDcell accounts for the stochastics of uptake of radioactivity by randomly assigning activity in any given cell according to the statistical distribution selected by the user, and the stochastics of death on a cell-by-cell basis given the absorbed dose calculated for each individual cell, using a Monte Carlo approach based on the probability of cell survival. However, the stochastics of decay and energy deposition are not specifically considered. Despite this, MIRDcell does a reasonable job of predicting effects observed in experiments with clusters of cells with nonuniform distributions of the alpha particle emitter ^{210}Po [1]. One can actually use MIRDcell to explore these stochastic effects by labelling a small percentage of cells in a cluster with few cells and then repeating the CALCULATE many times. Each time the activity is assigned to cells randomly according to the selected activity distribution, and each time a different cell survival curve emerges. Detailed information is provided in the OUTPUT tab that enables the user to see the changes in mean absorbed dose and surviving fraction that arise each time the activity distribution is reassigned. Nevertheless, there will be circumstances where microdosimetric considerations are essential to obtain a complete picture of the problem. Roeske and Stinchcomb's approaches to combining microdosimetry and S values through the use of microdosimetric moments will be very helpful in this regard [61, 78, 81, 91, 92].

Several comparisons between Monte Carlo track structure codes and MIRDcell V2 have been published that identified discrepancies in S values, particularly for cell surface and cytoplasmic activity distributions of radionuclides that emit electrons in the 25–30 keV range [55, 82]. Some of these publications have attributed these differences to the CSDA approximation used in MIRDcell V2. This issue could be investigated by adopting new analytical expressions created by the developers of the COOLER code [55]. While this is likely to offer a good solution, some believe that only Monte Carlo track structure methods are suited for cellular and multicellular dosimetry. While a full event-by-event approach is tantalizing, especially in the modern computing era, one must recognize that depending on the radionuclide and geometries selected, one may need to simulate hundreds of radiations per decay, thousands of decays per cell, in hundreds of thousands of cells. The computational overhead on this task is enormous and likely unsurmountable. Therefore, analytical approaches offer the best compromise. This same approach is taken routinely in external beam treatment planning systems where analytical algorithms are used.

15.8 TIME-INTEGRATED ACTIVITY

Assessment of the time-integrated activity in each cell of the population is necessary to calculate the distribution of absorbed doses that they receive from radiations emitted by the radiopharmaceutical. This is often achieved by a combination of measurements, assumptions, and modelling. A key ingredient of this assessment is an awareness that measurements are strongly influenced by the chemical properties of the radiopharmaceutical and the experimental techniques used to determine cell activity. The issue of radionuclides leaching from tissues, and its influence on assessing quantitatively the distribution of radioactivity in those tissues, has been known since the early 1950s [93]. More recently, these problems have been avoided by cryosectioning tissue blocks and then directly subjecting the tissue sections to quantitative measurements with beta cameras or alpha cameras [94]. Quantitative imaging of a sample is possible under these conditions for tissues such as tumours harvested at various time points (Figure 15.16). The spatial resolution of alpha cameras is of the order of several cell diameters.

Often, longitudinal studies of a sample are needed to assess effective uptake and clearance of a radiopharmaceutical at the cellular level. This is done often in cell culture models where aliquots of the sample can be acquired at different time points for quantitative assessment of cellular activity. Techniques have been developed to determine cellular activity accurately even for radiopharmaceuticals such as [^{201}T]thallous chloride that rapidly efflux when cells are washed [95]. These and other techniques can be used to determine cellular activity during various phases of experiments with experimental multicellular models. For example, Figure 15.17 shows the temporal change in cellular activity for a 3D multicellular cluster model [28, 29, 38]. Details on obtaining the time integrated activity during each phase of the experiment are contained within the referenced articles.

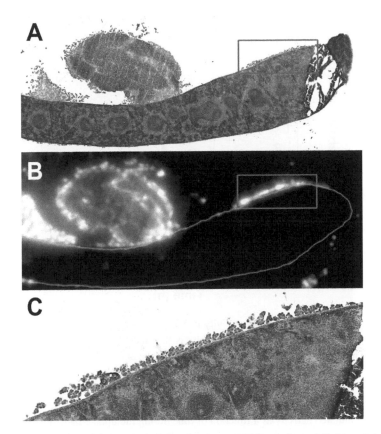

FIGURE 15.16 Alpha imaging of uptake in macro- and micro-tumours on the peritoneal lining of the spleen after i.p.-injection of ^{211}At-faretuzumab in a mice model of ovarian cancer. H&E-stained section of the the spleen (A), alpha image (B) with cyan ROI indicating periphery of the spleen and a zoom of an area (C, and red rectangles) with hot spot activity in areas corresponding to small tumour cell clusters. Figure and figure text from Chapter 30 in Volume I. Colour image available at www.routledge.com/9781138593299.

While mean activity per cell is an important quantity for calculating absorbed doses. The distribution about the mean can be equally important [39, 56]. Lognormal activity distributions are prevalent for radiopharmaceuticals and other drugs, which can have a profound impact on the response of a cell population [97].

15.9   EXAMPLES USING MIRDCELL V2

The remainder of this chapter is devoted to providing examples of how MIRDcell can be used to solve complex problems in single-cell and multicellular environments. Detailed instructions regarding program installation and the use of MIRDcell can be found in references [98] and [99], respectively.

15.9.1   Isolated Tumour Cells Labelled with ^{225}Ac (No Significant Cross-dose)

MIRDcell V2 can be used to predict the response of MDA-MB-231 cells labelled with an ^{225}Ac-labeled monoclonal antibody (^{225}Ac-Mab). Assume experimental procedures similar to those used in reference [100]. MDA-MB-231 cells are suspended in culture medium containing various concentrations of ^{225}Ac-Mab for 18 h, washed, and seeded into culture dishes to measure clonogenic cell survival. The radii of the cell and cell nucleus are 6 and 4 µm, respectively. The cellular activity corresponding to treatment with the highest concentration of ^{225}Ac-Mab is 0.5 mBq per cell and the activity is localized on the cell surface. The mean uptake of the radiochemical is linearly dependent on time, whereas the clearance is exponential with an effective half-time of 24 h. This yields a time-integrated activity coefficient for the incubation and colony-forming periods of 43.6 h (see reference [100] for details). In this example, assume that the cellular cross-dose is negligible during all stages of the experiment, so only the cellular self-dose needs to be considered [1, 10]. MIRDcell V2 can be used to plot a predicted cell survival curve.

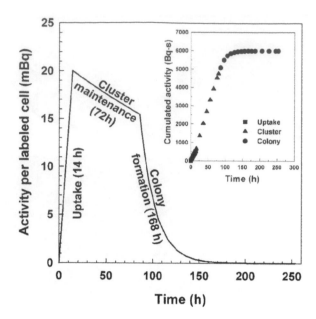

FIGURE 15.17 Temporal dependence of intracellular activity in V79 cells labelled with an average of 20 mBq/cell of [131]IdU is taken by the end of the uptake period. The time integrated activity is the area under the curve and proportional to the cumulated decays in the V79 cell nucleus. The time period of 0–14 h represents the uptake of the radiochemical into the labelled cells while they are incubated in culture medium containing [131]IdU. The time period of 14–86 h represents the 72-h period where the labelled cells were mixed in equal numbers with unlabelled cells and maintained at 10.5°C as a multicellular cluster. Finally, the curved region corresponds to the one-week colony-forming period where the cellular activity has an effective half-time of ~ 12 h [20, 96]. The inset shows the corresponding cumulated activity as a function of time during the uptake (■), cluster maintenance (▲) and colony formation (●) periods. This research was originally published in *JNM*. P. V. Neti and R. W. Howell, Isolating effects of microscopic nonuniform distributions of ^{131}I on labeled and unlabeled cells" J Nucl Med, vol. 45, no. 6, pp. 1050–8, 2004. © SNMMI [28].

a. Assume initially that the [225]Ac daughters do not contribute to the absorbed dose received by the cells. Click on the source radiation tab (Figure 15.18). Select [225]Ac from the drop-down list and click "β average energy spectrum". Note that the Input Data box filled in with the radiation data.

b. Click on the Cell Source/Target tab (Figure 15.18). Select Nucleus ← Cell Surface. Click on + to increase radius of cell to 6 μm and nucleus to 4 μm (ignore font problem (μ) in diagram below).

c. Click the Radiobiological Parameters tab (GUI not shown). Set the radiobiological parameters to values that are appropriate for alpha particles [20, 38]: $\alpha_{self} = 1.54$ Gy^{-1}, $\beta_{self} = 0$ Gy^{-2}, $\alpha_{cross} = 1.54$ Gy^{-1}, $\beta_{cross} = 0$ Gy^{-2}. The $\beta = 0$ corresponds to a monoexponential dose-response relationship for the surviving fraction of cells.

d. To satisfy dosimetric conditions wherein the cross-dose is negligible, create geometric conditions in MIRDcell V2 that will satisfy that requirement. Click the Multicellular Geometry tab and then click the 3-D Cluster tab. Increase distance between cells to 100 μm to simulate the suspension culture (Figure 15.20). This distance is larger than the range of the alpha particles emitted by [225]Ac, which will result in a negligible cross-dose. From the drop-down list of Shapes, select Sphere. Enter a radius that will contain enough cells to enable simulation of at least two logs of cell kill – start with a 500 μm radius. Select Labelling Method to be Uniform Distribution. Enter the Maximum mean Activity per Cell = 0.0005 Bq. Enter the Time-integrated activity coefficient = 43.6 h. Enter percentage of cells that are labelled = 100 per cent. Click Compute. Click the Surviving Fraction Curve tab.

e. Examine the resulting curve of Surviving Fraction mixed population of cells (in this case all cells are labelled so mixed = labelled) (Figure 15.20). Recall that this *does not* include the decays of [225]Ac daughters. To include the daughters with the assumption that daughters are in equilibrium with the parent [225]Ac, return to the Source Radiation tab and select [225]Ac+daughters (Figure 15.21). Leave all other parameters as they were.

f. Return to Multicellular Geometry tab and then click the 3-D Cluster tab. Click Compute. As expected, the plot of Surviving Fraction versus absorbed dose from [225]Ac gives essentially the same dose response as the case for [225]Ac+daughters (Figure 15.22). This is because, in this example, the dose response is dictated by the Radiobiological Parameter α_{self}.

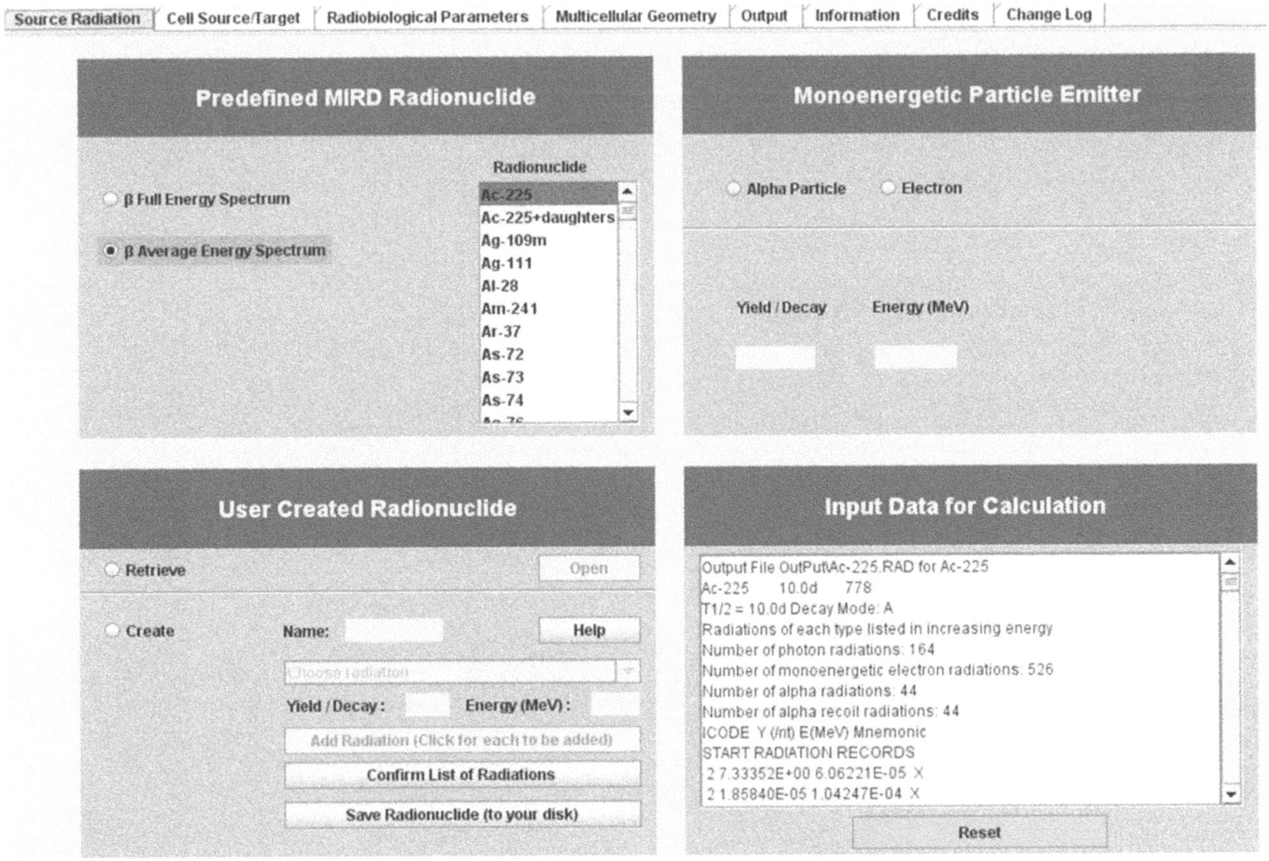

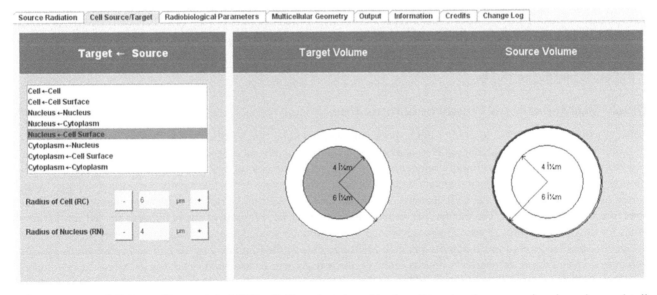

FIGURE 15.18 Source Radiation tab in MIRDcell. The database corresponding to β Average Energy Spectrum has been selected along with the radionuclide ^{225}Ac (upper left). The spectrum of radiations for ^{225}Ac is provided (lower right).

FIGURE 15.19 Cell Source/Target tab in MIRDcell. The selected combination of target and source regions is nucleus and cell surface, respectively. The radii of the cell and cell nucleus have been set to 6 and 4 μm, respectively.

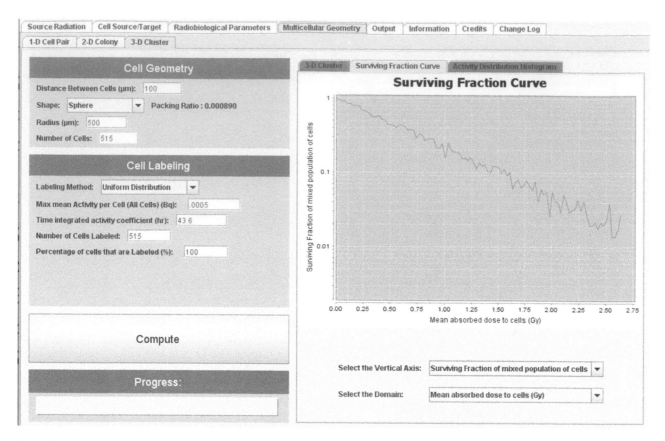

FIGURE 15.20   Multicellular Geometry < 3-D Cluster < Surviving Fraction Curve tab in MIRDcell. Simulation was performed for ²²⁵Ac-labeled cells spaced far apart (100 µm) and constrained within a sphere of radius 500 µm. The cells were labeled uniformly with up to a maximum of 0.0005 Bq/cell. The time integrated activity coefficient was 43.6 h. The surviving fraction as a function of absorbed dose is plotted on the right.

    g. To see how adding the daughters affects the surviving fraction, examine the plots below which are Surviving Fraction versus Mean Activity per Cell (Figures 15.23 and 15.24). As expected, note that considerably more activity per cell is required to achieve 10 per cent survival in the case of ²²⁵Ac alone.

    h. ²²⁵Ac+daughters (Figure 15.23).

    i. ²²⁵Ac alone (Figure 15.24).

15.9.2   3D MULTICELLULAR CLUSTER OF CULTURED CELLS

Consider using MIRDcell V2 to predict the response of a multicellular cluster of cells labelled with the alpha particle emitter, ²¹⁰Po. The experimental data of Neti and colleagues [38] are analysed as follows. Modelling is conducted analogous to that described in Howell and colleagues [88], except that the size of the cluster is decreased here to reduce computation time. The experimental cluster consists of cells, labelled with ²¹⁰Po, and tightly packed into a pellet at the bottom of a microcentrifuge tube. Cell clusters, containing various quantities of radioactivity, were maintained in these tubes to accumulate decays. The clusters were then dismantled, serial dilutions of the cells were seeded into culture dishes for the colony forming assay. The surviving fraction of initially seeded cells compared to controls was calculated and plotted as a function of mean activity per cell. Measurements of the diameters of the cell and cell nucleus yielded averages of 12 and 8 µm, respectively. In this example, the activity will be assumed to be distributed in the cytoplasm. As in Ref. [88], the cells will be constrained to a conical volume with a height equal to the diameter of the top surface. Here only a portion of the cells (68,883 out of 4x10⁶ cells) will be modelled to reduce CPU time and stay within the 1024 MB memory limit for 32 bit Java. Tests show that the 1024 MB setting in Java can accommodate up to about 10⁶ cells. As in Ref. (3), a lognormal distribution of activity will be selected with a shape factor of 2.0.

    a. Click on the source radiation tab. Select Po-210 from the drop-down list and click "β Average Energy Spectrum". Note that the Input Data box filled in with the appropriate radiation data (Figure 15.25).

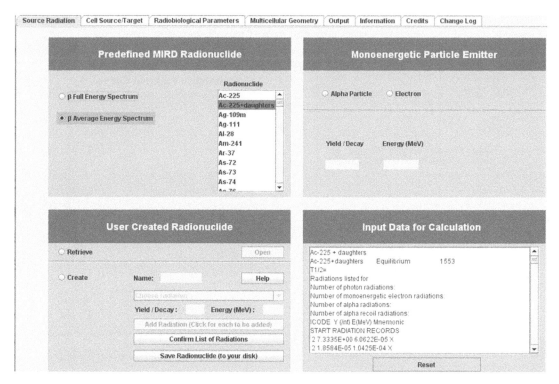

FIGURE 15.21 Source Radiation tab in MIRDcell. The database corresponding to β Average Energy Spectrum has been selected along with the ^{225}Ac+daughters (upper left). The spectrum of radiations for ^{225}Ac+daughters in equilibrium with parent is provided (lower right).

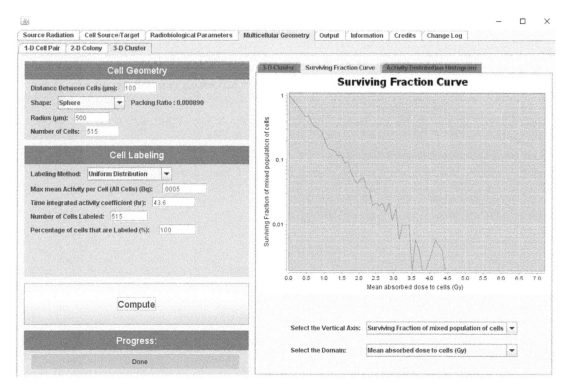

FIGURE 15.22 Multicellular Geometry < 3-D Cluster < Surviving Fraction Curve tab in MIRDcell. The simulation was repeated after replacing ^{225}Ac with ^{225}Ac+daughters. The surviving fraction as a function of absorbed dose is plotted on the right.

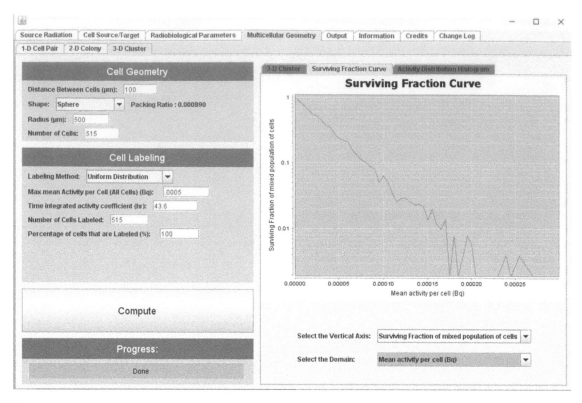

FIGURE 15.23 Multicellular Geometry < 3-D Cluster < Surviving Fraction Curve tab in MIRDcell. The simulation was for [225]Ac+daughters. The surviving fraction as a function of mean activity per cell is plotted on the right.

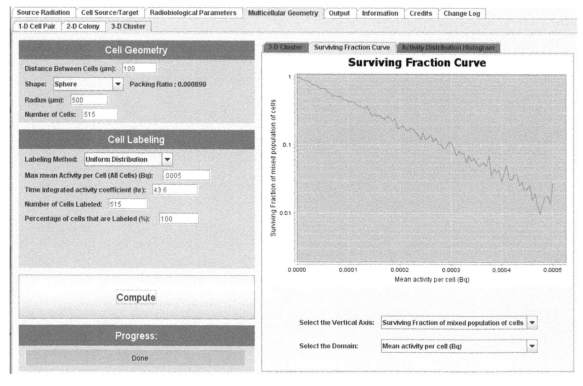

FIGURE 15.24 Multicellular Geometry < 3-D Cluster < Surviving Fraction Curve tab in MIRDcell. The simulation was for [225]Ac without daughters. The surviving fraction as a function of mean activity per cell is plotted on the right.

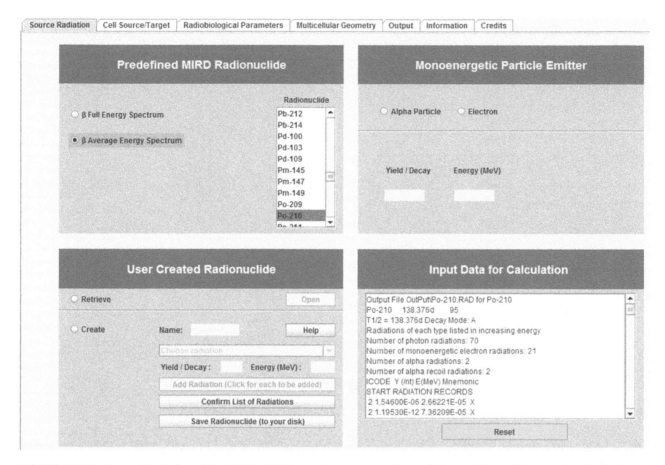

FIGURE 15.25 Source Radiation tab in MIRDcell. The database corresponding to β Average Energy Spectrum has been selected along with the radionuclide Po-210. The radiation spectrum data appears in the Input Data for Calculation box (lower right).

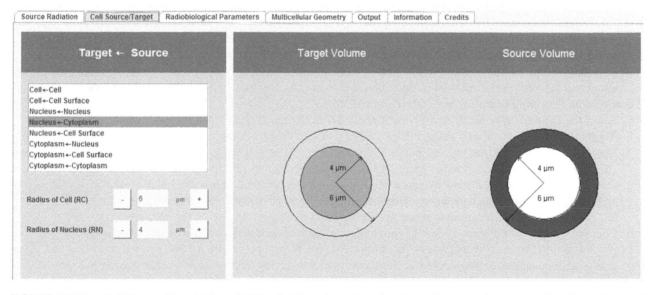

FIGURE 15.26 Cell Source/Target tab in MIRDcell. The selected combination of target and source regions is nucleus and cytoplasm, respectively. The radii of the cell and cell nucleus have been set to 6 and 4 µm, respectively.

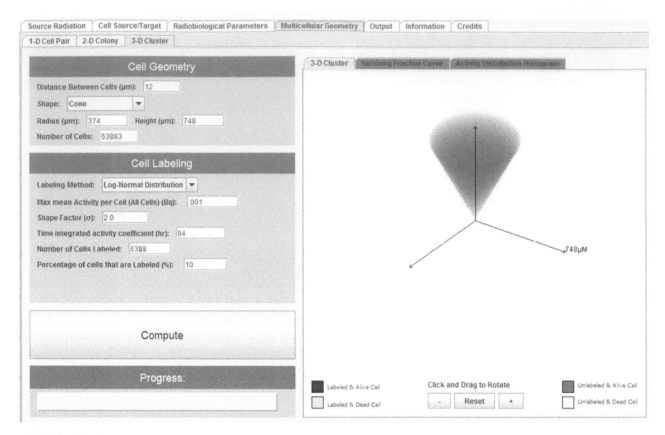

FIGURE 15.27 Multicellular Geometry < 3-D Cluster < 3-D cluster tab in MIRDcell. Cells were constrained within a cone of radius 374 μm and height of 748 μm. Only 10% of the cells were labeled with a log normal distribution. The maximum mean activity per cell entered was 0.001 Bq/cell. The time integrated activity coefficient was 94 h. The cluster geometry is presented on the right.

b. Click on the Cell Source/Target tab. Select Nucleus ← Cytoplasm. Click on + to increase radius of cell nucleus to 4 μm. Click on + to increase radius of cell to 6 μm (Figure 15.26).

c. Set the Radiobiological Parameters to (3): $\alpha_{self} = 1.54$ Gy^{-1}, $\beta_{self} = 0$ Gy^{-2}, $\alpha_{cross} = 1.54$ Gy^{-1}, $\beta_{cross} = 0$ Gy^{-2}. Click the Multicellular Geometry tab and then click the 3-D Cluster tab (Figure 15.27). From the drop-down list of Shapes, select Cone. Enter a radius of 374 μm radius and 748 μm height. Select Labelling Method to be Lognormal Distribution and the Shape Factor = 2.0. Enter the Maximum mean Activity per Cell = 0.001 Bq. Enter the Time-integrated activity coefficient = 94 h. Enter percentage of cells that are labelled = 10 per cent. Click Compute.

d. Click the Surviving Fraction Curve tab (Figure 15.28).

e. Select the Domain to be Mean Activity per Labelled Cell (Figure 15.29).

f. Right click on horizontal axis scale (Figure 15.29). Click on Properties tab. Click on Plot. In Other box, Click on Range. Unclick Auto-adjust range. Change Maximum range value to 0.0015. Click OK. The resulting plot (Figure 15.30) is a reasonable match with Figure 15.3 of Neti and colleagues [38].

g. Click the Activity Distribution Histogram tab. Right click on horizontal axis scale. Click on Properties tab. Click on Plot. In Other box, Click on Range. Unclick Auto-adjust range. Change Maximum range value to 0.025. Click OK. The lognormal distribution is apparent (Figure 15.31).

h. Click the Output Tab (Figure 15.32). Highlight data in columns of data in left box. Right click and copy.

i. Paste data into Excel using its Paste – Text Import Wizard. Repeat procedure for 100 per cent labelling and 1 per cent labelling and paste into Excel files. Use Excel to plot surviving fraction versus mean activity per cell (MAC) as shown in Figure 15.33. This demonstrates the MIRDcell V2 export capability.

15.9.3 3D MULTICELLULAR CLUSTERS IN VIVO

MIRDcell V2 can also be used to analyse data acquired at the cellular scale in vivo. Chouin and colleagues used their novel alpha camera to measure the cellular uptake of ^{211}At in multicellular clusters of human ovarian cancer cells NIH:OVCAR-3 growing in the peritoneal cavity of mice [44]. The D_{37} for these cells is 0.56 Gy ($\alpha = 1.79$ Gy^{-1}) when irradiated with alpha particles. Measurements were made for several cluster sizes; here the cluster with a radius of

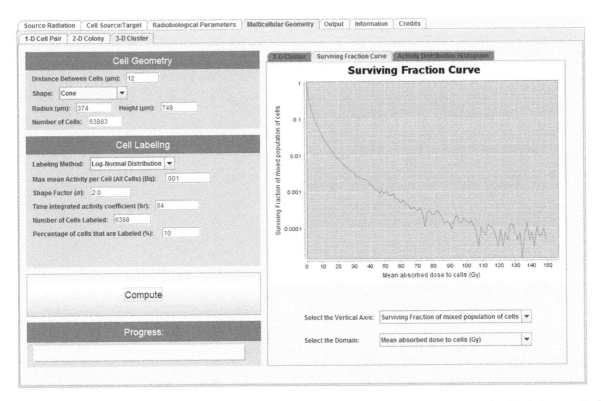

FIGURE 15.28 Multicellular Geometry < 3-D Cluster < Surviving Fraction Curve tab in MIRDcell. The simulation was for [210]Po with 10% of cells labeled lognormally within a cone-shaped geometry. The surviving fraction versus mean absorbed dose to cells is plotted on the right.

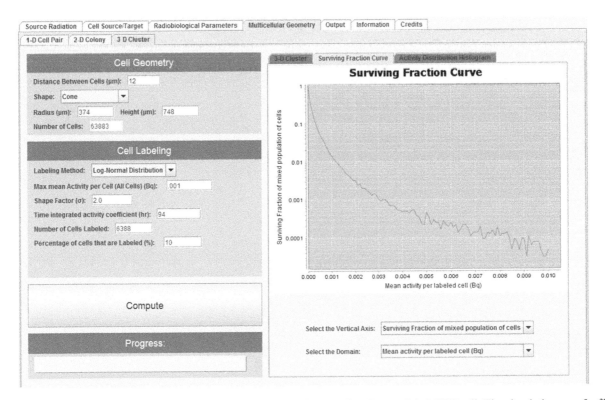

FIGURE 15.29 Multicellular Geometry < 3-D Cluster < Surviving Fraction Curve tab in MIRDcell. The simulation was for [210]Po with 10% of cells labeled lognormally within a cone-shaped geometry. The surviving fraction versus mean activity per labeled cell is plotted on the right.

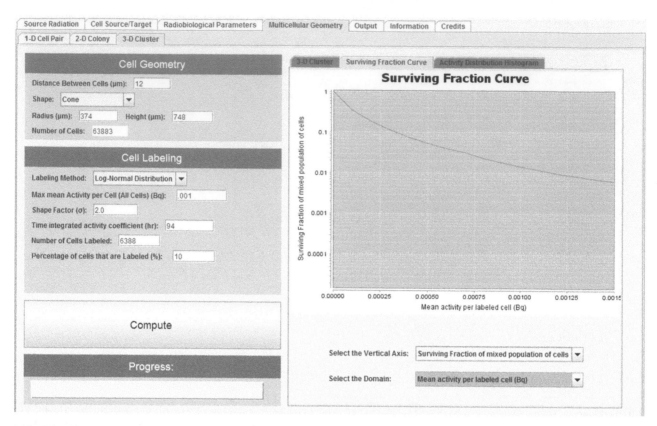

FIGURE 15.30   Same as Figure 15.29 with rescaled x-axis to permit comparison with data of Neti and colleagues [38].

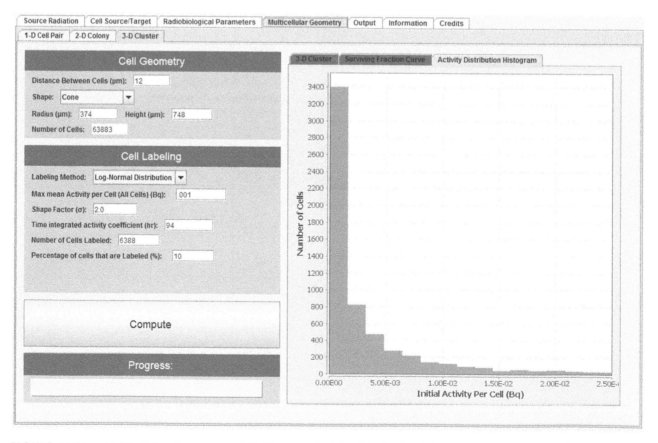

FIGURE 15.31   Multicellular Geometry < 3-D Cluster < Activity Distribution Histogram tab in MIRDcell. The lognormal distribution is apparent.

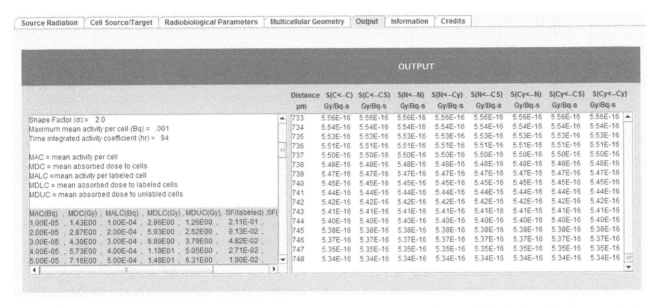

FIGURE 15.32 Output tab in MIRDcell. The left box contains information regarding the model details. The right box contains the cellular S values for self-dose and cross-doses.

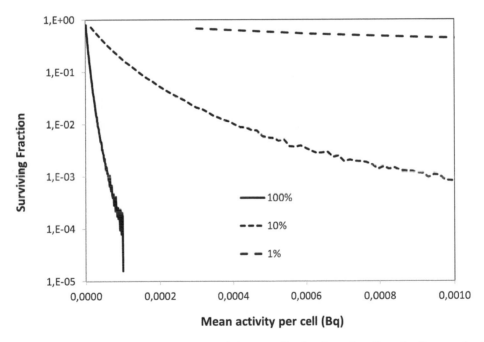

FIGURE 15.33 Plots of surviving fraction versus mean activity per cell using data taken from the Output tab of MIRDcell. The simulations were for [210]Po with either 1%, 10%, or 100% of cells labeled lognormally within a cone-shaped geometry.

42.8-μm will be considered (modelled by a spheroid containing 123 cells). The cell and cell nuclei had average radii of 6.9 and 5.5 μm, respectively. According to the second to last paragraph of the Results in Chouin and colleagues [44], "For 6-MBq injections, the activity per cell was constant from 1.5 h (~0.027 ± 0.010 Bq/cell) to 4 h (~0.034 ± 0.012 Bq/cell), then decreased slightly at 8 h (~0.015 ± 0.010 Bq/cell)". Therefore, the maximum [211]At uptake was 0.034 Bq/cell. The following paragraph in Chouin and colleagues [44] indicates that this activity delivers about 750 decays per cell. Therefore, the cellular time integrated activity coefficient $\tilde{a}$ can be approximated with $\tilde{a} = \tilde{A}/A_o$. The cumulated activity $\tilde{A}$ is simply 750 decays = 750 Bq s and A_o ~ 0.034 Bq, therefore $\tilde{a} = 6.1$ h.

a. The modelling process begins by first considering that ^{211}At decays to its daughter ^{211}Po, which decays in turn. If it is assumed that the parent and daughter are in equilibrium at all times, then radiations emitted by both parent and daughter need to be summed. Care must be taken to correct the ^{211}Po radiation yields for the ^{211}At $\rightarrow$ ^{211}Po branching ratio of 0.582. This can be accomplished by clicking the β Average Energy Spectrum database button and selecting ^{211}At from the list of Predefined Radionuclides on the Source Radiation tab. Copy the data in the Input Data for Calculation box and paste it into Excel. Repeat the process for ^{211}Po. Multiply all ^{211}Po yields by a factor of 0.582. Paste the corrected ^{211}Po data into a text file and then do the same for the ^{211}At data. Be sure to add header and footer data and format all numbers to match those in single radionuclide files. The resulting text file can be retrieved using the button in the User Created Radionuclide box (Figure 15.34). NOTE: The combined ^{211}At+daughters is available in MIRDcell V2.0.12 and later versions in the radionuclide choices in the Average β Spectrum category. However, this approach is used to demonstrate that decay chains can be modelled even when they are not present in the radionuclide choices.

b. Click the Cell Source/Target tab and select Nucleus < Cell Surface and set the radii of the cell and cell nucleus to 7 μm and 5 μm, respectively. Click the Radiobiological Parameters tab and set α_{self} = 1.79 Gy^{-1}, β_{self} = 0 Gy^{-2}, αcross = 1.79 Gy^{-1}, βcross = 0 Gy^{-2}. Click the Multicellular Geometry tab and then click the 3-D colony tab. From the drop-down list of Shapes, select Sphere. Enter a radius of 43 μm. Select Labelling Method to be Uniform Distribution. Enter the Maximum mean Activity per Cell = 0.034 Bq. Enter the Time integrated activity coefficient = 6.1 h. Enter Percentage of cells that are Labelled = 100 per cent. Click Compute (Figure 15.35).

c. Click the Output tab and scroll down to the bottom of the data in the left box (Figure 15.36). Note that the mean absorbed dose to the cells is 138 Gy when the mean activity per cell is 0.034 Bq. This is commensurate with the values of 125–245 Gy reported in [44].

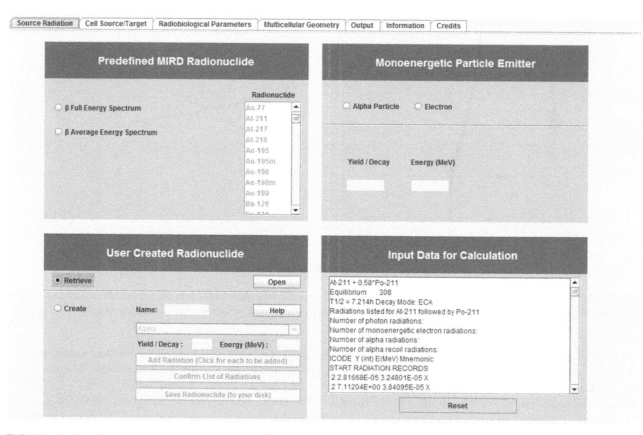

FIGURE 15.34 Source Radiation tab in MIRDcell. Here, the User Created Radionuclide feature (lower left) was used to create the radiation listing for ^{211}At and its daughter, ^{211}Po. The result appears in the Input Data for Calculation box (lower right).

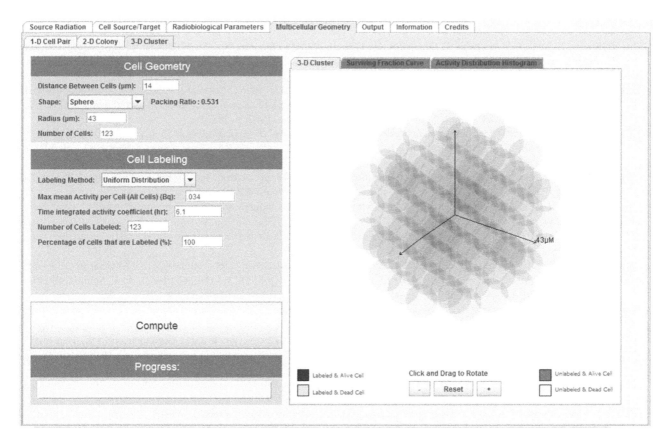

FIGURE 15.35 Multicellular Geometry < 3-D Cluster < 3-D Cluster tab in MIRDcell. The simulation was for [211]At in a spherical cluster of cells.

Distance μm	S(C<--C) Gy/Bq-s	S(C<--CS) Gy/Bq-s	S(N<--N) Gy/Bq-s	S(N<--Cy) Gy/Bq-s	S(N<--CS) Gy/Bq-s	S(Cy<--N) Gy/Bq-s	S(Cy<--CS) Gy/Bq-s	S(Cy<--Cy) Gy/Bq-s
28	1.95E-03	1.99E-03	1.91E-03	1.94E-03	1.96E-03	1.94E-03	2.00E-03	1.98E-03
29	1.79E-03	1.81E-03	1.75E-03	1.78E-03	1.79E-03	1.78E-03	1.83E-03	1.81E-03
30	1.64E-03	1.66E-03	1.61E-03	1.63E-03	1.65E-03	1.63E-03	1.67E-03	1.66E-03
31	1.51E-03	1.53E-03	1.48E-03	1.51E-03	1.52E-03	1.51E-03	1.54E-03	1.53E-03
32	1.40E-03	1.41E-03	1.37E-03	1.39E-03	1.40E-03	1.39E-03	1.42E-03	1.41E-03
33	1.29E-03	1.31E-03	1.27E-03	1.29E-03	1.30E-03	1.29E-03	1.32E-03	1.31E-03
34	1.20E-03	1.21E-03	1.18E-03	1.20E-03	1.20E-03	1.20E-03	1.22E-03	1.21E-03
35	1.12E-03	1.13E-03	1.10E-03	1.11E-03	1.12E-03	1.11E-03	1.13E-03	1.13E-03
36	1.04E-03	1.05E-03	1.03E-03	1.04E-03	1.05E-03	1.04E-03	1.06E-03	1.05E-03
37	9.75E-04	9.82E-04	9.63E-04	9.73E-04	9.77E-04	9.73E-04	9.85E-04	9.81E-04
38	9.12E-04	9.17E-04	9.03E-04	9.11E-04	9.14E-04	9.11E-04	9.18E-04	9.16E-04
39	8.54E-04	8.56E-04	8.48E-04	8.54E-04	8.56E-04	8.54E-04	8.57E-04	8.56E-04
40	7.99E-04	7.99E-04	7.97E-04	8.00E-04	8.00E-04	8.00E-04	7.99E-04	7.99E-04
41	7.47E-04	7.45E-04	7.49E-04	7.48E-04	7.47E-04	7.48E-04	7.45E-04	7.45E-04
42	6.97E-04	6.95E-04	7.03E-04	6.98E-04	6.96E-04	6.98E-04	6.94E-04	6.94E-04
43	6.50E-04	6.46E-04	6.58E-04	6.50E-04	6.47E-04	6.50E-04	6.46E-04	6.47E-04

Left box values:

2.92E-02	1.19E02	2.92E-02	1.19E02
2.96E-02	1.20E02	2.96E-02	1.20E02
2.99E-02	1.22E02	2.99E-02	1.22E02
3.03E-02	1.23E02	3.03E-02	1.23E02
3.06E-02	1.24E02	3.06E-02	1.24E02
3.09E-02	1.26E02	3.09E-02	1.26E02
3.13E-02	1.27E02	3.13E-02	1.27E02
3.16E-02	1.29E02	3.16E-02	1.29E02
3.20E-02	1.30E02	3.20E-02	1.30E02
3.23E-02	1.31E02	3.23E-02	1.31E02
3.26E-02	1.33E02	3.26E-02	1.33E02
3.30E-02	1.34E02	3.30E-02	1.34E02
3.33E-02	1.35E02	3.33E-02	1.35E02
3.37E-02	1.37E02	3.37E-02	1.37E02
3.40E-02	1.38E02	3.40E-02	1.38E02

FIGURE 15.36 Output tab in MIRDcell for the [211]At example problem. The left box contains information regarding the model details. The right box contains the cellular S values for self-dose and cross-doses.

REFERENCES

[1] B. Vaziri, H. Wu, A. P. Dhawan, P. Du, and R. W. Howell, "MIRD Pamphlet No. 25: MIRDcell V2.0 Software Tool for Dosimetric Analysis of Biologic Response of Multicellular Populations," *J Nucl Med,* vol. 55, no. 9, pp. 1557–64, 2014, doi: 10.2967/jnumed.113.131037.

[2] S. M. Goddu, R. W. Howell, L. G. Bouchet, W. E. Bolch, and D. V. Rao, *MIRD Cellular S Values: Self-absorbed dose per unit cumulated activity for selected radionuclides and monoenergetic electron and alpha particle emitters incorporated into different cell compartments.* Reston, VA: Society of Nuclear Medicine, 1997, p. 183.

[3] R. W. Howell, "The MIRD schema: From organ to cellular dimensions," *J. Nucl. Med.,* vol. 35, no. 3, pp. 531–33, 1994.

[4] R. W. Howell *et al.*, "The MIRD perspective 1999. Medical Internal Radiation Dose Committee," *J Nucl Med,* vol. 40, no. 1, pp. 3S-10S, 1999.

[5] J. Schuemann *et al.*, "TOPAS-nBio: An Extension to the TOPAS Simulation Toolkit for Cellular and Sub-cellular Radiobiology," *Radiat Res,* vol. 191, no. 2, pp. 125–38, 2019, doi: 10.1667/RR15226.1.

[6] L. J. Wu *et al.*, "Targeted cytoplasmic irradiation with alpha particles induces mutations in mammalian cells," *Proc. Natl. Acad. Sci. USA,* vol. 96, pp. 4959–64, 1999.

[7] J. P. Pouget *et al.*, "Cell membrane is a more sensitive target than cytoplasm to dense ionization produced by auger electrons," *Radiat Res,* vol. 170, no. 2, pp. 192–200, 2008, doi: 10.1667/RR1359.1.

[8] D. R. Fisher, "The microdosimetry of monoclonal antibodies labeled with alpha emitters," in *Proceedings of Fourth International Radiopharmaceutical Dosimetry Symposium,* vol. CONF-851113 – (DE86010102), A. T. Schlafke-Stelson and E. E. Watson, Eds. Springfield, VA: National Technical Information Service, 1986, pp. 26–36.

[9] J. S. Nettleton and R. Lawson, "Cellular dosimetry of diagnostic radionuclides for spherical and ellipsoidal geometry," *Phys. Med. Biol.,* vol. 41, no. 9, pp. 1845–54, 1996.

[10] S. M. Goddu, D. V. Rao, and R. W. Howell, "Multicellular dosimetry for micrometastases: dependence of self-dose versus cross-dose to cell nuclei on type and energy of radiation and subcellular distribution of radionuclides," *J Nucl Med,* vol. 35, pp. 521–30, 1994.

[11] A. Stenvall, E. Larsson, S. E. Strand, and B. A. Jönsson, "A small-scale anatomical dosimetry model of the liver," *Phys Med Biol,* vol. 59, no. 13, pp. 3353–71, 2014, doi: 10.1088/0031-9155/59/13/3353.

[12] H. H. Rossi and R. H. Ellis, Jr., "Distributed beta sources in uniformly absorbing media," *Nucleonics,* vol. 7, no. 2, pp. 19–25, 1950.

[13] H. H. Rossi and R. H. Ellis, Jr., "Distributed beta sources in uniformly absorbing media-1," *Nucleonics,* vol. 7, no. 1, pp. 18–25, 1950.

[14] W. K. Sinclair, "The dosimetry of beta radiation and its application to inhomogeneous distributions of radioactivity in cells," *Texas Reports on Biology and Medicine,* vol. 11, no. 4, pp. 745–54, 1953.

[15] R. B. Painter, R. M. Drew, and W. L. Hughes, "Inhibition of HeLa growth by intranuclear tritium," *Science,* vol. 127, pp. 1244–45, 1958.

[16] M. E. Wrenn, "The dosimetry of Fe-55," in *Proceedings of the First International Radiation Protection Association Congress,* vol. 2, W. S. Snyder, Ed. Rome, 1968, pp. 843–50.

[17] H. H. Ertl, L. E. Feinendegen, and H. J. Heiniger, "Iodine-125, a tracer in cell biology: Physical properties and biological aspects," *Phys. Med. Biol.,* vol. 15, pp. 447–56, 1970.

[18] K. G. Hofer and W. L. Hughes, "Radiotoxicity of intranuclear tritium, iodine-125 and iodine-131," *Radiat. Res.,* vol. 47, pp. 94–109, 1971.

[19] E. W. Bradley, P. C. Chan, and S. J. Adelstein, "The radiotoxicity of iodine-125 in mammalian cells. I. Effects on the survival curve of radioiodine incorporated into DNA," *Radiat. Res.,* vol. 64, pp. 555–63, 1975.

[20] R. W. Howell, V. R. Narra, D. V. Rao, and K. S. R. Sastry, "Radiobiological effects of intracellular polonium-210 alpha emissions: A comparison with Auger-emitters," *Radiat Prot Dosim,* vol. 31, pp. 325–28, 1990.

[21] D. V. Rao, V. R. Narra, R. W. Howell, G. F. Govelitz, and K. S. R. Sastry, "In-vivo radiotoxicity of DNA-incorporated I-125 compared with that of densely ionising alpha-particles," *Lancet,* vol. II, no. 8664, pp. 650–53, 1989.

[22] D. E. Charlton and J. Booz, "A Monte Carlo treatment of the decay of I-125," *Radiat. Res.,* vol. 87, pp. 10–23, 1981.

[23] R. W. Howell, "Radiation spectra for Auger-electron emitting radionuclides: Report No. 2 of AAPM Nuclear Medicine Task Group No. 6," *Med. Phys.,* vol. 19, no. 6, pp. 1371–83, 1992.

[24] J. L. Humm, R. W. Howell, and D. V. Rao, "Dosimetry of Auger electron emitting radionuclides: Report No. 3 of the AAPM Nuclear Medicine Task Group No. 6," *Med. Phys.,* vol. 21, no. 11, pp. 1901–15, 1994.

[25] A. I. Kassis, F. Fayad, B. M. Kinsey, K. S. R. Sastry, R. A. Taube, and S. J. Adelstein, "Radiotoxicity of I-125 in mammalian cells," *Radiat. Res.,* vol. 111, pp. 305–18, 1987.

[26] R. W. Howell, V. R. Narra, K. S. R. Sastry, and D. V. Rao, "On the equivalent dose for Auger electron emitters," *Radiat. Res.,* vol. 134, pp. 71–78, 1993.

[27] H. A. Wright, R. N. Hamm, J. E. Turner, R. W. Howell, D. V. Rao, and K. S. R. Sastry, "Calculations of physical and chemical reactions with DNA in aqueous solution from Auger cascades," *Radiat. Prot. Dosim.,* vol. 31, pp. 59–62, 1990.

[28] P. V. Neti and R. W. Howell, "Isolating effects of microscopic nonuniform distributions of ^{131}I on labeled and unlabeled cells," *J Nucl Med,* vol. 45, no. 6, pp. 1050–58, 2004.

[29] P. V. Neti and R. W. Howell, "When may a nonuniform distribution of ^{131}I be considered uniform? An experimental basis for multicellular dosimetry," *J Nucl Med,* vol. 44, no. 12, pp. 2019–26, 2003.

[30] C. Haydock and K. S. R. Sastry, "Physical basis of radioimmunotherapy: A theoretical study," University of Massachusetts for New England Nuclear Corporation, Amherst, MA, 1983.

[31] R. W. Howell, D. V. Rao, and C. Haydock, "Dosimetry techniques for therapeutic applications of incorporated radionuclides," in *Dosimetry of Administered Radionuclides*, S. J. Adelstein, A. I. Kassis, and R. W. Burt, Eds. Washington, DC: American College of Nuclear Physicians, 1990, pp. 215–56.

[32] D. E. Charlton, "Radiation effects in spheroids of cells exposed to alpha emitters," *Int J Radiat Biol,* vol. 76, no. 11, pp. 1555–64, 2000.

[33] Z. Cai, J. P. Pignol, C. Chan, and R. M. Reilly, "Cellular dosimetry of ^{111}In using Monte Carlo N-particle computer code: Comparison with analytic methods and correlation with in vitro cytotoxicity," *J Nucl Med,* vol. 51, no. 3, pp. 462–70, 2010, doi: 10.2967/jnumed.109.063156.

[34] E. Kalogianni, G. D. Flux, and A. Malaroda, "The use of BED and EUD concepts in heterogeneous radioactivity distributions on a multicellular scale for targeted radionuclide therapy," *Cancer Biotherapy and Radiopharmceuticals,* vol. 22, no. 1, pp. 143–50, 2007, doi: 10.1089/cbr.2007.308.

[35] A. Malaroda, G. Flux, and R. Ott, "The application of dose-rate volume histograms and survival fractions to multicellular dosimetry," *Cancer Biother. Radiopharm.,* vol. 20, no. 1, pp. 58–65, 2005.

[36] A. Malaroda, G. D. Flux, F. M. Buffa, and R. J. Ott, "Multicellular dosimetry in voxel geometry for targeted radionuclide therapy," *Cancer Biother. Radiopharm.,* vol. 18, no. 3, pp. 451–61, 2003.

[37] R. Spaic, R. Ilic, M. Dragovic, and B. Petrovic, "Generation of dose-volume histograms using Monte Carlo simulations on a multicellular model in radionuclide therapy," *Cancer Biother. Radiopharm.,* vol. 20, no. 3, pp. 320–24, 2005.

[38] P. V. S. V. Neti and R. W. Howell, "Biological response to nonuniform distributions of ^{210}Po in multicellular clusters," *Radiat Res,* vol. 168, no. 3, pp. 332–40, 2007.

[39] P. V. Neti and R. W. Howell, "Log normal distribution of cellular uptake of radioactivity: implications for biologic responses to radiopharmaceuticals," *J Nucl Med,* vol. 47, no. 6, pp. 1049–58, 2006, PMID: 16741316.

[40] R. W. Howell, P. V. Neti, M. Pinto, B. I. Gerashchenko, V. R. Narra, and E. I. Azzam, "Challenges and progress in predicting biological responses to incorporated radioactivity," *Radiat Prot Dosimetry,* vol. 122, no. 1–4, pp. 521–27, 2006, doi: 10.1093/rpd/ncl448.

[41] R. W. Howell and P. V. Neti, "Modeling multicellular response to nonuniform distributions of radioactivity: differences in cellular response to self-dose and cross-dose," *Radiat Res,* vol. 163, no. 2, pp. 216–21, 2005, doi: 10.1667/rr3290.

[42] R. W. Howell and A. Bishayee, "Bystander effects caused by nonuniform distributions of DNA-incorporated ^{125}I," *Micron,* vol. 33, pp. 127–32, 2002.

[43] E. Hindie *et al.*, "Calculation of electron dose to target cells in a complex environment by Monte Carlo code "CELLDOSE"," *Eur J Nucl Med Mol Imaging,* vol. 36, no. 1, pp. 130–36, 2009, doi: 10.1007/s00259-008-0893-z.

[44] N. Chouin *et al.*, "Ex vivo activity quantification in micrometastases at the cellular scale using the alpha-camera technique," *J Nucl Med,* vol. 54, no. 8, pp. 1347–53, 2013, doi: 10.2967/jnumed.112.113001.

[45] N. Chouin, S. Lindegren, H. Jensen, P. Albertsson, and T. Back, "Quantification of activity by alpha-camera imaging and small-scale dosimetry within ovarian carcinoma micrometastases treated with targeted alpha therapy," *The Quarterly Journal of Nuclear Medicine and Molecular Imaging: Official publication of the Italian Association of Nuclear Medicine,* vol. 56, no. 6, pp. 487–95, 2012.

[46] R. F. Hobbs, H. Song, D. L. Huso, M. H. Sundel, and G. Sgouros, "A nephron-based model of the kidneys for macro-to-micro alpha-particle dosimetry," *Phys Med Biol,* vol. 57, no. 13, pp. 4403–24, 2012, doi: 10.1088/0031-9155/57/13/4403.

[47] G. Sgouros, R. F. Hobbs, and H. Song, "Modelling and dosimetry for alpha-particle therapy," *Current Radiopharmaceuticals,* vol. 4, no. 3, pp. 261–65, 2011.

[48] R. F. Hobbs *et al.*, "A model of cellular dosimetry for macroscopic tumors in radiopharmaceutical therapy," *Med Phys,* Research Support, N.I.H., Extramural vol. 38, no. 6, pp. 2892–903, 2011.

[49] D. Emfietzoglou *et al.*, "Liposome-mediated radiotherapeutics within avascular tumor spheroids: Comparative dosimetry study for various radionuclides, liposome systems, and a targeting antibody," *J Nucl Med,* vol. 46, no. 1, pp. 89–97, 2005.

[50] D. Lee, M. Li, B. Bednarz, and M. K. Schultz, "Modeling Cell and Tumor-Metastasis Dosimetry with the Particle and Heavy Ion Transport Code System (PHITS) Software for Targeted Alpha-Particle Radionuclide Therapy," *Radiat Res,* vol. 190, no. 3, pp. 236–47, 2018, doi: 10.1667/RR15081.1.

[51] R. Raghavan, R. W. Howell, and M. R. Zalutsky, "A model for optimizing delivery of targeted radionuclide therapies into resection cavity margins for the treatment of primary brain cancers," *Biomedical Physics & Engineering Express,* vol. 3, no. 3, 2017, doi: 10.1088/2057-1976/aa6db9.

[52] S. Marcatili *et al.*, "Realistic multi-cellular dosimetry for (177)Lu-labelled antibodies: Model and application," *Phys Med Biol,* vol. 61, no. 19, pp. 6935–52, 2016, doi: 10.1088/0031-9155/61/19/6935.

[53] V. Reijonen *et al.*, "Multicellular dosimetric chain for molecular radiotherapy exemplified with dose simulations on 3D cell spheroids," *Physica Medica: PM: An international journal devoted to the applications of physics to medicine and biology: official journal of the Italian Association of Biomedical Physics,* vol. 40, pp. 72–78, 2017, doi: 10.1016/j.ejmp.2017.07.012.

[54] N. Falzone *et al.*, "Targeting micrometastases: The effect of heterogeneous radionuclide distribution on tumor control probability," *J Nucl Med,* 2018, doi: 10.2967/jnumed.117.207308.

[55] M. Siragusa *et al.*, "The COOLER Code: A novel analytical approach to calculate subcellular energy deposition by internal electron emitters," *Radiat Res,* vol. 188, no. 2, pp. 204–20, 2017, doi: 10.1667/RR14683.1.

[56] D. Rajon, W. E. Bolch, and R. W. Howell, "Lognormal distribution of cellular uptake of radioactivity: Monte Carlo simulation of irradiation and cell killing in 3-dimensional populations in carbon scaffolds," *J Nucl Med,* Research Support, N.I.H., Extramural vol. 52, no. 6, pp. 926–33, 2011, doi: 10.2967/jnumed.110.080044.

[57] D. Rajon, W. E. Bolch, and R. W. Howell, "Survival of tumor and normal cells upon targeting with electron-emitting radionuclides," *Med Phys,* vol. 40, no. 1, p. 014101, 2013, doi: 10.1118/1.4769409.

[58] A. I. Kassis, S. J. Adelstein, C. Haydock, and K. S. R. Sastry, "Thallium-201: An experimental and a theoretical radiobiological approach to dosimetry," *J. Nucl. Med.,* vol. 24, pp. 1164–75, 1983.

[59] A. I. Kassis, S. J. Adelstein, C. Haydock, and K. S. R. Sastry, "Thallium-201: an experimental and a theoretical radiobiological approach to dosimetry," *J Nucl Med,* vol. 24, no. 12, pp. 1164–75, 1983.

[60] J. C. Roeske and T. G. Stinchcomb, "The use of microdosimetric moments in evaluating cell survival for therapeutic alpha-particle emitters," *Radiat. Res.,* vol. 151, no. 1, pp. 31–38, 1999.

[61] J. C. Roeske and T. G. Stinchcomb, "Tumor control probability model for alpha-particle-emitting radionuclides," *Radiation Research,* vol. 153, no. 1, pp. 16–22, 2000.

[62] W. E. Bolch, "Further explorations of cellular uptake of radioactivity," *J Nucl Med,* vol. 49, no. 6, pp. 869–70, 2008, doi: 10.2967/jnumed.108.050567.

[63] P. Zanotti-Fregonara and E. Hindie, "Lognormal distribution of cellular uptake of radiopharmaceuticals: implications for biologic response in cancer treatment," *J Nucl Med,* vol. 52, no. 4, pp. 501–3, 2011, doi: 10.2967/jnumed.110.084590.

[64] P. Zanzonico, "Cell-level dosimetry and biologic response modeling of heterogeneously distributed radionuclides: A step forward," *J Nucl Med,* Comment vol. 52, no. 6, pp. 845–47, 2011, doi: 10.2967/jnumed.111.087841.

[65] ICRU, "ICRU Report No. 67. Absorbed-dose specification in nuclear medicine," *Journal of the ICRU,* vol. 2, no. 1, pp. 3–110, 2002.

[66] R. Loevinger and M. Berman, "MIRD Pamphlet No. 1: A schema for absorbed-dose calculations for biologically distributed radionuclides." *J Nucl Med,* vol. 9, Suppl. No. 1, pp. 7–14, 1968.

[67] R. Loevinger, T. F. Budinger, and E. E. Watson, *MIRD Primer for Absorbed Dose Calculations,* Revised ed. New York: The Society of Nuclear Medicine, 1991, p. 128.

[68] ICRU, "ICRU Report No. 85. Fundamental quantities and units for ionizing radiation," *Journal of the ICRU,* vol. 11, no. 1, pp. 1–30, 2011, doi: 10.1093/jicru/ndr012.

[69] W. E. Bolch, K. F. Eckerman, G. Sgouros, and S. R. Thomas, "MIRD pamphlet No. 21: A generalized schema for radiopharmaceutical dosimetry—standardization of nomenclature," *J Nucl Med,* vol. 50, no. 3, pp. 477–84, 2009, doi: 10.2967/jnumed.108.056036.

[70] S. M. Goddu, R. W. Howell, and D. V. Rao, "Cellular dosimetry: absorbed fractions for monoenergetic electron and alpha particle sources and S-values for radionuclides uniformly distributed in different cell compartments," *J Nucl Med,* vol. 35, no. 2, pp. 303–16, 1994.

[71] D. E. Charlton, J. Booz, J. Fidorra, T. Smit, and L. E. Feinendegen, "Microdosimetry of radioactive nuclei incorporated into the DNA of mammalian cells," in *Sixth Symposium Microdosimetry,* vol. I, J. Booz and H. G. Ebert, Eds., no. EUR6064). London: Harwood Academic, 1978, pp. 91–110.

[72] D. E. Charlton and R. Sephton, "A relationship between microdosimetric spectra and cell survival for high-LET irradiation," *Int. J. Radiat. Biol.,* vol. 59, pp. 447–57, 1991.

[73] D. R. Fisher, M. E. Frazier, and T. K. Andrews, Jr., "Energy distribution and the relative biological effects of internal alpha emitters," *Radiat. Prot. Dosim.,* vol. 13, no. 1–4, pp. 223–27, 1985.

[74] D. R. Fisher and R. Harty, "The microdosimetry of lymphocytes irradiated by alpha-particles," *Int. J. Radiat. Biol.,* vol. 41, no. 3, pp. 315–24, 1982.

[75] J. L. Humm, "Dosimetric aspects of radiolabeled antibodies for tumor therapy," *J. Nucl. Med.,* vol. 27, pp. 1490–97, 1986.

[76] J. L. Humm, L. M. Chin, L. Cobb, and R. Begent, "Microdosimetry in radioimmunotherapy," *Radiat. Prot. Dosim.,* vol. 31, pp. 433–36, 1990.

[77] T. G. Stinchcomb and J. C. Roeske, "Analytic microdosimetry for radioimmunotherapeutic alpha emitters," *Med. Phys.,* vol. 19, no. 6, pp. 1385–93, 1992.

[78] T. G. Stinchcomb and J. C. Roeske, "Values of "S," <z1>, and <(z1)2> for dosimetry using alpha-particle emitters," *Med. Phys.,* vol. 26, no. 9, pp. 1960–71, 1999.

[79] J. C. Roeske *et al.*, "Modeling of dose to tumor and normal tissue from intraperitoneal radioimmunotherapy with alpha and beta emitters," *Int J Radiat Oncol Biol Phys,* vol. 19, no. 6, pp. 1539–48, 1990.

[80] J. C. Roeske, B. Aydogan, M. Bardies, and J. L. Humm, "Small-scale dosimetry: challenges and future directions," *Semin Nucl Med,* vol. 38, no. 5, pp. 367–83, 2008, doi: 10.1053/j.semnuclmed.2008.05.003.

[81] J. C. Roeske and M. Hoggarth, "Alpha-particle Monte Carlo simulation for microdosimetric calculations using a commercial spreadsheet," *Phys. Med. Biol.,* vol. 52, no. 7, pp. 1909–22, 2007, doi: 10.1088/0031-9155/52/7/010.

[82] Z. Cai, Y. L. Kwon, and R. M. Reilly, "Monte Carlo N-Particle (MCNP) Modeling of the Cellular Dosimetry of 64Cu: Comparison with MIRDcell S Values and Implications for Studies of Its Cytotoxic Effects," *J Nucl Med,* vol. 58, no. 2, pp. 339–45, 2017, doi: 10.2967/jnumed.116.175695.

[83] K. S. R. Sastry, C. Haydock, A. M. Basha, and D. V. Rao, "Electron dosimetry for radioimmunotherapy: Optimal electron energy," *Radiat Prot Dosimetry,* vol. 13, pp. 249–52, 1985.

[84] N. Falzone, J. M. Fernandez-Varea, G. Flux, and K. A. Vallis, "Monte Carlo Evaluation of Auger Electron-Emitting Theranostic Radionuclides," *J Nucl Med,* vol. 56, no. 9, pp. 1441–46, 2015, doi: 10.2967/jnumed.114.153502.

[85] S. K. Kennel *et al.*, "Radiotoxicity of bismuth-213 bound to membranes of monolayer and spheroid cultures of tumor cells," *Radiat. Res.,* vol. 151, pp. 244–56, 1999.

[86] C. Zhu *et al.*, "Alpha-particle radiotherapy: For large solid tumors diffusion trumps targeting," *Biomaterials,* vol. 130, pp. 67–75, 2017, doi: 10.1016/j.biomaterials.2017.03.035.

[87] J. A. O'Donoghue, M. Bardies, and T. E. Wheldon, "Relationships between tumor size and curability for uniformly targeted therapy with beta-emitting radionuclides," *J Nucl Med,* vol. 36, no. 10, pp. 1902–09, 1995.

[88] R. W. Howell, D. Rajon, and W. E. Bolch, "Monte Carlo simulation of irradiation and killing in three-dimensional cell populations with lognormal cellular uptake of radioactivity," *Int J Radiat Biol,* vol. 88, no. 1–2, pp. 115–22, 2012, doi: 10.3109/09553002.2011.602379.

[89] B. Vaziri, H. Wu, J. M. Akudugu, V. S. Neti, and R. W. Howell, "Methods and systems for determining the distribution of radiation dose and response," USA Patent 9,623,262, April 18, 2017, 2017.

[90] J. L. Humm, J. C. Roeske, D. R. Fisher, and G. T. Y. Chen, "Microdosimetric concepts in radioimmunotherapy," *Med. Phys.,* vol. 20, Pt. 2, no. 2, pp. 535–41, 1993.

[91] J. C. Roeske and T. G. Stinchcomb, "The average number of alpha-particle hits to the cell nucleus required to eradicate a tumour cell population," *Phys. Med. Biol.,* vol. 51, no. 9, pp. N179–86, 2006, doi: 10.1088/0031-9155/51/9/N02.

[92] T. G. Stinchcomb *et al.*, "Binary methods for the microdosimetric analysis of cell survival data from alpha-particle irradiation," *Cancer Biotherapy and Radiopharmaceuticals,* vol. 18, no. 3, pp. 481–87, 2003, doi: 10.1089/108497803322285242.

[93] W. Norris and L. A. Woodruff, "The fundamentals of autoradiography," *Annu. Rev. Nucl. Sci.,* Review vol. 5, pp. 297–326, 1955.

[94] T. Back and L. Jacobsson, "The alpha-camera: a quantitative digital autoradiography technique using a charge-coupled device for ex vivo high-resolution bioimaging of alpha-particles," *J Nucl Med,* vol. 51, no. 10, pp. 1616–23, 2010, doi: 10.2967/jnumed.110.077578.

[95] A. I. Kassis and S. J. Adelstein, "A rapid and reproducible method for the separation of cells from radioactive media," *J. Nucl. Med.,* vol. 21, pp. 88–90, 1980.

[96] R. W. Howell, D. V. Rao, D.-Y. Hou, V. R. Narra, and K. S. R. Sastry, "The question of relative biological effectiveness and quality factor for Auger emitters incorporated into proliferating mammalian cells," *Radiat. Res.,* vol. 128, pp. 282–92, 1991.

[97] J. B. Pasternack, J. D. Domogauer, A. Khullar, J. M. Akudugu, and R. W. Howell, "The advantage of antibody cocktails for targeted alpha therapy depends on specific activity," *J Nucl Med,* vol. 55, no. 12, pp. 2012–19, 2014, doi: 10.2967/jnumed.114.141580.

[98] *MIRDcell – Installation Guide.* http://jnm.snmjournals.org/content/suppl/2014/09/02/jnumed.113.131037.DC1/131037_Supplemental_Data.pdf

[99] *MIRDcell – Users' Guide.* http://jnm.snmjournals.org/content/55/9/1557.

[100] R. W. Howell *et al.*, "Radiotoxicity of ^{195m}Pt labeled *trans*-platinum(II) in mammalian cells," *Radiat Res,* vol. 140, pp. 55–62, 1994.

16 Alpha-particle Dosimetry

Stig Palm

CONTENTS

16.1 INTRODUCTION

A new class of drugs for treatment of spread cancers is now introduced in the clinic. These novel radiopharmaceuticals are based on alpha-particle emitting radionuclides, targeted to cancer cells. Alpha particles offer potentially significant advantages over previously used beta particles, that is, electrons. Due to the high energy deposited, one single alpha-particle "hit", that is, traversals through the cell nucleus, can significantly reduce the cell's probability of surviving. For beta particles, several hundred "hits" are required for the same effect. Alpha particles have a range of ~100 μm in tissue and the deposited energy therefore also "conforms" better to the smallest microtumours (diameters <200 μm). The properties of alpha emitters therefore seem ideal for treatment of micrometastases that signify many disseminated cancers. For a more comprehensive review of the dosimetry and radiobiology of alpha emitters the reader is referred to [1].

To-date, alpha-emitters ^{225}Ac, ^{213}Bi, ^{212}Pb, ^{227}Th, ^{223}Ra and ^{211}At, linked to various targeting vectors, have been or are currently being evaluated in clinical trials. As more effort is being made to evaluate the efficacy of these compounds, a strategy is needed for selecting the most proper alpha-emitter with the best targeting vector for treating patients who will benefit the most from this type of therapy. Such a strategy should include some attempts to calculate absorbed dose to both tumour cells and critical healthy tissues.

An alpha-particle travels up to 0.1 mm in soft tissue. For dosimetry, it is often sufficient to model the track as a straight line and the track-end straggling can be ignored. The energy deposited along the track is described by the Stopping Power (keV/μm) and can be found from, for example, ICRU 49 [2]. Since the initial energy of all alpha emitters of clinical relevance are within a relatively small interval (4–9 MeV), a tabulation of Stopping Power values for 9 MeV down to a full stop will include the full spectrum of all Stopping Power values for all emitted alphas. This is illustrated in Figure 16.1 where the initial kinetic energy of alphas from ^{225}Ac and daughters ^{221}Fr, ^{217}At and ^{213}Bi are plotted against Stopping Power values in water.

DOI: 10.1201/9780429489549-16

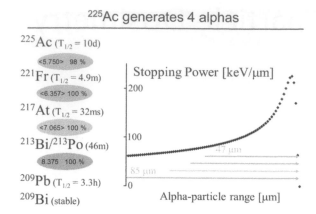

FIGURE 16.1   Schematic decay chain with LET and ranges in water of alphas emitted from ^{225}Ac and daughter decays. Colour image available at www.routledge.com/9781138593299.

16.2   RADIOACTIVITY MEASUREMENTS

Since detectors capable of direct measurement of alpha-particles are not commonly available in nuclear medicine departments, it is the photons associated with alpha-decay that allow more standard equipment to be used for radioactivity measurement. As for any radionuclide, proper settings for equipment such as radionuclide radioactivity calibrators ("dose calibrators") or gamma-well counters must be derived with particular attention being paid to any photon contribution from daughter radionuclides.

In addition to the sometimes-complex mixtures of gammas and characteristic x-rays from parent and daughter radionuclides, the decay data itself can carry large uncertainties. This must be accounted for when evaluating the errors involved in determining the radioactivity that forms the basis for dosimetry. An illustrative example is the 687 keV gamma from ^{211}At, where the primary standards laboratories provide its abundance (0.245%) with 5 per cent uncertainty. This uncertainty demonstrates the difficulty in providing an accurate radioactivity measurement for alpha-emitters. For more precise measurements, some other gammas or characteristic x-rays, with much lower uncertainty in the decay data, should be used.

16.3   TARGETING VECTOR

Alpha-particle emitters typically need to be attached to some vehicle for efficient targeting of malignant cells or tissues. Typical targeting vectors are monoclonal antibodies that bind to antigens on cancer cells. Several alternative vehicles, such as nanoparticles and liposomes, have been evaluated and many more proposed.

Regardless of targeting vector, for dosimetry it is important to find the biodistribution of the compound. This is often done in animal experiments, where mice are injected with the alpha-emitting compound and various organs dissected so that the time-varying biodistribution can be determined. The stability of the alpha-emitter/vehicle compound and any subsequent distribution of "free" alpha-emitters (and daughters) could also be evaluated in such experiments. Additional cell experiments can be designed to reveal the rate at which the vehicles bind to, and are released from, the target cells.

16.4   ABSORBED DOSE TO A SINGLE CELL

Even rough estimates of absorbed dose to a single cell can prove very useful for analysing the clinical potential of a proposed radiopharmaceutical. As illustrated in Figure 16.1, all alphas have roughly the same LET (~80 keV) at the beginning of their path. It is therefore relatively simple to provide a quick estimate of the specific energy (the microdosimetric equivalent to absorbed dose) to a cell nucleus if the alpha decay takes place on the cell surface. Cancer cells can have large nuclei, with diameters ~80 per cent that of the cell. If the cell and its nucleus are concentric spheres, then there is ~20 per cent probability that an alpha track originating on the cell surface will traverse the nucleus (Figure 16.2). For a 7 μm radius cell with a 5.6 μm radius nucleus, one alpha-particle traversal will result in ~0.2 Gy to the cell nucleus.

As a (made-up) illustration, consider an idea to target single-cell disease with an alpha emitter labelled antibody. Say a typical cell has, for example, 10,000 antigens for this antibody. Further, if the specific activity of the proposed radioimmunoconjugate translates to 1 in 1000 antibodies being radiolabelled with an alpha-emitter, then, at best, ten

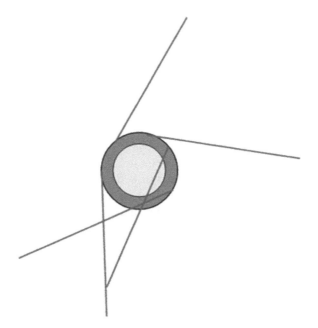

FIGURE 16.2 Illustration how 1 in 5 alpha decays occurring on a spherical cell surface results in a traversal through the nucleus.

alphas will originate from a cell surface and on average two will traverse the cell nucleus, resulting in ~0.4 Gy. This will not be an efficient therapy.

This type of quick dosimetric analysis often provides meaningful input when novel alpha-emitting agents are proposed for variable clinical indications and can serve to improve the planning of pre-clinical experiments. The biological reality is, however, far more complex, and any additional information on the distribution of alpha decays in relation to the targeted cells will improve the dosimetry. Further, cell and nuclei sizes vary, as do their shapes. Cells can be *crossfire* irradiated by alphas originating from a neighbouring cell. There may also be *by-stander* effects on cells not directly hit by an alpha-particle. The difficulty of including all biological complexity should, however, not prevent presenting some simplified dosimetry that can often serve to optimize the proposed therapies.

16.5 ABSORBED DOSE TO TUMOUR

Whole-body and some organ uptake may be provided by quantitative gamma-camera imaging. The absorbed dose to tumour is, however, more difficult to estimate, particularly for the small metastases or single tumour cells where targeted alpha therapy holds its most promise.

If the targeted tumours are too small to be detected with any method, it is obviously impossible to measure an absorbed dose to them. This should not hinder an attempt to at least estimate the absorbed dose. In doing so, some information needs to be acquired and sometimes translated to make it useful for such estimates.

Cell and cell nuclei sizes can often be directly measured using a microscope. One must be cautious that the cell shapes are the same as in the therapy setting and not flattened during the measurement.

The average number of targeted sites, for example, antigens, per cell can be derived from measurements of the antigen density by flow cytometry. If such results are not available, then immunohistochemistry which primarily produces results describing the fraction of the sample cells stained categorized as +, ++, or +++, can provide some information, if not only the fraction, but also the intensity of the stain is used.

A radiopharmaceutical is partly described by its specific activity. If, in addition, the molecular weight of the compound is known, then it is easy to calculate the fraction of targeting vector that carry a radionuclide. This immediately gives some insight into the therapeutic potential of the studied drug. As described earlier, if only 1 in 1000 antibodies carry an alpha-emitting radionuclide, it will be difficult to kill single cells with this drug. On the other hand, if this ratio is much higher, for example, 1-on-1, the mAbs may be *consumed* on first-encounter cells instead of being distributed to all tumour cells. This type of information can thus be used for optimizing the therapy.

For target tissues that are smaller than the range of the emitted alpha-particles, that is < 100 μm, it is clear that using an absorbed fraction of 1 will be grossly misleading. However, even for larger sizes, a more detailed analysis of the actual microdistribution should be sought. If, for example, a spherical microtumour with radii 500 μm, is irradiated by alphas from radionuclide decays occurring only on the tumour surface, the inner core of that tumour will consist of tumour cells that have not been irradiated at all. Even if they may be affected by possible by-stander effects, they will likely survive. If, instead, some large number of decays occur homogeneously distributed throughout the microtumour, all cells will be eradicated.

16.6 GAMMA-CAMERA IMAGING

Most alpha-emitters proposed for clinical use involve the emission of photons, either directly or through daughter decay. When the probability of gammas emitted per decay is too low for imaging, then often characteristic x-rays in the 70–100 keV range can be used. This makes it possible to image the distribution also of alpha-emitters on a gamma-camera, but several aspects must be considered when information is derived from such images. The most obvious is a low count-rate that will result in noisy images and difficulty in quantifying uptake. If characteristic x-rays are sampled, the energy window will typically include contamination from x-rays generated in the lead collimator. Other aspects include choice of camera, collimator, energy window, acquisition time, and method for reconstruction, including scatter correction.

The various considerations involved in ^{223}Ra gamma-camera imaging with energy windows covering the characteristic x-rays (81–84 keV; 39% abundance) and gammas at 154 keV (5.8%) and 269 keV (14.2%) using a medium-energy collimator were presented by Flux [3]. Alpha-emitter ^{211}At has been imaged using the 77–93 keV characteristic x-rays (43.3%) with corrections for the influence of the higher-energy gammas (i.e. 578 keV, 687 keV and 898 keV; all < 1%) (Figure 16.3) [4]. Gamma-camera images of ^{225}Ac distribution are typically acquired using gammas from daughters ^{221}Fr (218 keV) and ^{213}Bi (440 keV).

16.7 ORGAN AND WHOLE-BODY ABSORBED DOSE

Often, repeat measurements with a simple probe at some fixed distance from a patient will provide a reasonable estimate on the whole-body retention. Whole-body scans with a gamma-camera result in more precise measurements with

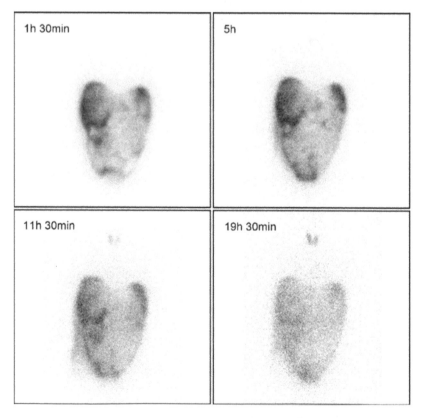

FIGURE 16.3   Gamma-camera images following intraperitoneal administration of ^{211}At-MX35 F(ab')2. At the later time-points, the uptake in the thyroid become visible. From J Nucl Med 2009 Jul;50(7):1153–60 © SNMMI (with permission) [4].

valuable distribution data, but comes at the cost of scheduling the patient for repeat scans. Any sampling of fluid and tissue will provide additional information about the biodistribution of the injected alpha-emitting compound. Repeat measurements of blood, urine, saliva, sweat, and faeces can provide valuable indirect information on the absorbed dose to critical organs such as the bone marrow and kidneys. Samples can typically be measured in gamma-well counters or with any calibrated probe.

Gross organ distribution in patients can sometimes be found from quantitative SPECT images. Since the amount of radioactivity, and the abundance of emitted photons, is typically much lower than for a diagnostic image, the uncertainty in estimating organ uptake using this approach is often very large. Suggestions for improving estimates on organ uptake include the use of gamma-emitting surrogate radionuclides (instead of alpha-emitters) for acquisition of SPECT images. It is also of value to translate biodistribution derived in animal experiments to what can be expected in a patient.

With an estimate of the biokinetics, time-activity curves can be generated for organs and possible targets. For dosimetry of organs and targets larger than the smallest cell clusters, an absorbed fraction of 1 can be assumed for the emitted alphas. Energy from emitted electrons or photons (gammas or characteristic x-rays) are often negligible in comparison. The only exception would be organs with zero uptake of the injected alpha-emitting compound where some fraction of the energy from the elsewhere emitted photons are absorbed in these organs.

16.8   PHARMACOKINETIC MODELLING

Construction of a pharmacokinetic model for intraperitoneally administered antibodies radiolabelled with alpha-emitters can serve as an example for how absorbed dose to microtumors and healthy tissues can be estimated.

First, the amount of radioactivity and the administered volume must be known. The specific activity must then be translated to the fraction of antibodies labelled with a radionuclide. For various alpha-emitters, this can be 1 in 50, or as low as 1 in 1000 antibodies being radiolabelled. A first assumption is that the radiolabel does not impact the antibody's binding properties to antigens expressed on a tumour cell surface. Once within the peritoneum, the main mechanisms that determine the position of the mAbs can be modelled.

One mechanism is the probability of being bound to a specific antigen expressed on a tumour cell and directly exposed to the peritoneal fluid. This time-dependent probability is modelled using the initial concentration of mAbs in the fluid together with the concentration of antigens in a single tumour cell or micrometastases. For a single cell ($r = 7$ μm) with 700 000 antigens, this translates to ~487 antigens μm^{-3}. The concentrations, typically expressed as mol/L, of mAbs and antigens can then be modelled globally to a reaction mechanism equation where the concentration of bound mAb is determined per time interval.

Additional parameters needed for the modelling include the fraction of mAbs with ability to bind to the antigens (immunoreactive fraction) and the rate with which binding and release occur (association k_{on} and dissociation k_{off} constants). These parameters and those describing the size and antigen density of the cancer cells are best derived from in-vitro experiments mimicking the patient therapy setting as closely as possible.

A dynamic compartment model was then constructed, which enabled the computation of the cumulated activity, that is, the total number of alpha decays, on a tumour cell. The model was constructed in the commercially available software STELLA (ISEE Systems Inc.). Originally, two compartments were defined – one representing the injected volume and the number of mAbs in the abdominal cavity, and one representing the number of mAbs bound to the antigenic sites of one selected tumour cell [5].

A more refined model (Figure 16.4) allowed for a varying mAb concentration in the peritoneal fluid [6]. This variation was due to departure of mAbs from the intraperitoneal fluid because of (a) direct absorption by the diaphragmatic lymphatics and (b) transcapillary absorption. If saline is i.p. infused, the transcapillary absorption will result in an additional absorption of water from the i.p. fluid.

If an icodextrin solution is instead used, the transcapillary absorption can be partially reversed. This lowers the mAb concentration in the i.p. fluid and therefore slightly lowers the number of mAbs bound to antigens. However, the benefits of securing a large i.p. fluid volume for a longer duration that also resulted in a large decrease in absorbed dose to healthy tissues, including the bone marrow, outweighed the slight reduction in absorbed dose to microtumours in a clinical phase I trial [4]. A later model [7] also includes penetration of antibodies into microtumours with radii up to 400 μm and evaluates the effect of adding unlabelled antibodies as a boost.

The described pharmacokinetic models provide results for the number of radiolabelled mAbs on and within microtumours as well as for healthy tissues at any time. The results are then used for microdosimetry. A custom Monte Carlo program, originally written in C, has been used for simulating absorbed dose, for example, ^{211}At-labelled mAbs [8]. The program allows for possible relocation of daughter ^{211}Po ($t_{1/2}$=0.52s) and generates results for specific energy (or absorbed dose) to cell nuclei of various sizes and shapes for a single cell or for microtumours.

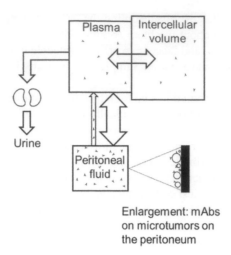

Enlargement: mAbs
on microtumors on
the peritoneum

FIGURE 16.4 Schematic illustration of the main transports included in model. Unidirectional arrow from peritoneal fluid symbolizes lymphatic absorption, which includes mAb transport. Two-headed arrow between peritoneal fluid and plasma reflects transcapillary absorption. From J Nucl Med 2016, 57 (4) 594–600 © SNMMI (with permission) [6].

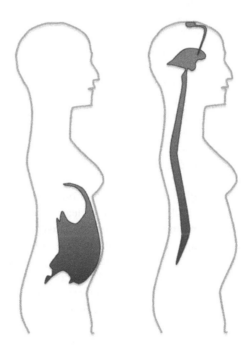

FIGURE 16.5 Illustration of local–regional therapy in the peritoneal fluid (left) or the cerebro-spinal fluid (right).

To complement all types of measurements, pharmacokinetic modelling may be used. Examples includes intraperitoneal infusion (Figure 16.4 and Figure 16.5-left) of radiolabelled antibodies for ovarian cancer [6, 7] and intra-thecal infusion (Figure 16.5-right) for neuroblastoma and medulloblastoma spread in the central nervous system [9–11].

16.9 CONCLUSION

While accurate dosimetry for all target cells and healthy tissue of a specific patient is a near-impossibility, some estimates from measurements involving common nuclear medicine equipment can provide very valuable information for evaluating and optimizing therapies with alpha-particle emitters.

REFERENCES

[1] G. Sgouros, Ed., *MIRD – Radiobiology and dosimetry for radiopharmaceutical therapy with alpha-particle emitters.* Reston, VA: Society of Nuclear Medicine and Molecular Imaging, 2015.

[2] M. J. Berger *et al.*, "Report 49," *Journal of the International Commission on Radiation Units and Measurements,* vol. os25, no. 2, pp. NP-NP, 2016, doi: 10.1093/jicru/os25.2.Report49%J Journal of the International Commission on Radiation Units and Measurements.

[3] G. D. Flux, "Imaging and dosimetry for radium-223: The potential for personalized treatment," *Br J Radiol,* vol. 90, no. 1077, p. 20160748, 2017, doi: 10.1259/bjr.20160748.

[4] H. Andersson *et al.*, "Intraperitoneal alpha-particle radioimmunotherapy of ovarian cancer patients: Pharmacokinetics and dosimetry of (211)At-MX35 F(ab')2 – a phase I study," *J Nucl Med,* vol. 50, no. 7, pp. 1153–60, 2009, doi: 10.2967/jnumed.109.062604.

[5] J. Elgqvist *et al.*, "Therapeutic efficacy and tumour dose estimations in radioimmunotherapy of intraperitoneally growing OVCAR-3 cells in nude mice with (211)At-labeled monoclonal antibody MX35," *J Nucl Med,* vol. 46, no. 11, pp. 1907–15, 2005.

[6] S. Palm, T. Back, B. Haraldsson, L. Jacobsson, S. Lindegren, and P. Albertsson, "Biokinetic Modeling and Dosimetry for Optimizing Intraperitoneal Radioimmunotherapy of Ovarian Cancer Microtumors," *J Nucl Med,* vol. 57, no. 4, pp. 594–600, 2016, doi: 10.2967/jnumed.115.167825.

[7] S. Palm, T. Back, S. Lindegren, R. Hultborn, L. Jacobsson, and P. Albertsson, "Model of Intraperitoneal Targeted Alpha-Particle Therapy Shows that Posttherapy Cold-Antibody Boost Enhances Microtumor Radiation Dose and Treatable Tumor Sizes," *J Nucl Med,* vol. 59, no. 4, pp. 646–51, 2018, doi: 10.2967/jnumed.117.201285.

[8] S. Palm, J. L. Humm, R. Rundqvist, and L. Jacobsson, "Microdosimetry of astatine-211 single-cell irradiation: role of daughter polonium-211 diffusion," *Med Phys,* vol. 31, no. 2, pp. 218–25, 2004, doi: 10.1118/1.1640951.

[9] P. He *et al.*, "Two-compartment model of radioimmunotherapy delivered through cerebrospinal fluid," *Eur J Nucl Med Mol Imaging,* vol. 38, no. 2, pp. 334–42, 2011, doi: 10.1007/s00259-010-1633-8.

[10] Y. Lv, N. K. Cheung, and B. M. Fu, "A pharmacokinetic model for radioimmunotherapy delivered through cerebrospinal fluid for the treatment of leptomeningeal metastases," *J Nucl Med,* vol. 50, no. 8, pp. 1324–31, 2009, doi: 10.2967/jnumed.108.060798.

[11] R. S. Yerrabelli *et al.*, "IntraOmmaya compartmental radioimmunotherapy using (131)I-omburtamab-pharmacokinetic modeling to optimize therapeutic index," *Eur J Nucl Med Mol Imaging,* 2020, doi: 10.1007/s00259-020-05050-z.

17 Staff Radiation Protection

Lena Jönsson

CONTENTS

17.1 INTRODUCTION

From a radiation protection point of view, nuclear medicine is a complex medical specialty that includes both radio-nuclide and radiopharmaceutical production and patient diagnostics and therapy. The practical work with radiation sources includes a variety of procedures, activity levels, dose rates, and risks of contamination. The procedures consist of, for example, cyclotron production of radionuclides; synthesis, radiochemistry, preparation, and transportation of radiopharmaceuticals; withdrawal of the activity; and patient injection. After injection, the patient is the radiation

DOI: 10.1201/9780429489549-17

source, and the staff have to keep this in mind while positioning the patient in the imaging system. In addition, there is also the handling of blood samples, urine samples, and radioactive waste.

Handling open radiation sources involves the risk of contamination and possible accidental inhalation or oral intake of radiopharmaceuticals, which can lead to internal irradiation to the worker. In addition, contamination can give rise to misleading examination results if patients, measuring equipment, or premises become contaminated. Hybrid imaging such as SPECT/CT and PET/CT combines different imaging modalities in an integrated system. The CT system introduces yet another risk of external irradiation from scattered radiation if someone has to be present in the room during exposure. The planning and design of the facility and the radiation shielding in walls, floor, and ceiling are also important issues to minimize the exposure to staff, patients, and the public.

The radiation dose to the worker is largely determined by the knowledge and awareness of health risks associated with working with unsealed sources. It is important to utilize time, distance, and radiation shielding to the extent possible to minimize the radiation dose to the staff.

17.2 LEGISLATION OF RADIATION PROTECTION

17.2.1 FUNDAMENTAL PRINCIPLES OF RADIATION PROTECTION

The fundamental principles of radiation protection defined by the International Commission on Radiological Protection, ICRP, [1] are justification, optimization, and individual dose limits, and these are reviewed in detail in Chapter 6 in this book. An overview of dose limits for workers is given below.

17.2.2 DOSE LIMITS

Occupational exposure is of no benefit to the exposed worker; therefore, dose limits are set at a level of acceptable risk to protect the individual. In addition, based on the linear-non-threshold (LNT) model, which assumes that the risk for stochastic effects increases with increasing dose, the radiation doses always should be kept as low as reasonably achievable (ALARA) to minimize the risk of these effects.

The ICRP recommendations [1] and the IAEA safety guide [2] provide occupational dose limits (Table 17.1). The dose limits are the maximum dose accepted for regulated sources in planned radiation situations.

Based on these dose limits, Euratom [4] has issued directives that have been implemented in the Member States of the European Union. The individual Member States have based their radiation protection legislation on the EU directive, but they may have decided on additional restrictions at a national level.

17.2.3 CLASSIFICATION OF WORKING AREAS AND OF EXPOSED WORKERS

As a tool in the radiation protection work to control radiation sources and occupational radiation protection, workplaces are classified as either controlled or supervised areas. The classification is based on radiation exposure levels or the risk of contamination and the spread of contamination the work may entail. The level of protective measures needed is adjusted with respect to these risks.

TABLE 17.1
Occupational Dose Limits in Planned Exposure Situations [1, 3]

Type of limit	Dose limit	Comments
Effective dose	20 mSv/year	Averaged over defined periods of 5 years. Should not exceed 50 mSv in any single year.
		Additional limitations for pregnant women.
Annual equivalent dose		
Lens of the eye	20 mSv/year	Averaged over defined periods of 5 years. Should not exceed 50 mSv in any single year.
Skin	500 mSv/year	Averaged over 1 cm^2 area of skin, regardless of the area exposed.
Hands and feet	500 mSv/year	

A controlled area requires a higher level of radiation protection than a supervised area [1]. In a supervised area, there is under normal working conditions no need for specific measures for protection and radiation safety, but exposure conditions are required to be kept under review [1]. Controlled areas might be, for example, rooms where radiopharmaceuticals are prepared, stored, and injected. In addition, according to Carlsson and Le Heron [5], gamma camera rooms and waiting areas could also be classified as controlled areas because of the potential risk of contamination.

Controlled and supervised areas should be identified, and signs at the entrance of the room or facility should indicate the type of area and the kind of radiation source. Working instructions appropriate to the radiological risk associated with the sources and the operations involved need to be laid down. Workers should have special training related to the radiation sources and working procedures. Access to a controlled area must be restricted, and visitors are only allowed access in company with a staff member who knows the protection and safety measures for the area [2, 4].

The Euratom [4] and the ICRP [1] have recommended the classification of working areas, while Euratom also provides a classification for exposed workers in different categories, that is, categories A and B. Workers at risk to receive an effective dose of more than 6 mSv per year or an equivalent dose to the lens of the eye of more than 15 mSv per year, or an equivalent dose to the skin and extremities greater than 150 mSv per year, should be placed in category A, according to Euratom [4]. Exposed workers not classified as category A are category B workers.

17.3 RADIONUCLIDES IN NUCLEAR MEDICINE

Nuclear medicine is a specialty that comprises the use of radioactive unsealed sources for a wide range of activities, from kBq levels for *in vitro* tests and calibrations of some test equipment to GBq levels for radionuclide therapies and cyclotron production of radionuclides. There is also a large variation in radionuclide selection with respect to decay mode and physical half-life depending on application. In nuclear medicine diagnostic imaging, it is desirable to use radionuclides that emit photons within an energy range adapted for gamma cameras or PET cameras, whereas the particle emission should be as small as possible to minimize patient radiation doses. Therapies with radiopharmaceuticals are performed with particle-emitting radionuclides to obtain the intended absorbed dose to the target cells. However, it is in most therapies desirable that the radionuclide also emits photons of detectable energy for imaging of the biodistribution of the radiopharmaceutical for localization and dosimetric purposes.

The majority of nuclear medicine procedures, approximately 80 per cent [6], are performed with ^{99m}Tc because of its favourable radiation characteristics, with 140-keV photons that are optimal for gamma camera detection. It also has a short half-life (6.01 h) and low particle emission, providing only a small contribution to the patient radiation dose in diagnostic nuclear medicine. Other radionuclides used in diagnostic nuclear medicine include ^{111}In, ^{123}I, ^{201}Tl, and ^{67}Ga. Some radionuclides in Table 17.2, such as ^{51}Cr and ^{125}I, are primarily used for non-imaging studies and are usually used at low activity levels. ^{75}SeHCAT, which is used for *in vivo* investigation of the enterohepatic circulation of bile salts, is

---

TABLE 17.2

Photon Energy, Half-Value Layer (HVL) in Lead and Tungsten, Respectively, and Attenuation in 0.5-mm Lead for a Selection of Single-Photon-Emitting Radionuclides Used in Nuclear Medicine Diagnostic Procedures

Radionuclide	Decay mode	Half-life	Principal gamma energies (keV)	HVL lead (mm)[a, b]	HVL tungsten (mm)[a, b]	Attenuation in 0.5-mm lead[a, b] (%)
^{51}Cr	E.C.	27.7 d	320	1.66	1.21	19
^{67}Ga	E.C.	3.26 d	93, 185, 300	1.52	1.11	20
^{75}Se	E.C.	120 d	136, 265, 280	1.17	0.87	26
^{99m}Tc	I.T.	6.01 h	140	0.22	0.17	79
^{111}In	E.C.	2.81 d	171, 245	0.84	0.62	34
^{123}I	E.C.	13.2 h	159	0.33	0.25	65
^{125}I	E.C.	59.4 d	27[c], 35	0.027	0.022	100
^{133}Xe	β^-	5.25 d	81	0.26	0.05	74
^{201}Tl	E.C.	3.04 d	69–83[c], 167	0.37	0.27	61

[a] Calculated from data obtained from [7].

[b] HVL and attenuation calculated for the highest of the given photon energies for each radionuclide respectively.

[c] Characteristic X-rays.

TABLE 17.3
Physical Data for a Selection of Positron-Emitting Radionuclides Used in Nuclear Medicine Diagnostic Procedures. Photon Energy, Half-Value Layer (HVL) in Lead and Tungsten, Respectively, and Attenuation in 0.5-mm Lead Are Given. The CSDA Range Is Given for the Maximum Positron Energy for the Given Radionuclides

Radio-nuclide	Half-life[a,b]	Principal photon energy (keV)	HVL lead (mm)[b,c]	HVL tungsten (mm)[c]	Attenuation in 0.5-mm lead[c] (%)	Maximum positron energy [a,d] (keV)	Positron range i water[e] (mm)	Positron range in tungsten[e] (mm)
^{11}C	20.4 min	511	3.9	2.7	8.5	961	4.2	0.38
^{13}N	9.97 min	511	3.9	2.7	8.5	1198	5.4	0.50
^{15}O	2.04 min	511	3.9	2.7	8.5	1735	8.4	0.72
^{18}F	109.77 min	511	3.9	2.7	8.5	634	2.4	0.23
^{68}Ga	67.8 min	511, 1077	6	N/A	8.5	1899	9.2	0.79
^{82}Rb	1.27 min	511, 777	N/A	N/A	N/A	3381	17	1.4
^{124}I	4.18 d	511, 603, 1691	8	N/A	8.5	2137	11	0.89

[a] www.nucleide.org/DDEP_WG/DDEPdata.htm.
[b] Delacroix et al. [8].
[c] https://physics.nist.gov/PhysRefData/Xcom/html/xcom1.html.
[d] http://nucleardata.nuclear.lu.se/toi/radSearch.aspe.
[e] https://physics.nist.gov/PhysRefData/Star/Text/ESTAR.html.

also administered with low activity because the imaging is performed with an uncollimated gamma camera. Physical data for commonly used radionuclides in diagnostic nuclear medicine are given in Table 17.2.

Positron emission tomography (PET) is a fast-growing diagnostic method. Currently, ^{18}F is the most used radionuclide for PET because of its fairly long half-life, approximately 110 min. Other positron emitters of interest include ^{82}Rb, ^{68}Ga, ^{11}C, ^{13}N, ^{15}O, and ^{124}I. The short half-life for these radionuclides, on the order of minutes (except for ^{124}I), results in fairly low radiation doses to the patients, despite the positron decay. However, a very short half-life means that the staff has to handle higher activities during withdrawal and administration to the patient to obtain adequate statistics in the PET images. PET radionuclides are also more difficult to shield because of the high photon energy of 511 keV. Physical data for commonly used positron emitting radionuclides in diagnostic nuclear medicine are given in Table 17.3. The CSDA range in water and tungsten, respectively, is given for the maximum positron energy for the radionuclides. Ranges in soft tissue, plastic, and acrylic glass are comparable with the range in water.

Treatment of the thyroid with ^{131}I started in the 1940s and is still used. The emission of both beta particles for the treatment itself and gamma photons for localization and quantification of the uptake makes this iodine isotope a good treatment alternative. Other radionuclides for radionuclide therapies include ^{177}Lu, ^{90}Y, ^{32}P, and ^{153}Sm (Table 17.4).

The use of alpha emitting radionuclides has increased in nuclear medicine therapy. In recent years, for instance, ^{223}RaCl$_2$ (Xofigo®, Bayer), has entered the market to be used for treatment of bone metastases. Unlike many other radionuclide therapies, only a low activity, 55 kBq / kg body weight, is used (Xofigo Package leaflet: Information for the patient. Bayer). The external radiation protection of the staff is only a minor problem for this alpha emitter. The CSDA range in air for 10 MeV alpha particles is less than 11 cm, and in water, it is 0.11 mm. Instead, concerning the alpha particles, the focus is on minimizing the risk of contamination of the skin and intake of the radionuclide for the staff.

17.4   RADIATION PROTECTION IN NUCLEAR MEDICINE

The large variation in radioactive decay and energies for the emitted radiation types requires good knowledge by the staff regarding radiation safety and the risks associated with the work.

Appropriate education, training, and information should be given to all individuals working with tasks that require radiation protection [4]. Knowledge and understanding of health risks linked to work with ionizing radiation is an important part of radiation protection. Procedures to be used and measures to be taken to minimize radiation exposure should be well known and understood. Regular, continuing training of staff is important to maintain competence and to disseminate information regarding new methods and routines and information about new equipment.

TABLE 17.4
Photon Energy, Half-Value Layer (HVL) in Lead and Tungsten, Respectively, and Attenuation in 0.5-mm Lead for a Selection of Radionuclides Used for Radionuclide Therapies. Data for the Emitted Energies Are Limited to Those with Highest Yield

Nuclide	Decay mode	Half-life	Principal gamma energy (keV)	HVL lead (mm)[a]	HVL tungsten (mm)[a]	Attenuation in 0.5-mm lead[a] (%)	Principal alpha energy (MeV)	Maximum β− energy[c,d] (keV)	Electron range in water[e] (mm)	Electron range in tungsten[e] (mm)
32P	β−	14.3 d	N/A	N/A	N/A	N/A	N/A	1711	8.2	0.71
89Sr	β−	50.6 d	N/A	N/A	N/A	N/A	N/A	1495	7.0	0.62
90Y	-	2.67 d	N/A	N/A	N/A	N/A	N/A	2279	11	0.95
131I	β−	8.02 d	364, 637, 723	2.08	1.50	15	N/A	606	2.3	0.22
153Sm	β−	1.93 d	70, 103	0.11	0.084	95	N/A	635, 705, 808	3.3	0.31
177Lu	β−	6.65 d	208	0.64	0.48	42	N/A	498	1.8	0.17
213Bi+	α (2.09%) β− (97.91%)	45.6 min	440	3.0	2.1	11	5.9–8.4	644, 983, 1423	6.7	0.59
223Ra+	α	11.4 d	144–832, 351	1.9	1.4	16	5.5–7.4	535, 1367, 1418	6.6	0.59
225Ac+	α	10.0 d	218, 440,	3.0	2.1	11	5.6–8.4	644, 983, 1423	6.7	0.59
227Th+	α	18.7 d	144–832, 351	1.9	1.4	16	5.5–7.4	535, 1367, 1418	6.6	0.59

a https://physics.nist.gov/PhysRefData/Xcom/html/xcom1.html.
b Delacroix et al. [8].
c www.nucleide.org/DDEP_WG/DDEPdata.htm.
d http://nucleardata.nuclear.lu.se/toi/radSearch.asp.
e https://physics.nist.gov/PhysRefData/Star/Text/ESTAR.html.
f HVL calculated for 364-keV photons.
+ Particle energies and photon energies for the daughter radionuclides are included.

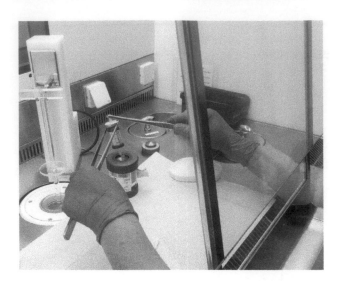

FIGURE 17.1 Withdrawal of activity can be performed with a syringe shield and long tweezers to minimize the doses to fingers and hands. Disposable gloves should be used to minimize the risk of contamination. (Because of local hygiene rules, work clothes with short sleeves are used.)

The tasks related to the management of radionuclides and patients in nuclear medicine can be distributed among various personnel groups, such as technologists, nurses, physicians, physicists, and others in different countries. The radiation protection work is discussed here in relation to situations and tasks where exposure to ionizing radiation can occur without regard to who is potentially exposed.

17.5 RADIATION PROTECTION IN PRACTICE

The magnitude of the external radiation dose is determined by several factors, including time, distance, and radiation shielding. Practical working rules based on these three basic factors are given by, for example, IAEA [2]. In addition to the risk of external irradiation, work with unsealed radiation sources also involves the potential risk of contamination, which should be considered when establishing local rules and monitoring programs.

17.5.1 TIME

It is obvious that the radiation dose is directly proportional to the time spent in the radiation field. Thus, the time spent close to the radiation source should be kept as short as possible, taking the tasks into account. It is important to work fast and, at the same time, safely and without the risk of contamination. Training for particularly difficult work can be done with non-radioactive materials to reduce the risk of problems and unnecessary irradiation. Working with patients injected with positron emitting radionuclides usually means a higher annual dose for the staff compared with those working with conventional diagnostic nuclear medicine only. At facilities working with diagnostic nuclear medicine using both gamma emitters and positron emitters, the staff can alternate between the different tasks to reduce the individual radiation dose.

17.5.2 DISTANCE

The dose rate from a point source decreases with the distance to the radiation source according to the inverse square law;

$$\dot{D} \propto \frac{1}{d^2} \qquad (17.1)$$

where $\dot{D}$ is the dose rate and d is the distance to the point source. This relationship is only truly valid for a point source. However, maintaining a distance from any type of radiation source is always advisable, as it reduces the dose. During preparation, withdrawal, and injection of radiopharmaceuticals, the finger doses can become high if working procedures are not optimized. Direct contact with the source should be avoided. Using distance tools such as long tweezers and forceps, in combination with syringe shields and other radiation shields, the finger doses can be minimized (Figure 17.1). Long tweezers can also be used to connect and detach the syringe from the cannula or peripheral vein catheter during the injection of the radiopharmaceutical. Various withdrawal techniques are discussed in ICRP [9].

After injection of the radiopharmaceutical, the patient is the radiation source, and it is thus important to minimize the time spent close to the patient after injection. Therefore, all interviewing should be conducted, information given, and the patient should be given the opportunity to ask questions before the injection. The distance to the patient should be maintained in a considerate manner after injection so as to not worry the patient.

The distance becomes even more important during work with radionuclides emitting high-energy photons, such as positron-emitting radionuclides, because of the difficulty of achieving effective radiation shielding. This is important for work with PET patients because lead aprons only provide a minor dose reduction. The use of automatic injection systems for injection of PET tracers reduces both the whole-body dose as a result of the increased distance to the patient and the finger dose because of the reduced handling of the PET radiopharmaceuticals [10].

17.5.3 Radiation Shielding

17.5.3.1 Shielding of Facilities

The ICRP [1] recommends an annual effective dose limit of 1 mSv for public exposure in planned situations. It is also stated that if the average dose over a 5-year period does not exceed 1 mSv per year, higher effective dose values could be accepted under special conditions. The legislation differs in different countries. Within the European Union member

TABLE 17.5
Dose Rate Data for Some Selected Photon Emitters in a Vial and a Syringe, Respectively, and Data for the Dose Rate from a Patient. *Note the Different Dose Rate Units*

Nuclide	Dose rate from a 10-ml glass vial at 1 m[a] (μSv h^{-1} MBq^{-1})	Dose rate from contact with 5-ml syringe[a] (mSv h^{-1} MBq^{-1})	Dose rate from a patient at 1 m (μSv h^{-1} MBq^{-1})	References for dose rate data for patients or phantoms
Single-photon-emitting radionuclides				
^{67}Ga	0.0254	0.402	0.014–0.0186	[11, 12]
^{99m}Tc	0.0224	0.354	0.01–0.0174	[11–13]
^{111}In	0.0717	1.22	0.02–0.06	[11, 14, 15]
^{123}I	0.0343	0.605	0.0179–0.03	[11, 14, 15]
^{201}Tl	0.0185	0.285	0.0159–0.02	[11, 14]
Positron-emitting radionuclides				
^{11}C	0.163	6.41	0.114–0.129	[11]
^{13}N	0.163	12.9	0.117	[11]
^{15}O	0.167		0.117	[11]
^{18}F	0.158	2.88	0.0517–0.121	[14] [11–13, 15–17]
^{68}Ga	0.16	31.4	0.0394–0.124	[11, 15]
^{82}Rb	N/A	N/A	0.133	[11]
Radionuclides used for radiotherapy				
^{90}Y	0.0711	43.5	0.000525–0.00519	[11, 12]
^{131}I	0.0636	1.13	0.038–0.054	[11–13]
^{153}Sm	0.0148	0.241	0.0117	[11]
^{177}Lu	N/A	N/A	0.00698	[11]
^{223}Ra	N/A	N/A	0.0216	[11]

[a] Delacroix et al. [8].

states, the effective dose for public exposure is limited to 1 mSv in a year. This dose limit should not be exceeded for a member of the public when different and allowed exposures are annually summed up. The planning and design of a facility and the radiation shielding in the walls, floor, and ceiling are important to minimize the exposure to staff, patients, and the public. It is important to shield in all directions to prevent unnecessary radiation doses to the surrounding floors above or below. The shielding has to be calculated taking into account the radionuclides to be used, the administered activities, the number of patients, and the length of time they will spend at the department. The shielding must be checked with measurements after construction to verify that the radiation protection requirements are fulfilled.

In nuclear medicine facilities, the camera rooms have to be shielded from the ambient radiation to ensure correct measurements as well as to protect the people outside the room. In many departments, patient examination is controlled via a control room adjacent to the camera room. The surveillance of the patient can be performed via a window of lead glass or via a surveillance camera. Most modalities have a built-in system for communication between staff and patients.

Special rules may exist for premises where work with unsealed radioactive sources takes place, concerning, for example, pressure conditions to reduce the risk of any airborne spread to other premises [2, 18].

The design and planning of nuclear medicine facilities, cyclotron units, PET facilities, and facilities for radionuclide therapy are not covered by this chapter but are described elsewhere [5, 16, 19-21].

17.5.3.2   Shielding of Radioactive Sources

Shielding in walls can for some applications possibly be replaced by local shielding; for example, by the use of lead bricks or L-shields in a fume hood. Lead bricks should be placed so as to avoid gaps in the protection. The more localized the protection is, the smaller the volume of shielding material that is needed, and thus a lower weight is possible. The weight of all shielding, even a lead-shielded fume hood, has to be considered when planning a facility.

All handling of radioactive substances during withdrawal should be performed behind shields of lead, lead glass, or tungsten of sufficient thickness. Shielding of vials and syringes is essential to reduce the radiation dose to the staff. All radioactive substances should be kept in lead, lead glass, or tungsten shields with adequate thickness. Also, all kinds of waste material that have been in contact with a radiopharmaceutical, such as syringes, cannulas, catheters, and swabs, have to be stored in a lead shielded container and handled as radioactive waste. The dose calibrators may require extra radiation shielding around the ionization chamber to avoid misleading contributions from external radiation sources and to ensure correct activity measurements.

High activities can be administered for nuclear medicine therapies, and possibly also radionuclides with higher photon energies (^{131}I), which requires more radiation shielding. The time spent close to the patient should be minimized, and the distance should be increased to keep the dose as low as possible. Treatment of children or patients in need of extra care may require mobile radiation shields to achieve acceptable radiation protection for the parents or caring staff.

The relatively high photon energy of ^{131}I, 364 keV, as well as higher energies (Table 17.4) of lower yield, requires thicker radiation shielding than that required for ^{99m}Tc. Also, the electrons from ^{131}I entail the risk of inducing bremsstrahlung in lead because of the high atomic number. The combination of beta particle emission and high-energy photons requires thick lead shielding or lead-shielded acrylic glass to minimize the production of bremsstrahlung.

Pure beta emitters are shielded using material of low atomic number, such as acrylic glass or similar material, or a lead-shielded acrylic glass, to minimize the production of bremsstrahlung.

The higher photon energy of 511 keV used in PET puts even greater demands on the radiation shielding. The half-value layer (HVL) in lead and tungsten is 3.9 and 2.7 mm, respectively, for 511-keV photons (Table 17.3). Some of the commonly used positron emitters, for example, ^{68}Ga, ^{82}Rb, and ^{124}I, also emit photons with higher energies, making the shielding even more demanding. Tungsten shielding of sufficient thickness is required when preparing and handling PET radiopharmaceuticals. The dose rate from positron emitting radionuclides is 2–10 times higher at 1 m compared with the dose rate from single photon emitters (Table 17.5). Time and distance are of particular importance when working with patients undergoing PET examinations to minimize the dose contribution to the staff.

17.5.3.3   Shielding of Syringes

In nuclear medicine, it is likely that fingers and hands may receive the highest radiation dose for the staff when managing radiopharmaceuticals, particularly when handling positron emitters, and the equivalent dose to the hands may exceed the annual dose limit of 500 mSv [22–25].

Tools for maximizing the distance from the source, in combination with shielded syringes, are necessary to keep the doses as low as possible. In addition, the doses can be reduced by placing the fingers as far as possible from the volume of activity in the syringe. This is especially important when handling radionuclides emitting electrons or positrons. As

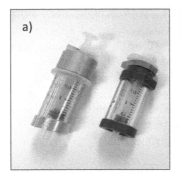
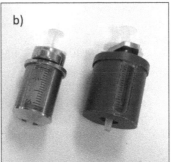

FIGURE 17.2 Syringe shielding made of (a) lead glass, used for single-photon-emitting radionuclides, and (b) tungsten, used for positron-emitting radionuclides.

a rule of thumb, the syringe should not be filled with more than half the maximum volume to enable the fingers to be placed far from the activity.

Syringe shields of lead, lead glass, or tungsten (Figure 17.2) should be used when possible to bring down the finger doses. Photon energies for radionuclides used in conventional nuclear medicine diagnostics are in general so low that lead or lead glass shielding with an effective thickness of a few millimetres has a good shielding effect, shown as low values of the HVL in Tables 2–4. In contrast, PET radionuclides require thick syringe shields of tungsten to achieve a sufficient dose reduction. The doses to fingers and hands are determined not only by the withdrawn activity but also by the total shielding of the vial, and the total activity in the vial contributes to exposure of fingers and hands.

17.6 RADIATION PROTECTION APRONS

Radiation doses for the whole body, extremities, and the lens of the eye are i.a. depending on working methods, the use of radiation shields, lead aprons, and syringe shields, as well as vial activity during preparation and withdrawal of the radiopharmaceutical.

The use of lead aprons in nuclear medicine is somewhat controversial, as there are both advantages and disadvantages associated with their use. The weight of the lead apron can be 8.45 kg for a 0.5-mm lead equivalent apron. This weight increases the pressure on intervertebral discs and may present a risk of back pain if used over long periods [26]. This risk may be balanced against the benefit of reduced dose to the worker. The dose reduction depends on the material of the apron and the radionuclide used. Lightweight aprons designed for X-ray shielding can provide lower protection for photon energies in nuclear medicine. These aprons can also provide a lower risk of back pain, but the dose savings should be investigated for different radionuclides to ensure sufficient good effect [12, 26, 27].

Lead aprons with an effective lead thickness of 0.5 mm provide a theoretical photon attenuation of 79 per cent for the 140-keV photons of [99m]Tc. For radionuclides emitting photons with higher energies, a lead apron is less effective. The theoretical attenuation for the 364 keV-photons from ^{131}I is 15 per cent, and for annihilation photons (511 keV), it is 8.5 per cent. Measurements have shown that lead aprons of 0.5-mm effective lead thickness can reduce the effective dose by at least a factor of two for photon energies of 140 keV and lower [5, 12, 28], but of only 3 per cent for the 364 keV-photons from [131]I [12]. The difference between theoretical calculations and measurements is explained by the dose contribution of the produced characteristic X-ray photons in the lead. Also, the electrons from ^{131}I entail a risk of inducing bremsstrahlung in the lead apron because of the high atomic number of lead.

A lead apron of 0.5-mm lead thickness reduces the whole-body dose by half or more for radionuclides emitting low-energy photons, for example, ^{99m}Tc, and could be used when working close to the patient and the radiation source. For radionuclides emitting photons with higher energies, for example, ^{131}I and positron emitters, the lead apron does not provide sufficient attenuation of these high-energy photons. Using lead aprons can in these situations give a false sense of safety, leading to longer time spent close to the radiation source.

17.6.1 CONTAMINATION RISKS

Working with unsealed sources in nuclear medicine entails a risk of internal exposure to staff. Handling of radioactive gases, aerosols, or volatile substances may present a risk of accidental intake, inhalation, and possibly external contamination of skin, hair, and clothing. The handling of open radioactive sources must be done in a safe way to avoid spillage and contamination. Contamination can give rise to an accidental intake of the radionuclide, resulting in unnecessary internal irradiation. It is therefore not allowed to eat, drink, or smoke when handling radioactive solutions, and contact with the mouth, eyes, and nose should be avoided to minimize the risk of intake. Contamination can also cause an absorbed dose to the skin or the lens of the eye.

If imaging equipment has become contaminated, an incorrect or misleading diagnostic result can be obtained. In addition, if the patient becomes contaminated, it also may give rise to an unnecessary radiation dose. For a safe nuclear medical diagnosis and therapy and to avoid internal contamination, good working practices and awareness and good radiation protection skills are required of the staff, as well as adequate control programs for radiation protection for staff and premises.

Suitable personal protective clothing, gloves, safety glasses, and shoe covers / overshoes may be needed when working in a controlled area to prevent contamination and spread of contamination to other premises. Other requirements, such as the use of caps and masks for aseptic work, may also apply. In addition to working with disposable gloves, the working surface should be protected with plastic-lined absorbent paper to easily remove any spills.

Contamination control of hands and work surfaces can easily be done using radiation protection instruments after completion of work.

To minimize the risk of contamination of hands and fingers, it is important to use disposable gloves when working with radionuclides. Minimizing the risk of contamination also reduces the risk of accidental ingestion of the radionuclide. The gloves should be changed regularly to avoid penetration of a contaminant through the glove material, and the gloves should be removed such that the contamination is not transferred to the hands [29]. However, there are different types of gloves with different thicknesses, showing a variation in permeability depending on radiopharmaceutical and time after contamination. Ridone and colleagues [30] suggest that gloves should be tested for permeability before starting to use a new type of glove in clinical routines.

The skin dose is determined by the decay of the radionuclide, that is, the emitted radiation, its energy, and the half-life of the radionuclide. In addition, the skin dose is also affected by the permeability of the radiopharmaceutical through the skin. Hands should be checked for contamination after completion of work. Early detection of contamination and a quick and effective decontamination as soon as the contamination is obtained is important to reduce the skin dose. The efficiency of the decontamination depends on the radiopharmaceutical, the solutions, the binding to, and the permeability of the skin [31]. Covens and colleagues [32] reported that ^{99m}Tc-pertechnetate and ^{18}F-FDG were easily removed from the skin by handwashing with soap and water. If the activity was allowed to remain on the skin, ^{99m}Tc-pertechnetate was found to permeate quickly and to a high degree [31].

Several studies have reported on the effectiveness of decontamination of the skin using various dedicated decontamination fluids or just soap and water. The results vary depending on radiopharmaceutical and decontamination agent, but gently washing with soap and lukewarm water is recommended by many [10, 31, 33–35]. Some decontamination fluids are not supposed to be used on the skin and can even be harmful and possibly damage the skin barrier [33]. The skin must not be damaged, as the radioactive substance can cause greater damage if it penetrates deeper into the skin [10].

In some situations, there is a higher risk of internal contamination. Working with gases, aerosols, or volatile substances such as iodine solutions involves a certain risk of inhalation of the radionuclide. The volatility of solutions containing sodium iodide depends on the pH and additives in the solution [36]. It is important to, as far as possible, work in fume hoods with dedicated exhaust systems to minimize the risk of accidental inhalation of the iodine. Another potential risk of internal contamination is when patients examined by lung scintigraphy undergo a ventilation examination. At the ventilation, for example, ^{99m}Tc-Technegas can be inhaled by the patient via a hose system. In this context, there is a certain risk of leakage if the patient has difficulty keeping the mouth tightly closed around the mouthpiece. A plastic hood with air extraction can be placed over the patient's head while ventilation is performed to minimize the risk of inhalation of the radionuclide for people other than the patient.

Working with radionuclide therapies where high activity and / or alpha- or beta-emitting radionuclides are used are situations where extra precautions may need to be taken. For therapies using high activities of photon-emitting radionuclides, the same precautions must be taken as at nuclear medicine diagnostics; however, more careful measurements and calculations of dose rates and shielding have to be performed to ensure a safe working place.

For alpha-emitting radionuclides such as ^{223}Ra and ^{227}Th, the risk of internal contamination must be addressed. Lassman and Eberlein [37] have summarized available studies regarding radiation protection for staff and relatives to patients who have received radionuclide therapies with ^{223}Ra. They noted that there are no significant risks related to either external or internal contamination in addition to the use of ^{223}Ra for therapy.

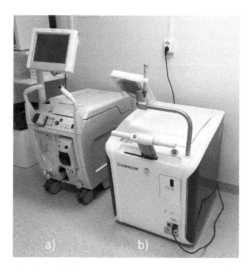

FIGURE 17.3 Two examples of automatic injection systems for administration of PET-radiopharmaceuticals: (a) MEDRAD® Intego™ PET Infusion system and (b) IRIS Radiopharmaceutical Multidose Injector (Comecer).

17.6.2 HYBRID TECHNIQUES

In hybrid imaging, for example, SPECT/CT and PET/CT, there is a risk of external exposure from scattered radiation from the patient during the CT examination. Most of the time, staff is outside the examination room during the CT exposure. Personnel who must be inside the examination room during exposure should use a radiation protection apron because it gives an effective dose reduction. The staff should also remain at as large a distance to the patient as the work allows. If possible, it is advisable to stand with the CT gantry as a radiation shield. It is important to be aware that in PET / CT examinations, although the lead apron does not provide adequate shielding regarding the annihilation photons from the positron-emitting radionuclide, it is a good protection for the scattered radiation from the CT examination.

17.7 RADIATION DOSES TO NUCLEAR MEDICINE STAFF

17.7.1 WHOLE-BODY RADIATION DOSE

Dose rates for different radionuclides at a distance of 1 m are presented in Table 17.5 for the radionuclide in a 10-ml glass vial, as well as for the radionuclide injected in patients. The measurements for the bottle and the patient differ somewhat, partly because of differences in attenuation and measurement geometry. A certain variation is found between the different measured dose rates for the patients for each radionuclide. This can partly be explained by the fact that the measurements were conducted for different radiopharmaceuticals with different distributions in the body. The measurements were also performed at slightly different time points after injection. The dose rates from positron-emitting radionuclides are up to 10 times higher per activity unit than those from single-photon emitters (Table 17.5). This, in combination with the high photon energy, causes a greater radiation protection problem in PET. Exposure rate constants for a point source are given for over 1100 radionuclides in a work by Smith and Stabin [38].

Manual withdrawal and injection of PET tracers can be replaced by automatic injection systems (Figure 17.3) to reduce both whole-body doses and finger doses [10]. Reduction of whole-body doses of 38 per cent [39] and 50 per cent [40] during the injection of ^{18}F-FDG have been reported.

17.7.2 RADIATION DOSES TO FINGERS AND HANDS

ICRP [9] gives a review of several studies of hand exposure during dispensing of radiopharmaceuticals labelled with ^{99m}Tc and conclude that a wide range of doses were reported, from a few μGy/GBq to over 100 μGy/GBq. When dealing with positron-emitting radionuclides, it is also of interest to note the energy and range of the positrons (Table 17.3). A large amount of the positrons will penetrate the syringe wall and contribute to a high absorbed dose if the fingers are placed close to the active volume of an unshielded plastic syringe. Fingers placed over the activity in an unshielded plastic syringe containing 300 MBq ^{68}Ga will obtain an equivalent dose of 500 mSv in a little more than 3 min [8].

A combination of using a radiation protection syringe shield, placing the fingers far from the activity, and using distance tools are effective working methods to reduce the doses to fingers and hands when handling radiopharmaceuticals and especially positron emitters. Skill and speed are also important factors in minimizing radiation dose. Again, it is advisable to practice difficult steps to work safely.

Finger doses can be significantly reduced using automatic injection systems for PET pharmaceuticals, and several different systems are currently available. Reduction of finger doses of 94 per cent [39] and 95 per cent [40] compared with manual withdrawal and injection of ^{18}F-FDG have been reported.

17.7.3 Radiation Dose to the Lens of the Eye

Management of open radiation sources involves a risk of irradiation of the whole body, hands, and fingers, as well as the eye lens. A detailed review of the radiobiology and dosimetry for the eye lens is provided by Dietze [41] and the ICRP [1, 3]. If there is a risk of contamination of the eyes, protective goggles should be used. Contamination of the eye can result in a relatively high radiation dose to the lens of the eye, depending on various factors, including the type of emitted radiation and its energy, the half-life of the radionuclide, and the duration of the irradiation. The position of the lens in the eye, approximately 3–3.5 mm from the cornea [41], means that low-energy particle radiation does not reach the lens. The ICRP [1] recommend that the dose assessments for the lens are made for a depth of 3 mm. With this distance from the cornea, the emitted particles from, for example, ^{99m}Tc, ^{123}I, and ^{18}F, do not contribute to the dose; only photons will. In contrast, the positron energies from, for example, ^{11}C, ^{15}O, and ^{68}Ga, are high enough for the particles to reach the lens and contribute to the dose.

Several authors have reported doses to the eye lens for various situations; however, published data can be given for several different radionuclides, specific or combined working procedures, divided into different occupational groups with different work tasks, or reported as annual doses for a particular activity [42]. The handling and the activity levels are not always presented in a way that makes comparisons possible. A range of equivalent doses between 0.48 and 34 μSv / GBq [42–44] is given for combined work with ^{99m}Tc, ^{131}I, and ^{153}Sm. For ^{18}F equivalent doses between 1.1 and 56 μSv / GBq [23, 42] have been reported. Wrzeisen and Albiniak [45] have made measurements for elution, labelling, and injection of [^{68}Ga] Ga-DOTA-TATE, reporting 207 μSv / GBq as the highest equivalent dose to the eye lens. It has been suggested that the effective dose measured by a personal dosimeter can be used as a conservative measure of dose to the eye lens [42, 46, 47], provided that the measurement is done without the influence of a lead apron. With the new annual dose limit of 20 mSv for the eye lens [3], it is advisable to make measurements for the working conditions at each workplace to ensure that the dose limit is not exceeded.

17.7.4 Skin Radiation Doses

The radiation-sensitive cells of the skin are located at a depth of between 0.020 and 0.16 mm, depending on the body part [3]. The ICRP [1] recommend that the dose assessments for the skin is made at a depth of 0.07 mm ($H_p(0.07)$).

Covens and colleagues [32, 48, 49] have studied skin contaminations of technologists during nuclear medicine work. They measured a wide range of contamination levels, up to several hundreds of kBq [49]. According to their measurements and calculations, skin contamination can result in doses that may exceed the annual dose limit. The same group also has published skin dose rate conversions factors for 39 radionuclides of medical interest; some of these factors are given in Table 17.6. The data in Table 17.6 show that the skin doses from the positron- and beta-emitters in the table are up to 8 times higher than that from ^{99m}Tc.

17.7.5 Radiation Dose to Pregnant or Breastfeeding Staff

Children and foetus are more sensitive to radiation and should be protected as much as possible. When a woman has declared to her employer that she is pregnant, the foetus should be protected at the same level as the public, that is, a maximum of 1 mSv during the remainder of the pregnancy [1]. In the United States, 5 mSv has been set for the entire pregnancy [50].

It is difficult to make reliable measurements of the foetal dose. The measured dose from the woman's personal dosimeter during a month is low, and the uncertainty becomes large when determining the foetal dose based on this measurement [51]. Mountford and Steele [52] have made estimates and found that a dosimeter value of 1.3 mSv corresponds to a foetal dose of 1 mSv for ^{99m}Tc and ^{131}I. For higher photon energies, for example, positron emitters, the foetal dose should be more comparable to the surface dose of the abdomen [51].

TABLE 17.6
Skin Absorbed Doses After a Contaminated Skin Area of 0.01 cm² [48]

Radionuclide	Skin dose (mGy h⁻¹ kBq⁻¹)
Single-photon-emitting radionuclides	
⁵¹Cr	0.0118
⁶⁷Ga	0.344
⁹⁹ᵐTc	0.22
¹¹¹In	0.316
¹²³I	0.323
¹²⁵I	0.0121
²⁰¹Tl	0.254
Positron-emitting radionuclides	
¹¹C	1.69
¹³N	1.73
¹⁵O	1.74
¹⁸F	1.65
⁶⁸Ga	1.78
⁸²Rb	1.75
¹²⁴I	0.419
Radionuclides used for radionuclide therapy	
³²P	1.73
⁸⁹Sr	1.68
⁹⁰Y	1.72
¹³¹I	1.40
¹⁵³Sm	1.56
¹⁷⁷Lu	1.28
²¹³Bi+	2.14
²²³Ra⁺	3.88

⁺ Decay products included.

In case of an internal contamination, measurements of activity uptake and biokinetics can be made with, for example, whole-body measurements and / or with urine samples to estimate the radiation dose. To determine the foetal dose, placental transfers must also be known.

If a member of the staff is breastfeeding, she should not participate in work that poses a significant risk of internal contamination. Some radiopharmaceuticals are excreted via the breast milk and can give an unnecessary radiation dose to the child. Radioiodine is known to be excreted to the milk and may give a high dose to the thyroid of the child. The excretion to the breast milk must be known or determined by measurements to be able to calculate the dose to the child [53, 54].

To minimize the irradiation of a pregnant woman, suitable and less appropriate tasks can be identified, and guidelines can be set up for each facility. Almén and Mattsson [51] have made an overview of various tasks based on radiation dose per administered activity and the risk of accidents within the business. Work with ⁹⁹ᵐTc examinations generally gives a low dose, while work with PET examinations, radionuclide therapies, radiochemistry, and cyclotron work can be considered less suitable for pregnant and breastfeeding women.

17.8 MONITORING PROGRAMS

The purpose of monitoring the external and internal radiation exposure of workers is to monitor and document radiation doses and ensure regulatory compliance.

Equivalent dose and effective dose are not measurable quantities; instead, operational quantities are used. For measurements in external radiation fields, equivalent ambient dose equivalent $H^*(10)$ and directional dose equivalent $H'(0.07, \Omega)$ are used for area measurements. The operational quantity for individual monitoring is the personal dose equivalent, $H_p(d)$, where d is a specific depth in soft tissue. A depth of $d=10$ mm is chosen for the assessment of the effective dose, $d=0.07$ mm for the equivalent dose to the skin and to the hands and feet, and $d=3$ mm for the lens of the eye. For internal exposure, the equivalent and effective dose has to be calculated from uptake measurements and biokinetic models [1].

All systems used for measurements and monitoring have to be adequately calibrated for the types of radiation and energies and for the specific measurement geometries. Detector systems used for measurements of internal contamination of workers should also be calibrated for the radionuclides to be investigated, and the minimum detectable activity should be known [55].

Individual monitoring of workers should be performed by a dosimetry service approved by the regulatory body [4, 18].

17.8.1 Monitoring Program for External and Internal Exposure of Staff

The licensee, in cooperation with the employer, has the responsibility to ensure that appropriate personal monitoring is provided to staff [18]. Area monitoring or workplace monitoring means that measurements of radiation levels must be made at predefined locations in the facility. For category A workers, individual dose is systematically monitored, and if there is a risk of significant external or internal exposure or contamination, this must be monitored with an adequate monitoring system. For category B workers, dose monitoring should be performed to confirm that the category classification is correct [4]. Because equivalent dose and effective dose are not directly measurable quantities, the International Commission on Radiation Units (ICRU) [56] has defined operational quantities for radiation protection purposes. Personal dose equivalent is used for individual monitoring and ambient dose equivalent and directional dose equivalent are used for area monitoring.

Individual monitoring for external radiation should be used for all who work in controlled areas, category A workers [57]. Personal dosimeters are used to monitor and to make a reasonable estimate of personnel radiation doses. There are different opinions about whether the measurements should be made outside or under the lead apron or both using two dosimeters [18, 58]. Clear guidelines on how to use the dosimeter must be provided at the workplace. The Council of the European Union states that monitoring of category B workers should be performed to ensure that they are correctly classified. Individual measurements could be performed if necessary [4].

The new reduced dose limit for the eye lens means that measurement of the eye doses may be needed to verify that the dose limit is not exceeded.

Finger doses are a greater problem than whole-body doses for certain tasks in nuclear medicine. In many cases, continuous finger dose measurements are not made; rather, only occasional measurements are conducted. Ring dosimeters work well for monitoring individual changes in finger dose caused by, for example, increased work-load, changed routines, or new tasks. The ring dosimeter should be placed on the same hand, finger, and position and be turned in the same direction during all measurements to ensure reliable results. Methods and techniques determine which finger and whether it is the dominant or non-dominant hand that receives the highest exposure and thus on which finger it should be placed [9]. The measured dose obtained by a ring dosimeter underestimates the finger doses and can give a value 2.5–10 [24, 58–61] times too low, depending on how it is carried and the kind of work. Ring dosimeters are preferred to wrist dosimeters, which underestimate the maximum finger dose to an even greater extent, up to a factor of 20 according to Ginjaume [61]. ICRP [9] states that finger dosimeters should be used in therapies with high-energy beta-radiation, as ring dosimeters will underestimate the dose by up to 100 times.

In nuclear medicine diagnostics and therapy, radiopharmaceuticals are used as liquids, radioactive gases, or aerosols, which entails a certain risk of external and internal contamination. The radiation dose from an internal contamination can be determined with individual monitoring of the activity uptake and distribution and information regarding the biokinetics. External measurements can be performed on the whole body or specific organs or tissues using a whole-body counter, or smaller calibrated detectors. A dual-head scintillation camera system without collimators [55] can also be used for a simple and quick overview in case of suspected internal contamination.

Indirect methods for monitoring occupational intake of radionuclides emitting non-penetrating radiation can also be applied, such as measurements of blood, urine, faeces, and breath. Air samples can be taken in the working environment to determine the activity concentration in the air breathed by the worker. The radiation dose is determined by the results of samples taken and biokinetic models

REFERENCES

[1] ICRP, 2007. *The 2007 Recommendations of the International Commission on Radiological Protection.* ICRP Publication 103, Ann. ICRP (2–4).

[2] *Radiation Protection and Safety in Medical Uses of Ionizing Radiation. Specific Safety Guide, No. SSG-46.* Vienna: International Atomic Energy Agency, 2018.

[3] ICRP, 2012. *ICRP statement on tissue reactions / Early and late effects of radiation in normal tissues and organs – Threshold doses for tissue reactions in a radiation protection context.* ICRP Publication 118, Ann. ICRP 41 (1/2).

[4] E. Commission, *Directives council directive 2013/59/EURATOM of 5 December 2013 laying down basic safety standards for protection against the dangers arising from exposure to ionizing radiation. Official J Eur Union L,* 2014.

[5] S. T. Carlsson and J. C. Le Heron, "Radiation protection," in *Nuclear Medicine Physics. A Handbook for Teachers and Students,* D. L. Bailey, J. H. Humm, and A. Todd-Pokropek Eds. Vienna: IAEA, 2014.

[6] "World Nuclear Association, May 2020." www.world-nuclear.org/information-library/non-power-nuclear-applications/radioisotopes-research/radioisotopes-in-medicine.aspx

[7] M. J. Berger et al. "XCOM: Photon Cross Sections Database." https://www.nist.gov/pml/xcom-photon-cross-sections-database

[8] D. Delacroix, J. P. Guerre, P. Leblanc, and C. Hickman, *Radionuclide and Radiation Protection Data Handbook,* 2nd ed. (2002), *Radiat Prot Dosimetry,* vol. 98, no. 1, pp. 9–168, 2002, doi: 10.1093/oxfordjournals.rpd.a006705.

[9] ICRP, 2008. *Radiation Dose to Patients from Radiopharmaceuticals – Addendum 3 to 53.* ICRP Publication 106, Ann. ICRP 38 (1–2).

[10] R. Reiman, "Radiation protection of technologists and ancillary personnel," in *Clinical PET-CT in Radiology,* P. Shreve and D. Townsend, Eds. New York: Springer, 2011.

[11] A. D. Soares, L. Paixão, and A. Facure, "Determination of the dose rate constant through Monte Carlo simulations with voxel phantoms," *Med Phys,* vol. 45, no. 11, pp. 5283–92, 2018, doi: 10.1002/mp.13181.

[12] A. M. Young, "Dose rates in nuclear medicine and the effectiveness of lead aprons: updating the department's knowledge on old and new procedures," *Nucl Med Commun,* vol. 34, no. 3, pp. 254–64, 2013, doi: 10.1097/MNM.0b013e32835c91d5.

[13] F. Sudbrock, K. Uhrhan, A. Rimpler, and H. Schicha, "Dose and dose rate measurements for radiation exposure scenarios in nuclear medicine," *Radiation Measurements,* vol. 46, no. 11, pp. 1303–06, 2011, doi: https://doi.org/10.1016/j.radmeas.2011.06.074.

[14] P. J. Mountford and M. J. O'Doherty, "Exposure of critical groups to nuclear medicine patients," *Appl Radiat Isot,* vol. 50, no. 1, pp. 89–111, 1999, doi: 10.1016/s0969-8043(98)00074-8.

[15] J. Zhang-Yin et al., "Equivalent dose rate 1 meter from neuroendocrine tumor patients exiting the nuclear medicine department after undergoing imaging," *J Nucl Med,* vol. 58, no. 8, pp. 1230–35, 2017, doi: 10.2967/jnumed.116.187138.

[16] M. T. Madsen et al., "AAPM Task Group 108: PET and PET/CT shielding requirements," *Med Phys,* vol. 33, no. 1, pp. 4–15, 2006, doi: 10.1118/1.2135911.

[17] S. Leide-Svegborn, "Radiation exposure of patients and personnel from a PET/CT procedure with 18F-FDG," *Radiat Prot Dosimetry,* vol. 139, no. 1–3, pp. 208–13, 2010, doi: 10.1093/rpd/ncq026.

[18] *Occupational Radiation Protection. General Safety Guide, GSG-7.* Vienna: International Atomic Energy Agency, 2018.

[19] *Cyclotron Produced Radionuclides: Guidance on Facility Design and Production of Fluorodeoxyglucose (FDG).* Vienna: International Atomic Energy Agency, 2012.

[20] *Nuclear Medicine Resources Manual.* Vienna: International Atomic Energy Agency, 2006.

[21] L. Dauer, "Management of therapy patients," in *Nuclear Medicine Physics. A Handbook for Teachers and Students,* D. L. Bailey, J. H. Humm, and A. Todd-Pokropek, Eds. Vienna: IAEA, 2014.

[22] S. Mattsson, M. Andersson, and M. Soderberg, "Technological advances in hybrid imaging and impact on dose," *Radiat Prot Dosimetry,* vol. 165, no. 1–4, pp. 410–15, 2015, doi: 10.1093/rpd/ncv024.

[23] S. Leide-Svegborn, "External radiation exposure of personnel in nuclear medicine from 18F, 99mTC and 131I with special reference to fingers, eyes and thyroid," *Radiat Prot Dosimetry,* vol. 149, no. 2, pp. 196–206, 2012, doi: 10.1093/rpd/ncr213.

[24] G. J. Kemerink, F. Vanhavere, I. Barth, and F. M. Mottaghy, "Extremity doses of nuclear medicine personnel: A concern," *Eur J Nucl Med Mol Imaging,* vol. 39, no. 3, pp. 529–32, 2012, doi: 10.1007/s00259-011-1973-z.

[25] M. Wrzesien and K. Napolska, "Investigation of radiation protection of medical staff performing medical diagnostic examinations by using PET/CT technique," *J Radiol Prot,* vol. 35, no. 1, pp. 197–207, 2015, doi: 10.1088/0952-4746/35/1/197.

[26] H. Warren-Forward et al., "A comparison of dose savings of lead and lightweight aprons for shielding of 99m-Technetium radiation," *Radiat Prot Dosimetry,* vol. 124, no. 2, pp. 89–96, 2007, doi: 10.1093/rpd/ncm176.

[27] L. S. Fog and P. Collins, "Monte Carlo simulation of the dose to nuclear medicine staff wearing protective garments," *Australas Phys Eng Sci Med,* vol. 31, no. 4, pp. 307–16, 2008, doi: 10.1007/BF03178600.

[28] X. He, R. Zhao, L. Rong, K. Yao, S. Chen, and B. Wei, "Answers to if the lead aprons are really helpful in nuclear medicine from the perspective of spectroscopy," *Radiat Prot Dosimetry,* vol. 174, no. 4, pp. 558–64, 2017, doi: 10.1093/rpd/ncw255.

[29] IAEA, *Radiation Protection and Safety in Medical Uses of Ionizing Radiation. Specific Safety Guide, No. SSG-46.* Vienna: IAEA. 9789201111043, 2018, https://books.google.se/books?id=U05RAAAAMAAJ

[30] S. Ridone, R. Matheoud, S. Valzano, R. Di Martino, L. Vigna, and M. Brambilla, "Permeability of gloves used in nuclear medicine departments to [(99m)Tc]-pertechnetate and [(18)F]-fluorodeoxyglucose: Radiation protection considerations," *Phys Med,* vol. 29, no. 5, pp. 545–48, 2013, doi: 10.1016/j.ejmp.2013.01.005.

[31] M. A. Bolzinger, C. Bolot, G. Galy, A. Chabanel, J. Pelletier, and S. Briançon, "Skin contamination by radiopharmaceuticals and decontamination strategies," *Int J Pharm,* vol. 402, no. 1–2, pp. 44–49, 2010, doi: 10.1016/j.ijpharm.2010.09.027.

[32] P. Covens, D. Berus, V. Caveliers, L. Struelens, and D. Verellen, "Skin contamination of nuclear medicine technologists: Incidence, routes, dosimetry and decontamination," *Nucl Med Commun,* vol. 33, no. 10, pp. 1024–31, 2012, doi: 10.1097/MNM.0b013e32835674d9.

[33] A. Tazrart, P. Bérard, A. Leiterer, and F. Ménétrier, "Decontamination of radionuclides from skin: An overview," *Health Phys,* vol. 105, no. 2, pp. 201–7, 2013, doi: 10.1097/HP.0b013e318290c5a9.

[34] L. Dominguez-Gadea and L. Cerezo, "Decontamination of radioisotopes," *Rep Pract Oncol Radiother,* vol. 16, no. 4, pp. 147–52, 2011, doi: 10.1016/j.rpor.2011.05.002.

[35] S. Rana *et al.,* "Scintigraphic evaluation of decontamination lotion for removal of radioactive contamination from skin," *Disaster Med Public Health Prep,* pp. 1–6, 2014, doi: 10.1017/dmp.2014.17.

[36] L. W. Luckett and R. E. Stotler, "Radioiodine volatilization from reformulated sodium iodide I-131 oral solution," *J Nucl Med,* vol. 21, no. 5, pp. 477–79, 1980.

[37] M. Lassmann and U. Eberlein, *Targeted alpha-particle therapy: imaging, dosimetry, and radiation protection.* Ann ICRP, vol. 47, no. 3–4, pp. 187–95, 2018, doi: 10.1177/0146645318756253.

[38] D. S. Smith and M. G. Stabin, "Exposure rate constants and lead shielding values for over 1,100 radionuclides," *Health Phys,* vol. 102, no. 3, pp. 271–91, 2012, doi: 10.1097/hp.0b013e318235153a.

[39] M. Lecchi, G. Lucignani, C. Maioli, G. Ignelzi, and A. Del Sole, "Validation of a new protocol for ^{1}-F-FDG infusion using an automatic combined dispenser and injector system," *Eur J Nucl Med Mol Imaging,* vol. 39, no. 11, pp. 1720–29, 2012, doi: 10.1007/s00259-012-2174-0.

[40] P. Covens, D. Berus, F. Vanhavere, and V. Caveliers, "The introduction of automated dispensing and injection during PET procedures: A step in the optimisation of extremity doses and whole-body doses of nuclear medicine staff," *Radiat Prot Dosimetry,* vol. 140, no. 3, pp. 250–58, 2010, doi: 10.1093/rpd/ncq110.

[41] G. Dietze, "Radiobiology and Radiation Dosimetry for the Lens of the Eye," in *Radiation Protection in Nuclear Medicine,* C. Hoeschen and S. Mattsson, Eds. Berlin and Heidelberg: Springer-Verlag, 2013.

[42] R. Kopec *et al.,* "On the relationship between whole body, extremity and eye lens doses for medical staff in the preparation and application of radiopharmaceuticals in nuclear medicine," *Radiation Measurements,* vol. 46, no. 11, pp. 1295–98, 2011, doi: 10.1016/j.radmeas.2011.07.036.

[43] M. Wrzesień, L. Królicki, Ł. Albiniak, and J. Olszewski, "Is eye lens dosimetry needed in nuclear medicine?" *J Radiol Prot,* vol. 38, no. 2, pp. 763–74, 2018, doi: 10.1088/1361-6498/aabef5.

[44] H. Piwowarska-Bilska, A. Supinska, J. Iwanowski, and B. Birkenfeld, "Should personnel of nuclear medicine departments use personal dosimeters for eye lens dose monitoring?" *Radiat Prot Dosimetry,* vol. 183, no. 3, pp. 393–96, 2019, doi: 10.1093/rpd/ncy118.

[45] M. Wrzesien and L. Albiniak, "^{68}Ga-DOTA-TATE-a source of eye lens exposure for nuclear medicine department workers," *J Radiol Prot,* vol. 38, no. 4, pp. 1512–23, 2018, doi: 10.1088/1361-6498/aaea8e.

[46] S. Demeter, A. L. Goertzen, and J. Patterson, "Demonstrating compliance with proposed reduced lens of eye dose limits in nuclear medicine settings," *Health Phys,* vol. 117, no. 3, pp. 313–18, 2019, doi: 10.1097/HP.0000000000001059.

[47] J. Dabin, R. Kopec, L. Struelens, A. Szumska, M. Tomaszuk, and F. Vanhavere, "Eye lens doses in nuclear medicine: A multicentric study in Belgium and Poland," *Radiat Prot Dosimetry,* vol. 170, no. 1–4, pp. 297–301, 2016, doi: 10.1093/rpd/ncv538.

[48] P. Covens, D. Berus, V. Caveliers, L. Struelens, F. Vanhavere, and D. Verellen, "Skin dose rate conversion factors after contamination with radiopharmaceuticals: Influence of contamination area, epidermal thickness and percutaneous absorption," *J Radiol Prot,* vol. 33, no. 2, pp. 381–93, 2013, doi: 10.1088/0952-4746/33/2/381.

[49] P. Covens, D. Berus, V. Caveliers, L. Struelens, and D. Verellen, "The contribution of skin contamination dose to the total extremity dose of nuclear medicine staff: First results of an intensive survey," *Radiation Measurements,* vol. 46, no. 11, pp. 1291–94, 2011, doi: 10.1016/j.radmeas.2011.07.007.

[50] "Dose equivalent to an embryo/fetus." www.nrc.gov/reading-rm/doc-collections/cfr/part020/part020-1208.html

[51] A. Almén and S. Mattsson, "Radiological protection of foetuses and breast-fed children of occupationally exposed women in nuclear medicine: Challenges for hospitals," *Phys Med,* vol. 43, pp. 172–77, 2017, doi: 10.1016/j.ejmp.2017.08.010.

[52] P. J. Mountford and H. R. Steele, "Fetal dose estimates and the ICRP abdominal dose limit for occupational exposure of pregnant staff to technetium-99m and iodine-131 patients," *Eur J Nucl Med,* vol. 22, no. 10, pp. 1173–79, 1995, doi: 10.1007/BF00800600.

[53] M. G. Stabin and H. B. Breitz, "Breast milk excretion of radiopharmaceuticals: mechanisms, findings, and radiation dosimetry," *J Nucl Med,* vol. 41, no. 5, pp. 863–73, 2000.

[54] M. G. Stabin, "Radiation dose concerns for the pregnant or lactating patient," *Semin Nucl Med,* vol. 44, no. 6, pp. 479–88, 2014, doi: 10.1053/j.semnuclmed.2014.06.003.

[55] M. D. Short, A. R. Richards, and H. I. Glass, "The use of a gamma-camera as a whole-body counter," *Br J Radiol,* vol. 45, no. 532, pp. 289–93, 1972, doi: 10.1259/0007-1285-45-532-289.

[56] ICRU, *Quantities and Units in Radiation Protection Dosimetry. ICRU Report 51,* 1993.

[57] ICRP, 2007. *Radiological Protection in Medicine. ICRP Publication 105,* Ann. ICRP 37 (6).

[58] P. Covens, D. Berus, N. Buls, P. Clerinx, and F. Vanhavere, "Personal dose monitoring in hospitals: global assessment, critical applications and future needs," *Radiat Prot Dosimetry,* vol. 124, no. 3, pp. 250–59, 2007, doi: 10.1093/rpd/ncm418.

[59] N. Stritt and R. Linder, "Measures taken by the supervisory authority to reduce extremity doses in nuclear medicine facilities in Switzerland," *Radiation Measurements,* vol. 46, no. 11, pp. 1315–20, 2011, doi: 10.1016/j.radmeas.2011.06.002.

[60] C. J. Martin, "Strategies for assessment of doses to the tips of the fingers in nuclear medicine," *J Radiol Prot,* vol. 36, no. 3, pp. 405–18, 2016, doi: 10.1088/0952-4746/36/3/405.

[61] *Guidelines to Optimize Extremity Monitoring and to Reduce Skin Doses in Nuclear Medicine. Results of the ORAMED Project.* www.irpa.net/members/TS2a.3.pdf.

18 IAEA Support to Nuclear Medicine

Gian Luca Poli

CONTENTS

18.1 INTRODUCTION

The International Atomic Energy Agency (IAEA) is an independent international organization related to the United Nations (UN) system, promoting the safe, secure and peaceful uses of nuclear science and technology. It serves as the world's central intergovernmental forum for scientific and technical cooperation in the nuclear field, which includes the medical use of radiation and radionuclides. Figure 18.1 shows one of the buildings at the headquarters of the International Atomic Energy Agency in Vienna.

The Division of Human Health, part of the Department of Nuclear Sciences and Applications (see Figure 18.2), aims at enhancing the capabilities of the IAEA Member States [1] to address needs related to the prevention, diagnosis, and treatment of diseases through the application of nuclear techniques. Within this division, the Nuclear Medicine and Diagnostic Imaging Section promotes the use of nuclear medicine techniques, both in imaging and therapeutic applications to address health needs in Member States. In the same Division of Human Health, the Dosimetry and Medical Radiation Physics section has the objective to assure controlled radiation dosages in radiation medicine in Member States.

DOI: 10.1201/9780429489549-18

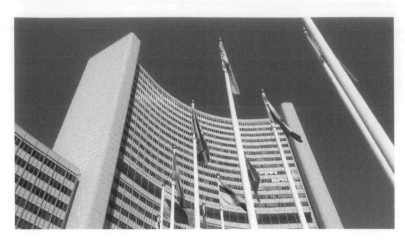

FIGURE 18.1 Headquarters of the International Atomic Energy Agency in Vienna, Austria. Colour image available at www.routledge.com/9781138593299.

The IAEA has a long tradition in assisting its Member States in the field of nuclear medicine. The main activities in this field are the production of guidance documents and educational material, the coordination of research projects, and the support to Member States for establishing and safely operating nuclear medicine facilities through the Technical Cooperation programme. Activities related to medical physics include Quality Assurance (QA) and Quality Control (QC) of nuclear medicine equipment, education and clinical training, professional recognition of the role of medical physicists in nuclear medicine, the coordination of research activities, and the development and dissemination of image quantification and internal dosimetry techniques.

This chapter will describe how the IAEA supports the practice of nuclear medicine, with a focus on the medical physics aspects.

18.2 STANDARDS AND GUIDANCE DOCUMENTS

The IAEA plays an important role in leading the development of standards and guidance documents related to nuclear medicine practice. To achieve this goal, renowned international experts in various fields are invited to contribute to the development of such documents. The electronic version of every IAEA publication is always made freely available for download, representing a vital source of information for the nuclear medicine community.

18.2.1 CLINICAL NUCLEAR MEDICINE

The section of Nuclear Medicine and Diagnostic Imaging of the IAEA has produced a variety of publications to support the enhancement, standardization and harmonization of clinical nuclear medicine. The *Nuclear Medicine Resources Manual* [2], for example, provides guidance to decision makers on the different applications of nuclear medicine and on the prerequisites and resources needed to establish this service. The *Human Health Series No. 11* presents an overview of the steps and requirements that are needed to establish a cyclotron and clinical PET centre [3]. Guidance documents have also been published on cardiac imaging [4, 5], clinical applications of SPECT/CT [6], the use of PET/CT in oncology [7, 8], radionuclide therapies [9], as well as atlases of images in the clinical use of gamma cameras [10], SPECT/CT [11] and PET/CT [12].

18.2.2 QUALITY ASSURANCE AND DOSIMETRY

Among the activities of the Dosimetry and Medical Radiation Physics (DMRP) section of the IAEA, the project on Clinical Medical Radiation Physics and Quality Assurance includes all clinical aspects of medical physics practices in radiation therapy and diagnostic radiology, as well as nuclear medicine [13]. This project aims at developing guidance and associated material to facilitate implementation of best clinical practice of medical physics in hospitals.

In the field of nuclear medicine medical physics, the IAEA has a long tradition of publishing guidance documents on quality assurance and quality control of equipment [14]. The IAEA TECDOC 602 covered QA/QC procedures

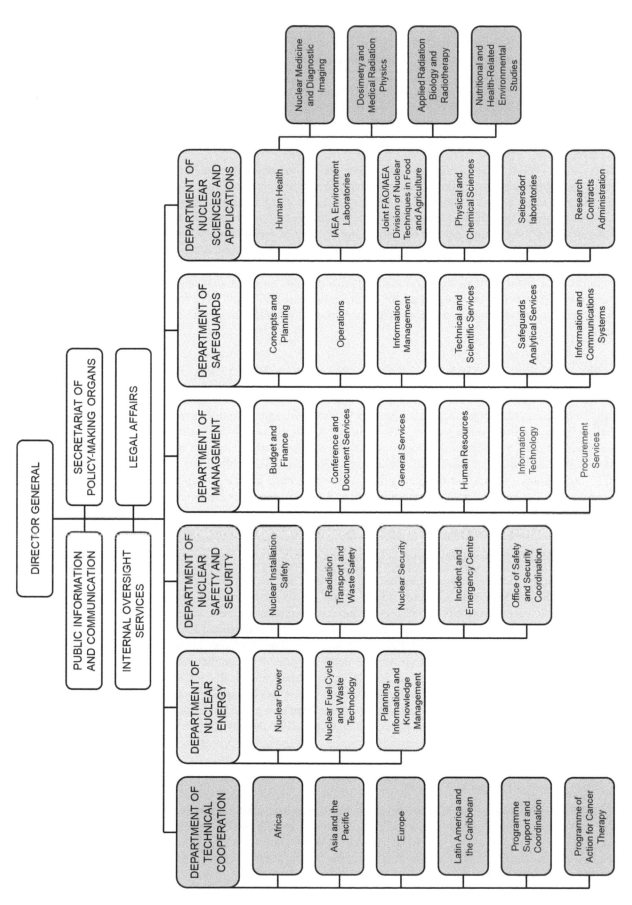

FIGURE 18.2 Organizational chart of the International Atomic Energy Agency. On the far right of the chart the four sections of the division of Human Health. Colour image available at www.routledge.com/9781138593299.

of non-imaging equipment used in nuclear medicine and gamma cameras [15]. Guidance on QA and proper activity measurements, both at the hospital and at the secondary radioactivity standards laboratory level, was published in 2006 [16]. Following the technological evolution of imaging equipment, separate recommendations on QA/QC of SPECT [17] PET and PET/CT [18] and more recently SPECT/CT systems [19] have been produced.

For the accurate interpretation of nuclear medicine images, it is vital to understand the principles of image formation and be aware of the artefacts that can arise from nuclear medicine imaging systems. Atlases have been produced to support the end-user to recognize image artefacts and understand their causes. These documents are available for SPECT [20], PET/CT [21] and SPECT/CT [19], and guide the reader with techniques to suppress these errors and avoid their recurrence.

The International Basic Safety Standards [22] requires the optimization of protection and safety for each medical exposure, including the administration of radiopharmaceuticals for therapeutic purposes. In recent years the DMRP section has increased its efforts to produce guidance documents in the field of dosimetry for radiopharmaceutical therapy, which would be beneficial in the international standardization of procedures for dosimetry in radionuclide therapy and in filling the existing gaps in education and training of medical physicists for patient-specific dosimetry. As a first step in this direction, and because of its vital application in radionuclide therapy, the IAEA published a report on quantitative nuclear medicine imaging in 2014 [23]. This report presents the current state of the art of image quantification and describes the physical effects that degrade image quality and affect the accuracy of quantification, proposing methods to compensate for them in planar, SPECT and PET imaging. These efforts set the stage for patient-specific dosimetry, a requirement for therapeutic nuclear medicine but also useful for diagnostic procedures.

18.2.3 Radiopharmacy

Radiopharmacy is an essential part of the activities in nuclear medicine and is a basic component of diagnostic and therapeutic procedures. Radiopharmaceuticals need to be produced under controlled conditions and tested for their quality before being administered to patients. The Industrial Applications and Chemistry Section, within the Division of Physical and Chemical Sciences of the Department of Nuclear Sciences and Applications, supports activities related to production of diagnostic and therapeutic radiopharmaceuticals [24]. Publications on radiopharmaceutical production [25–30], quality control and usage, regulatory aspects related to new radiopharmaceuticals [31], audits of radiopharmaceutical production facilities, implementation of Quality Management System, and Good Manufacturing Practice (GMP) have been produced.

18.2.4 Radiation Protection and Safety

The IAEA plays an important role in the development of safety standards and supporting their implementation in Member States. The IAEA Safety Standards are based, to the extent possible, on the recommendations of the International Commission on Radiological Protection (ICRP). These standards represent an international consensus on safety aspects for protecting people and the environment from harmful effects of ionizing radiation [22] and are often adopted by international sister organizations like WHO, ILO, IEC, and ICRU as well as regulatory bodies and other relevant national authorities for radiation protection purposes in various fields. To provide recommendations and guidance on how to comply with safety requirements, safety guides have been developed specifically for medical uses of ionizing radiation [32], including nuclear medicine, and addressing all three categories of exposure: medical exposure, occupational exposure and exposure of members of the public. Reports have been also published on topics of interest for the nuclear medicine community, such as the release of patients after radionuclide therapy [33] and radiation protection in PET/CT [34].

18.2.5 Education and Clinical Training

Training in nuclear medicine is vital for the development of adequate capacities in Member States. The IAEA has developed guidance documents on education and clinical training in different disciplines related to nuclear medicine. Moreover, training of health professionals is supported in different forms, such as the production of training material (handbooks, slides, e-learning modules, webinars, etc.), the organization of training courses and individual training (fellowships and scientific visits).

18.2.6 RECOMMENDATIONS FOR EDUCATION AND CLINICAL TRAINING

One of the IAEA's priorities in the field of nuclear medicine is the development of standardized syllabi for academic education, as well as clinical training guides. For example, guidelines to support Member States in establishing national postgraduate education programmes in medical physics have been produced [35]. In addition to academic education, a structured in-service specialized clinical training is required, providing a better preparation for medical physicists and ensuring that they are capable of independent, safe, and effective practice. For this reason, the IAEA has published Training Course Series publications with guidance and references to training material for clinical training programmes for medical physicists in radiation medicine, including nuclear medicine [36].

More recently, to raise the level of knowledge and competencies of nuclear medicine specialists worldwide, guidance has been provided to harmonize training programmes for nuclear medicine physicians [37]. This document addresses all the competencies required for a nuclear medicine physician to be able to provide adequate care to patients and ensure safety and quality of clinical practice.

18.2.7 SUPPORT TO EDUCATION AND CLINICAL TRAINING

Understanding the physics of nuclear medicine is crucial for all health professionals involved in this discipline. The basic concepts and practice of nuclear medicine physics are covered in a publication [38] that aspires to serve as a textbook for students attending medical physics academic programmes. To support teachers and students, sets of teaching slides have also been produced to complement this handbook. The slides are freely available on the Human Health Campus website [39]. A gamma camera laboratory is also available in Seibersdorf, near Vienna, where practical training courses on topics considered essential for medical physicists specializing in nuclear medicine are organized.

The IAEA also organizes several training activities, both under the regular budget and through the Technical Cooperation programme. Training courses are organized in collaboration with the Abdus Salam International Centre for Theoretical Physics (ICTP) in Italy. Joint IAEA/ICTP events are regularly organized on different topics of common interest. In the field of nuclear medicine medical physics, for example, an advanced school on internal dosimetry provided participants with a comprehensive review of the basics and recent developments in the fields of nuclear medicine image quantification and dosimetry in radiopharmaceutical therapy. Another event on quality assurance and dose optimization in hybrid imaging provided advanced knowledge on the best use of SPECT/CT and PET/CT. Physics and technological innovations, quality assurance program, procedures for quality control and dosimetry, and optimization strategies aiming to achieve diagnostic image quality at lower radiation doses were discussed. Each one of these events hosts tens of participants from countries throughout the world, with several participants from low-and-middle-income countries (LMIC) being financially supported. Similarly, other training courses are organized in collaboration with Argonne National Laboratories in the United States.

Because of the lack of medical physicists in many countries, particularly in LMIC, the IAEA encourages education and clinical training of medical physicists also through the Technical Cooperation programme, for example, by supporting students attending the MSc in Medical Physics of the ICTP [40]. This programme adopts the regional curriculum specifically developed to allow students to complete the academic and clinical training, either in radiotherapy or in imaging medical physics, in a time frame of two years. This rapidly puts students in a condition to practice independently in a clinical environment in their country of origin.

18.2.8 ON-LINE RESOURCES

In the current digital era one of the obvious methods to deliver capacity-building efforts is the use of on-line resources. Internet and communications technology is progressively becoming available worldwide, and digital tools are more and more effective in reaching out to a large number of health professional at a low cost. The IAEA Human Health Campus [41] is designed to serve as an informative resource for health professionals in various fields, including nuclear medicine, radiopharmacy, and medical physics. Lectures and educational material from IAEA's training courses are made available for the enhancement of the nuclear medicine profession. The Campus includes guidelines, publications, and teaching cases for different clinical applications that can be consulted by the nuclear medicine community. This educational material can be accessed at any time anywhere in the world.

Webinars offer the opportunity of interaction between the presenter and the learners – facilitated thanks to the use of slides and live streaming. The Human Health Campus hosts a collection of recorded webinars on various topics relevant to nuclear medicine, often organized through partnership with professional societies and other international organizations. E-learning modules are available on various clinical applications of nuclear medicine, expanding educational opportunities in the field [42]. The interactive environment enhances the self-directed learning experience that can be undertaken at one's own pace. Mobile applications for smartphones are also available, designed to support health professionals in the diagnosis and management of patients [43].

In the field of nuclear medicine medical physics, tutorial videos have been produced on quality control both for SPECT and PET/CT scanners [44, 45]. These videos demonstrate all the steps that need to be carried out to perform a quality-control test, starting with the phantom preparation, data acquisition, image reconstruction, and manipulations, concluding with data analysis and reporting of results. These videos are available to the nuclear medicine community and have been widely used during various training courses.

In an effort to standardize documentation and reporting of biodistribution data for internal dosimetry calculations, the IAEA Radiotracer Biodistribution Template (RaBiT) [46] has been developed and made freely available on the Human Health Campus [47]. As a sequel to the EANM recommendation on Good Dosimetry Reporting [48], the RaBiT supports summary reporting of tracer biodistribution within a patient, as this is a common/central point in most organ-level dose calculations protocols. The template is a structured format file that can be disseminated, interpreted, and used for method development widely across the field.

Proper quality control procedures in SPECT play an essential role in ensuring optimized performance of imaging equipment and are a requisite for providing high-quality clinical care. Since QC procedures are implemented routinely, streamlining them with automated software may offer several benefits: improved speed, reduced errors, and the standardization of calculation methods across centres. The IAEA Nuclear Medicine Quality Control (NMQC) Toolkit is a set of ImageJ (Fiji edition)-based codes that allow the processing and analysis of nuclear medicine images acquired for quality control tests of gamma cameras and SPECT systems. The IAEA-NMQC toolkit is a free resource developed to support common SPECT QC data-analysis procedures for several QC tests and is available with further documentation and instructions for use on the Human Health Campus [49].

The DATOL is a comprehensive online set of training resources, dedicated to nuclear medicine technologists, that provides information on nuclear medicine procedures and easy to understand science that underlines these procedures [50]. The material is available, both as open-access and as part of an instructor-led course, for use under direct supervision in the workplace, with formal assessment and certification [51].

One section of the Human Health Campus is dedicated to radiopharmacy with a virtual course for practitioners in the field that provides information on radiopharmaceutical preparation, radionuclide generators, and quality control of radiopharmaceuticals. The purpose of the course is to ensure that practitioners can perform a complete radiopharmaceutical preparation without error or assistance, understand issues regarding patient, personnel, and environment safety when working with radioactive materials, and are able to apply that knowledge in practice when preparing a radiopharmaceutical.

18.3 NUCLEAR MEDICINE MEDICAL PHYSICS

Medical physics dedicated to nuclear medicine plays a major role on the quality of exams and the outcomes of a department of nuclear medicine with several fields of applications: calibration, diagnostic, internal dosimetry, therapy, QC/QA programs, and radiation safety.

18.3.1 ROLES AND RESPONSIBILITIES OF MEDICAL PHYSICISTS IN NUCLEAR MEDICINE

Medical physicists are members of the multidisciplinary team involved in a nuclear medicine department and ensure the safe and effective delivery of radiation to achieve a diagnostic or therapeutic result as prescribed in patient care.

According to the definition of the International Basic Safety Standards (BSS) [22], a medical physicist working in a clinical environment is a "health professional with specialist education and training in the concepts and techniques of applying physics in medicine and competent to practice independently in one or more of the subfields (specialties) of medical physics". The BSS clearly states that the requirements for calibration, dosimetry, and QA, including the acceptance and commissioning of medical radiological equipment, should be fulfilled by or under the supervision of a medical physicist. Medical physicists in nuclear medicine are responsible for dosimetric and quantitative aspects in all clinical procedures. In particular, they advise or assist physicians and other health-care professionals in optimizing the balance between the beneficial and deleterious effects of radiation.

Medical physics's support to nuclear medicine is limited by the insufficient number of clinically qualified medical physicists in many countries. Challenges include not only the paucity of postgraduate programmes in medical physics and clinical training, but also the lack in many countries of professional recognition and regulation of the role of medical physicists in nuclear medicine. To fill these gaps, the various responsibilities and involvements of medical physicists in a nuclear medicine department are appropriately and unequivocally described in the *IAEA Human Health Series No. 25* [52]. This document also establishes internationally harmonized criteria on the minimum recommendations for academic and clinical training of medical physicists and promotes the recognition and professionalism of medical physics as a profession internationally.

18.3.2 Staffing Requirements

The safe and effective use of radiation in medicine depends also on the availability of well-trained clinical medical physicists. However, in many countries there is still a shortage of these health professionals, especially in diagnostic radiology and nuclear medicine. In order to determine the appropriate staffing levels for clinical medical physics services needed to ensure safe, effective, and efficient diagnostic imaging and radionuclide treatment of patients, the IAEA has developed an algorithm described in the *Human Health Reports No. 15* [53]. The algorithm has been developed by a group of experts from professional societies based on the roles and responsibilities of the medical physicist as they follow from the requirements of good clinical practice. The algorithm was validated and tested under a variety of field conditions to ensure its general applicability. The total number of medical physicists required is calculated considering factors which are dependent or related to equipment, patients, radiation protection, service, training, and academic teaching and research. An accompanying spreadsheet is also available to facilitate calculations of the staffing needs following these recommendations.

18.4 COORDINATED RESEARCH ACTIVITIES

The IAEA Coordinated Research Projects (CRPs) bring together research institutions throughout the world to collaborate on a well-defined research topic related to the acquisition and dissemination of new knowledge and technology in the various fields related to the peaceful use of atomic energy [54]. Institutions and scientists from all around the world are selected to exchange information and work together on some relevant aspect related to the main topic, thus creating international scientific networks and enhancing capabilities of participating countries to be involved in state-of-the-art scientific research. The results are made freely available to the Member States and the scientific community, usually through IAEA publications, training material, or articles published in peer-reviewed journals.

The IAEA also encourages training at the doctoral level of highly skilled physicists through the design and implementation of Doctoral CRPs. In this case, PhD students are enrolled to work on a specific research topic, with a supervisor from the host country bearing full responsibility for the progress of the graduate student. Students are also paired with highly experienced scientists in other countries with appropriate specialized knowledge in the selected research topic, who will assist in guiding the project to a successful completion.

CRPs are sponsored and coordinated by the IAEA and typically have a duration of 3 to 5 years. Research, technical, and doctoral contracts and cost-free research agreements are awarded to institutes that are selected for participating to the research project. Contracts and agreements are signed usually with 10 to 15 institutes, with one team member for each institute being designated as chief scientific investigator. These research activities are sometimes the first of their kind in a given Member State, and the participating researchers often act as the core group able to support future research in the country.

In the field of nuclear medicine, the work done in the frame of CRPs is related, for example, to clinical applications for the diagnosis and treatment of diseases, the enhancement or introduction of modern imaging techniques, and the improvement of the efficiency of existing modalities for paediatric medical imaging. Other CRPs are focused on the technological solutions for radioisotope production and separation, development and use of novel radiopharmaceuticals for diagnostic or therapeutic purposes.

Research activities in the field of nuclear medicine medical physics support, for example, the harmonization of quality practices for clinical radioactivity measurements in radiopharmacies and hospitals [55, 56], the standardization and dissemination of quantitative imaging [23, 57], and dosimetric methods in radionuclide therapy, or the implementation and enhancement of optimization techniques and methodologies for paediatric medical imaging.

18.5 COMPREHENSIVE CLINICAL AUDITS

With its three comprehensive clinical audit programmes in radiotherapy [58], nuclear medicine [59], and diagnostic radiology [60], the IAEA encourages a quality management approach for obtaining best results in radiation medicine practices.

The document on *Quality Management Audits in Nuclear Medicine Practices* (QUANUM) describes the methodology and tools needed to perform a comprehensive clinical audit in a nuclear medicine department. It can be used by end users as a reference document to perform self-reviews on their nuclear medicine practice. The document provides guidance on the preparation of the audit, including the composition of the auditing team, and all the following steps that lead to the final audit report. Checklists and spreadsheets [61] are also available as working tools to support the auditing team in the assessment of requirements for quality and safety of the department. The auditing team usually includes a nuclear medicine physician, a medical physicist, a radiopharmacist, and a nuclear medicine technologist.

The IAEA organizes, through the Technical Cooperation programme, several QUANUM audits yearly [62], assisting the audited centres and the auditing team in the implementation process. These audits are conducted on a voluntary basis and are always initiated upon the request of a facility in a Member State. Many nuclear medicine departments throughout the world have benefited from this peer-reviewed process, during which an independent and multidisciplinary auditing team has the task to assess the level against existing standards of the clinical practice quality and safety, providing recommendations for improvement.

18.6 TECHNICAL COOPERATION PROGRAMME

The Technical Cooperation (TC) programme is one of the mechanisms through which the IAEA directly helps its Member States to build, strengthen, and maintain capacities for the safe, peaceful, and secure use of nuclear technology in support of sustainable socioeconomic development. The TC programme addresses wide-ranging development objectives, which include greater food productivity, better health and nutrition services, improved energy development, and sustainable energy production.

TC projects can be national, driven by the development priorities of a single Member State, or regional, when a group of Member States belonging to the same geographical area cooperate to create regional sustainability and self-reliance in the effective use of nuclear technologies. All Member States are eligible for support through TC projects, although in practice technical cooperation activities is focused on the needs and priorities of low-and-middle-income countries.

Through TC projects, the IAEA supports Member States by coordinating several activities aiming to build human resource capacity, and transfer know-how and technology. These activities include fellowships for individuals, scientific visit opportunities for more experienced professionals, training courses, meetings, missions of experts in the field, as well as procurement of technology and equipment.

TC projects related to nuclear medicine focus, for example, on the establishment of a nuclear medicine service (often the first in the country), the upgrade of existing departments with newer hybrid imaging modalities, such as SPECT/CT or PET/CT, the enhancement of the clinical practice or the introduction of new diagnostic or therapeutic methodologies [63]. Establishing nuclear medicine practice requires planning and construction of the facility, licensing, training of staff, developing protocols and procedures, as well as all the activities related to equipment (specifications, procurement, installation, acceptance testing and commissioning). Because of the multidisciplinarity of nuclear medicine, these projects usually include other components related to radiopharmacy, medical physics, and safety. For example, medical physics aspects can be related to the development and implementation of QA/QC programs for radioactivity measurements or imaging equipment, the use of dosimetry in radionuclide therapy, or the introduction of strategies for optimization of diagnostic procedures.

Within TC, project fellowships are granted to health professionals to foster capacity building. These candidates are supported to spend an adequate period of time, in a well-established nuclear medicine service, for specialized and supervised hands-on training. The training programme is agreed with the hosting institute and is usually focused on a specific topic, for example, on the establishment and standardization of clinical protocols, the use of SPECT for cardiological and oncological studies, the therapeutic use of a certain radiopharmaceutical, the practical aspects of QA/QC of instrumentation and radiation protection, or the preparation of radiopharmaceuticals.

Education and training activities are key components of TC projects, and training courses are often included in the workplan to reach out to a larger number of health professionals. The use of international experts is another very effective means for the transfer of know-how. These experts are recruited by the IAEA and asked to support the project's counterparts on a specific aspect of the project. Being delivered locally, this kind of support is particularly important for solving specific issues and therefore for achieving the project's objectives. Finally, as one of the means for achieving their objectives, TC projects often include the procurement of important equipment or services based on the general aspects of sustainability and ownership.

18.7 NUCLEAR DATA SERVICES

The IAEA supports nuclear research activities by providing atomic and nuclear data and serving as the central authority for data collection and worldwide dissemination of such data. Having reliable data is of paramount importance for performing calculations and evaluations in nuclear research. In the field of nuclear medicine, for example, the interest is in information such as cross sections and yields for the production of radioisotopes used for medical applications, or data useful for accurate dosimetric calculations in the use of radiopharmaceuticals [64] (like those summarized in ICRP *Publication 107* [65]).

The compilation and evaluation of new atomic and nuclear data are performed by different networks of scientists worldwide. The Nuclear Data section of the IAEA initiates different research projects to further develop these data libraries, providing recommendations to the laboratories involved on the data deemed to be of interest, as well as support and coordination. Many of these CRPs are focused on radionuclides used in diagnostic or therapeutic nuclear medicine, with the results made freely available through IAEA publications [66, 67]. On-line databases are also maintained as support to the nuclear medicine community [64].

18.8 CONFERENCES AND TECHNICAL MEETINGS

One of the roles of the IAEA is to constantly appraise the state of the art and trends in various fields of nuclear technology, including nuclear medicine practices in Member States. This is done through the organization of technical meetings, where experts in the field and representatives of scientific societies, professional, and international organizations are consulted to share experience and information on highly specialized technical matters and advice the IAEA on the status, trends, and gaps in this area. For example, technical meetings have been organized on hybrid imaging and its role in the clinical practice, on the production and use of alpha emitters in therapeutic nuclear medicine [68], on guidance on prevention of unintended and accidental radiation exposures in nuclear medicine [32]. Another meeting was arranged to review the status of internal dosimetry and identify gaps to be addressed in this field, leading to a report prepared and published as a working document on the IAEA Human Health Campus website [69].

The IAEA organizes also various international conferences on topics of interest in nuclear medicine. Examples are conferences on Molecular Imaging and Clinical PET-CT (IPET), on Integrated Medical Imaging in Cardiovascular Diseases (IMIC), or on Trends in Radiopharmaceuticals (ISTR). Other conferences that are relevant to nuclear medicine are organized on radiation protection, radiopharmacy, and dosimetry (IDOS) [70, 71]. Sessions of these conferences are often livestreamed to reach out to a larger number of health professionals worldwide.

REFERENCES

[1] "List of IAEA Member States." www.iaea.org/about/governance/list-of-member-states.

[2] *Nuclear Medicine Resources Manual*. Vienna: International Atomic Energy Agency, 2020.

[3] *Planning a Clinical PET Centre*. Vienna: International Atomic Energy Agency, 2010.

[4] *Nuclear Cardiology: Guidance on the Implementation of SPECT Myocardial Perfusion Imaging*. Vienna: International Atomic Energy Agency, 2016.

[5] *Nuclear Cardiology: Its Role in Cost Effective Care*. Vienna: International Atomic Energy Agency, 2012.

[6] *Clinical Applications of SPECT/CT: New Hybrid Nuclear Medicine Imaging System*. Vienna: International Atomic Energy Agency, 2008.

[7] *Standard Operating Procedures for PET/CT: A Practical Approach for Use in Adult Oncology*. Vienna: International Atomic Energy Agency, 2013.

[8] *Appropriate Use of FDG-PET for the Management of Cancer Patients*. Vienna: International Atomic Energy Agency, 2010.

[9] *Practical Guidance on Peptide Receptor Radionuclide Therapy (PRRNT) for Neuroendocrine Tumours*. Vienna: International Atomic Energy Agency, 2013.

[10] *Atlas of Bone Scintigraphy in the Developing Paediatric Skeleton: The Normal Skeleton Variants and Pitfalls*. Vienna: International Atomic Energy Agency, 2011.

[11] *Atlas of Skeletal SPECT/CT Clinical Images*. Vienna: International Atomic Energy Agency, 2016.

[12] *Clinical PET/CT Atlas: A Casebook of Imaging in Oncology*. Vienna: International Atomic Energy Agency, 2015.

[13] A. Meghzifene and G. Sgouros, "IAEA support to medical physics in nuclear medicine," *Semin Nucl Med,* vol. 43, no. 3, pp. 181–7, 2013, doi: 10.1053/j.semnuclmed.2012.11.008.

[14] *Quality Control of Nuclear Medicine Instruments,* IAEA, Vienna, 1984.

[15] *Quality Control of Nuclear Medicine Instruments 1991,* IAEA, Vienna, 1991.

[16] *Quality Assurance for Radioactivity Measurement in Nuclear Medicine,* IAEA, Vienna, 2006.

[17] *Quality Assurance for SPECT Systems,* IAEA, Vienna, 2009.

[18] *Quality Assurance for PET and PET/CT Systems,* IAEA, Vienna, 2009.

[19] *SPECT/CT Atlas of Quality Control and Image Artefacts,* IAEA, Vienna, 2019.

[20] *IAEA Quality Control Atlas for Scintillation Camera Systems,* IAEA, Vienna, 2003.

[21] *PET/CT Atlas on Quality Control and Image Artefacts,* IAEA, Vienna, 2014.

[22] *Radiation Protection and Safety of Radiation Sources: International Basic Safety Standards General Safety Requirements Pt 3,* IAEA, Vienna, 2015.

[23] *Quantitative Nuclear Medicine Imaging: Concepts, Requirements and Methods,* IAEA, Vienna, 2014.

[24] A. Duatti and U. Bhonsle, "Strengthening radiopharmacy practice in IAEA Member States," *Semin Nucl Med,* vol. 43, no. 3, pp. 188–94, 2013, doi: 10.1053/j.semnuclmed.2012.11.009.

[25] *Cyclotron Produced Radionuclides: Emerging Positron Emitters for Medical Applications: ^{64}Cu and ^{124}I.* Vienna: International Atomic Energy Agency, 2016.

[26] *Radiopharmaceuticals for Sentinel Lymph Node Detection: Status and Trends.* Vienna: International Atomic Energy Agency, 2015.

[27] *Yttrium-90 and Rhenium-188 Radiopharmaceuticals for Radionuclide Therapy.* Vienna: International Atomic Energy Agency, 2015.

[28] *Technetium-99m Radiopharmaceuticals: Status and Trends.* Vienna: International Atomic Energy Agency, 2010.

[29] *Production of Long Lived Parent Radionuclides for Generators: ^{68}Ge, ^{82}Sr, ^{90}Sr and ^{188}W.* Vienna: International Atomic Energy Agency, 2010.

[30] *Cyclotron Produced Radionuclides: Guidance on Facility Design and Production of Fluorodeoxyglucose (FDG).* Vienna: International Atomic Energy Agency, 2012.

[31] *Good Practice for Introducing Radiopharmaceuticals for Clinical Use.* Vienna: International Atomic Energy Agency, 2016.

[32] C. J. Martin, M. Marengo, J. Vassileva, F. Giammarile, G. L. Poli, and P. Marks, "Guidance on prevention of unintended and accidental radiation exposures in nuclear medicine," *J Radiol Prot,* vol. 39, no. 3, pp. 665–95, 2019, doi: 10.1088/1361-6498/ab19d8.

[33] *Release of Patients After Radionuclide Therapy,* IAEA, Vienna, 2009.

[34] *Radiation Protection in Newer Medical Imaging Techniques: PET/CT,* IAEA, Vienna, 2008.

[35] *Postgraduate Medical Physics Academic Programmes.* Vienna: International Atomic Energy Agency, 2014.

[36] *Clinical Training of Medical Physicists Specializing in Nuclear Medicine.* Vienna: International Atomic Energy Agency, 2011.

[37] *Training Curriculum for Nuclear Medicine Physicians,* IAEA, Vienna, 2019.

[38] *Nuclear Medicine Physics: A Handbook for Teachers and Students,* IAEA, Vienna, 2014.

[39] "Nuclear Medicine Handbook slides." https://humanhealth.iaea.org/HHW/MedicalPhysics/e-learning/Nuclear_Medicine_Handbook_slides/index.html

[40] "ICTP Master of Advanced Studies in Medical Physics." www.ictp.it/programmes/mmp.aspx

[41] "IAEA Human Health Campus." https://humanhealth.iaea.org/

[42] T. N. Pascual, M. Dondi, D. Paez, R. Kashyap, and R. Nunez-Miller, "IAEA programs in empowering the nuclear medicine profession through online educational resources," *Semin Nucl Med,* vol. 43, no. 3, pp. 161–6, 2013, doi: 10.1053/j.semnuclmed.2012.11.005.

[43] "Mobile Applications." https://humanhealth.iaea.org/HHW/NuclearMedicine/MobileApps/index.html

[44] "Quality Assurance e-learning module for SPECT systems." https://humanhealth.iaea.org/HHW/MedicalPhysics/e-learning/QA_SPECT/index.html

[45] "Tutorial videos for Quality Control tests on PET/CT scanners." https://humanhealth.iaea.org/HHW/MedicalPhysics/e-learning/QC_PETCT/index.html

[46] A. L. Kesner, G. L. Poli, S. Beykan, and M. Lassmann, "The IAEA Radiotracer Biodistribution Template – A community resource for supporting the standardization and reporting of radionuclide pre-dosimetry data," *Physica Medica,* vol. 44, pp. 83–5, 2017, doi: 10.1016/j.ejmp.2017.07.022.

[47] "IAEA Radiotracer Biodistribution Template (RaBiT)." https://humanhealth.iaea.org/HHW/MedicalPhysics/NuclearMedicine/InternalDosimetry/iaeaBioDistributionTemplate/index.html

[48] M. Lassmann, C. Chiesa, G. Flux, and M. Bardies, "EANM Dosimetry Committee guidance document: Good practice of clinical dosimetry reporting," *Eur J Nucl Med Mol Imaging,* 2010, doi: 10.1007/s00259-010-1549-3.

[49] "IAEA-NMQC Toolkit." https://humanhealth.iaea.org/HHW/MedicalPhysics/NuclearMedicine/QualityAssurance/NMQC-Plugins/index.html

[50] H. E. Patterson, M. Nunez, G. M. Philotheou, and B. F. Hutton, "Meeting the challenges of global nuclear medicine technologist training in the 21st century: The IAEA Distance Assisted Training (DAT) Program," *Semin Nucl Med,* vol. 43, no. 3, pp. 195–201, 2013, doi: 10.1053/j.semnuclmed.2012.11.010.

[51] "Distance Assisted Training for Nuclear Medicine Professionals." www.datnmt.org

[52] *Roles and Responsibilities, and Education and Training Requirements for Clinically Qualified Medical,* IAEA, Vienna, 2013.

[53] *Assessing Medical Physics Staffing Needs in Diagnostic Imaging and Radionuclide Therapy: An Activity Based Approach,* IAEA, Vienna, 2018.

[54] "Coordinated Research Activities." www.iaea.org/services/coordinated-research-activities

[55] B. E. Zimmerman, A. Meghzifene, and K. R. Shortt, "Establishing measurement traceability for national laboratories: Results of an IAEA comparison of ^{131}I," *Appl Radiat Isot,* vol. 66, no. 6–7, pp. 954–9, 2008, doi: 10.1016/j.apradiso.2008.02.067.

[56] B. E. Zimmerman and S. Palm, "Results of an international comparison of ^{57}Co," *Appl Radiat Isot,* vol. 68, no. 7–8, pp. 1217–20, 2010, doi: 10.1016/j.apradiso.2009.12.021.

[57] B. E. Zimmerman *et al.*, "Multi-centre evaluation of accuracy and reproducibility of planar and SPECT image quantification: An IAEA phantom study," *Zeitschrift für Medizinische Physik,* vol. 27, pp. 98–112, 2017, doi: 10.1016/j.zemedi.2016.03.008.

[58] *Comprehensive Audits of Radiotherapy Practices: A Tool for Quality Improvement.* Vienna: International Atomic Energy Agency, 2007.

[59] *Quality Management Audits in Nuclear Medicine Practices.* Vienna: International Atomic Energy Agency, 2015.

[60] *Comprehensive Clinical Audits of Diagnostic Radiology Practices: A Tool for Quality Improvement.* Vienna: International Atomic Energy Agency, 2010.

[61] "QUANUM 3.0, Excel Tool and QNUMED." https://humanhealth.iaea.org/HHW/NuclearMedicine/QUANUM_2.0_Excel_Tool_and_QNUMED/index.html

[62] M. Dondi, R. Kashyap, T. Pascual, D. Paez, and R. Nunez-Miller, "Quality management in nuclear medicine for better patient care: the IAEA program," *Semin Nucl Med,* vol. 43, no. 3, pp. 167–71, 2013, doi: 10.1053/j.semnuclmed.2012.11.006.

[63] J. A. Casas-Zamora and R. Kashyap, "The IAEA technical cooperation programme and nuclear medicine in the developing world: objectives, trends, and contributions," *Semin Nucl Med,* vol. 43, no. 3, pp. 172–80, 2013, doi: 10.1053/j.semnuclmed.2012.11.007.

[64] "IAEA Nuclear Data Services." www-nds.iaea.org/

[65] K. Eckerman and A. Endo, "ICRP Publication 107. Nuclear decay data for dosimetric calculations," *Annals of the ICRP,* vol. 38, no. 3, pp. 7–96, 2008, doi: 10.1016/j.icrp.2008.10.004.

[66] *Nuclear Data for the Production of Therapeutic Radionuclides.* Vienna: International Atomic Energy Agency, 2012.

[67] *Charged Particle Cross-Section Database for Medical Radioisotope Production: Diagnostic Radioisotopes and Monitor Reactions.* Vienna: International Atomic Energy Agency, 2001.

[68] *Report of a Technical Meeting on "Alpha emitting radionuclides and radiopharmaceuticals for therapy,"* IAEA, Vienna, 2013.

[69] "Report of a Consultants' Meeting on Internal Dosimetry." https://humanhealth.iaea.org/HHW/MedicalPhysics/NuclearMedicine/InternalDosimetry/Consultants_report/index.html

[70] "International Symposium on Standards, Applications and Quality Assurance in Medical Radiation Dosimetry (IDOS 2019)." www.iaea.org/events/idos2019

[71] A. Meghzifene, D. Followill, Y. K. Dewaraja, P. J. Allisy, C. Kessler, and D. van der Merwe, "International symposium on standards, applications and quality assurance in medical radiation dosimetry (IDOS 2019): Highlights of an IAEA meeting," *Medical Physics International,* vol. 7, no. 3, pp. 342–60, 2019.